Management of Endodontic Complications

From Diagnosis to Prognosis

One book, one tree: In support of reforestation worldwide and to address the climate crisis, for every book sold Quintessence Publishing will plant a tree (https://onetreeplanted.org/).

Library of Congress Control Number: 2023933014

A CIP record for this book is available from the British Library.
ISBN: 978-1-64724-052-3

QUINTESSENCE PUBLISHING
USA

Quintessence Publishing Co, Inc
411 N Raddant Rd
Batavia, IL 60510
www.quintpub.com

5 4 3 2 1

Editor: Zachary Kocanda
Design: Sue Zubek
Production: Sue Robinson

Printed in Croatia

Management of Endodontic Complications

From Diagnosis to Prognosis

Edited by

Mahmoud Torabinejad, DMD, MSD, PhD
Professor of Endodontics
Loma Linda University School of Dentistry
Loma Linda, California

Research Professor
University of Minnesota
Minneapolis, Minnesota

Mohammad Sabeti, DDS, MA
Professor of Endodontics
University of California, San Francisco
San Francisco, California

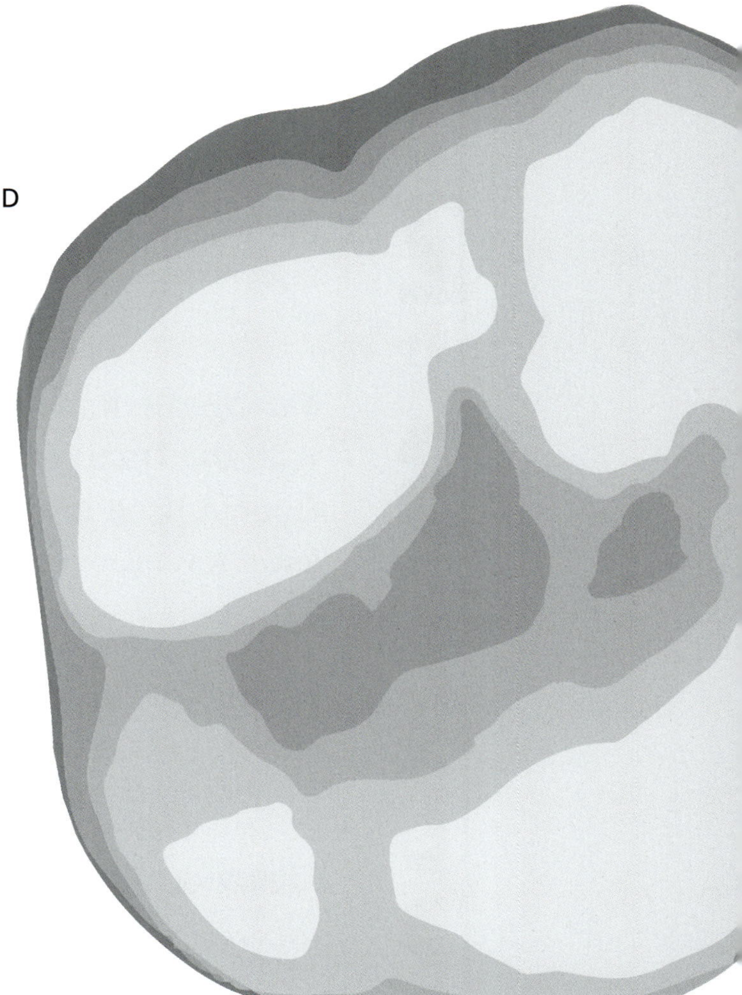

QUINTESSENCE PUBLISHING

Berlin | Chicago | Tokyo
Barcelona | London | Milan | Mexico City | Paris | Prague | Seoul | Warsaw
Beijing | Istanbul | Sao Paulo | Zagreb

Contents

Preface

Endodontics is a field of dentistry that deals with the biologic and technical aspects of root canal treatment. Root canal treatment is a well-established procedure that has provided pain relief, function, and esthetics to patients for decades. The main goal of this discipline is to preserve the natural dentition.

Like other dental and medical specialties, the practice of endodontics consists of two inseparable components: science and art. The science of endodontics covers the didactic and clinical aspects of this field as they relate to the biologic and pathologic conditions. The art of endodontics deals with proper execution of the technical aspects of this field.

Similar to other fields of dentistry, root canal treatment can have unwanted or unforeseen challenges that can affect its prognosis. These unwanted and unforeseen challenges are collectively termed *procedural accidents or errors*. The procedural accidents can occur during diagnosis, access preparation, shaping and cleaning, obturation, restoration, surgical and nonsurgical retreatments, and assessment of outcomes of root canal treatment. The principal objective of *Management of Endodontic Complications: From Diagnosis to Prognosis* is to discuss the etiology, prevention, and treatment of procedural errors before, during, and after root canal treatment.

This book presents clear and concise guidance on all aspects of both minor and major complications encountered in endodontic practice. Each chapter provides complete descriptions of the etiologic factors, explains the prevention of complications, and recommends treatment options associated with these complications. The main features of this book include learning objectives and key references; a systematic approach to each complication, including prevention, recognition, and management; and more than 500 high-quality clinical and radiographic images that demonstrate the discussed concepts.

During the writing and editing of this book, we noticed there are many areas within the field of endodontics that continue to need to be researched and investigated. We believe practitioners should be up to date regarding the latest scientific evidence in the field and know how to contribute their own research. As a result, we put together an online chapter that explains the proper methods to write and publish research protocols and focuses on the common errors in various steps of writing and publishing research findings. Scan the QR code here to access this supplementary information.

Having knowledge regarding the etiologic factors involved in procedural accidents and the methods to prevent and treat them properly should save millions of teeth throughout the world. We firmly believe most procedural errors can be avoided by adhering to the basic principles of diagnosis, case selection, treatment planning, access preparation, shaping and cleaning, obturation, restoration, nonsurgical and surgical retreatments, and outcomes assessment.

We would like to thank sincerely our contributing authors for sharing their valuable knowledge and experiences with us and our readers as well as the Quintessence staff for their assistance with the publication of this book.

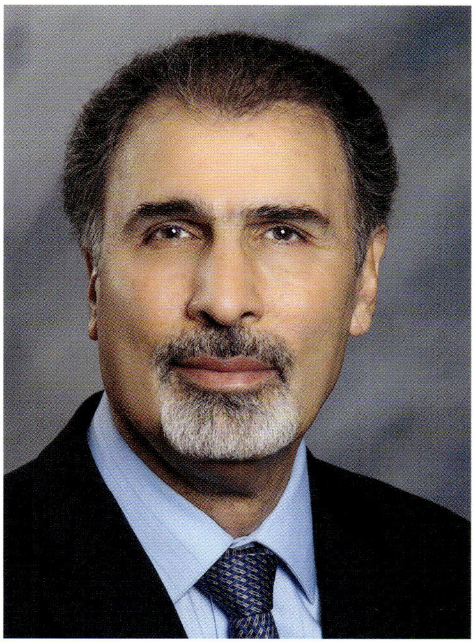

Mahmoud Torabinejad

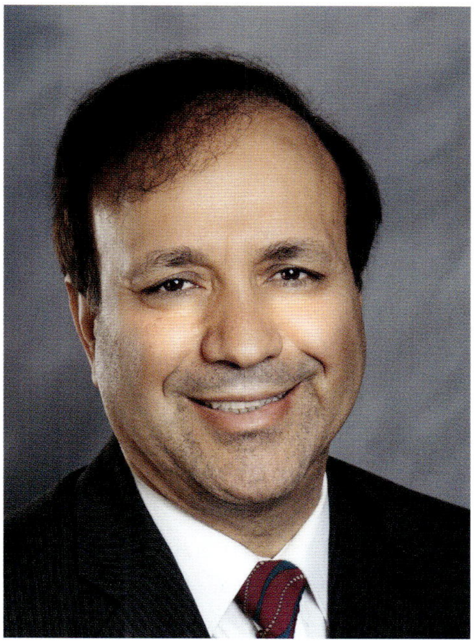

Mohammad Sabeti

Contributors

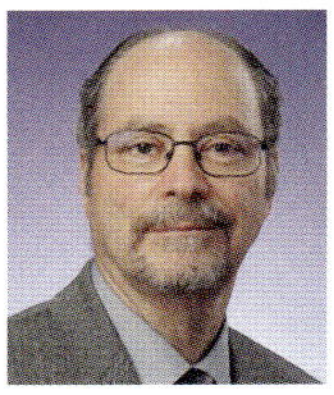

Kenneth Abramovitch, DDS, MS
Professor and Chair
Department of Oral Pathology, Radiology and Medicine
University of Missouri—Kansas City, School of Dentistry
Kansas City, Missouri

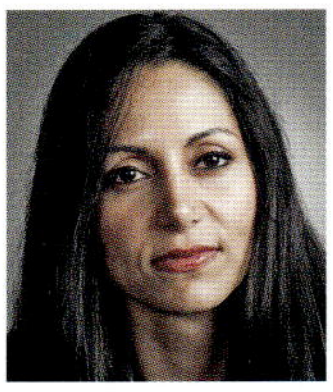

Anita Aminoshariae, DDS, MS
Professor
Department of Endodontics
Case Western Reserve University School of Dental Medicine
Cleveland, Ohio

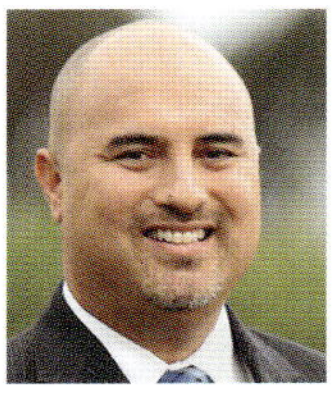

Daniel J. Boehne, DDS
Assistant Professor
UCLA School of Dentistry
Los Angeles, California

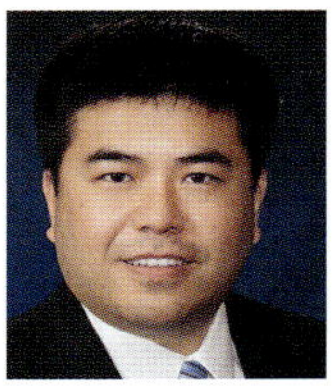

Yujie Huang, DDS, PhD
Assistant Professor
Division of Endodontics
University of California, San Francisco
San Francisco, California

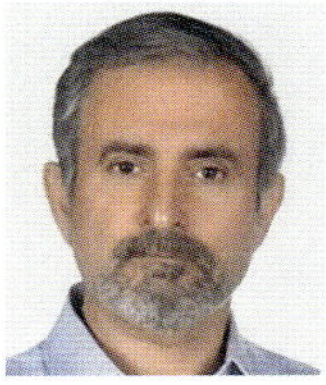

Kiumars Nazari Moghadam, DDS, MSc
Associate Professor
Department of Endodontics
Shahed University Dental School
Tehran, Iran

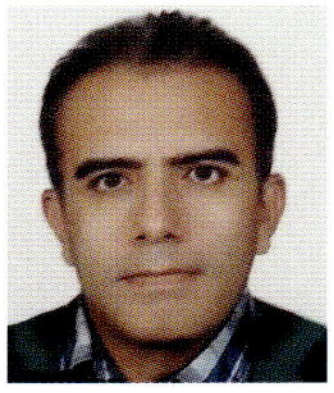

Zahed Mohammadi, DMD, MSD
Distinguished Clinical Scientist
Iranian Center for Endodontic Research
Universal Scientific Education and Research Network
Tehran, Iran

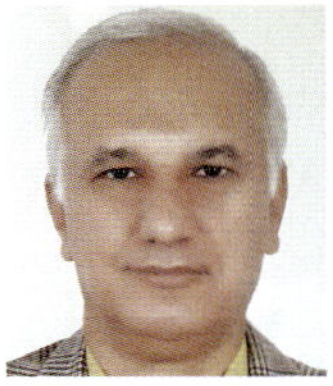

Masoud Parirokh, DMD, MSc
Distinguished Professor
Endodontology Research Center
Kerman University of Medical Sciences
Kerman, Iran

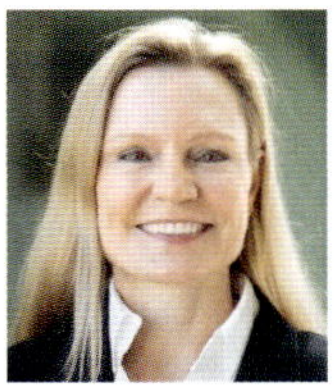

Christine I. Peters, DMD
Professor of Endodontics
The University of Queensland School of Dentistry
Herston, Queensland
Australia

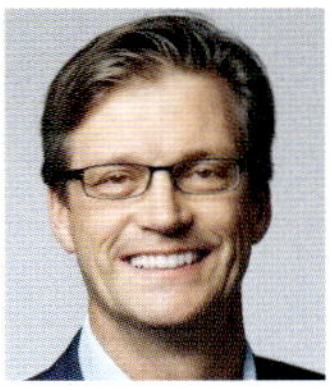

Ove A. Peters, DMD, MS, PhD
Professor of Endodontics
The University of Queensland School of Dentistry
Herston, Queensland
Australia

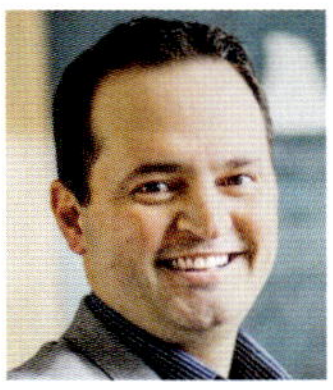

Joseph A. Petrino, DDS, MS
Private Practice Limited to Endodontics
Missoula, Montana

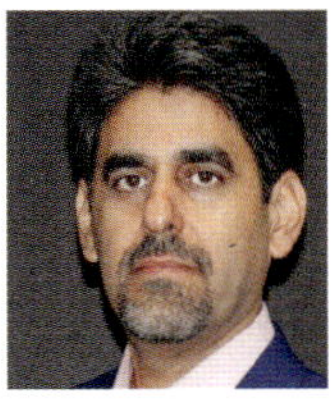

Mohsen Ramazani, DDS, MSc
Assistant Professor
Department of Endodontics
Mazandaran University of Medical Sciences School of Dentistry
Sari, Iran

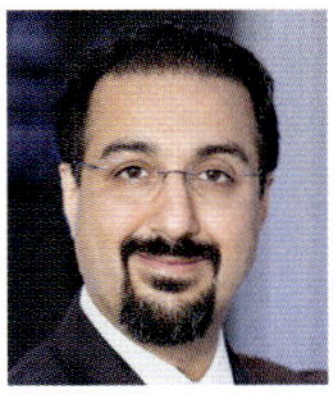

Seyed Aliakbar (Ali) Vahdati, DDS, MSD
Lecturer
Division of Endodontics
UCLA School of Dentistry
Los Angeles, California

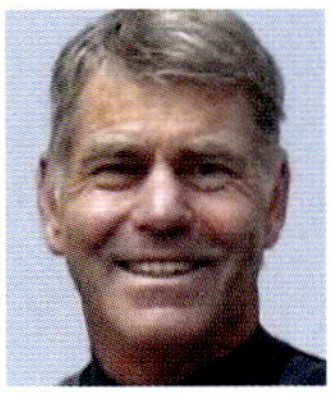

Shane N. White, BDentSc, MS, MA, PhD
Professor
UCLA School of Dentistry
Los Angeles, California

1

Complications During Diagnosis and Treatment Planning

MAHMOUD TORABINEJAD
ANITA AMINOSHARIAE

Objectives

After reading this chapter, the reader should be able to:

1. Differentiate between pulpal pain and other pains.
2. Identify the characteristics of pain with or without periapical pathology.
3. Describe the characteristics of nonpulpal pain with or without periapical pathology.
4. Discuss mishaps during the following:
   - Patient interview
   - Addressing the chief complaint
   - Recording medical history
   - Recording dental history
   - Clinical examination:
     - Extraoral examination
     - Intraoral examination
     - Clinical tests
     - Percussion
     - Palpation
     - Pulp sensitivity tests
     - Probing
     - Mobility
   - Radiographic examination
     - Radiolucencies simulating periapical pathosis
   - Additional diagnostic tests

Introduction

The discipline of endodontics deals with the biologic aspects of the human dental pulp and periapical tissues as well as treatment of diseases related to these tissues. Additionally, the scope of endodontics includes diagnosis and treatment of pulpal pain with or without periapical pathology, vital pulp therapy, regenerative endodontic procedures, nonsurgical root canal treatment, and surgical and nonsurgical retreatment of cases with persistent disease. When indicated and properly performed, root canal treatment is safe, alleviates pain and suffering, and preserves natural dentition with a favorable and predictable outcome.[1] Like other medical and dental procedures, the practice of endodontics has two components: art and science. The *art* of endodontics consists of executing technical procedures for root canal treatment, which is often subjective. The *science* of endodontics is objective and includes an understanding of the biologic and pathologic conditions related to the art of endodontics through the principles and methods of evidence-based treatment. One of the most important parts of the application of both the art and science is the accurate diagnosis of pulpal and periapical diseases. Lack of attention to detail in application of the science of endodontics can easily result in diagnostic mishaps and subsequent inappropriate treatment.

Mishaps can often occur outside of the technical components of root canal treatment—during diagnosis. Mistakes during diagnosis can result in improper and unnecessary treatment and increased costs, creating unsatisfied patients and leading to legal action against a provider. Furthermore, misdiagnosis can result in serious consequences to the systemic health of the patient and may affect the prognosis of future treatment(s). In short, an unnecessary—although well-executed—root canal treatment should be avoided because it can cause frustration for both the patient and the clinician. There are a number of clinical and radiographic normal and pathologic conditions that mimic endodontic pathosis.[2] To avoid misdiagnosis, the clinician should use a systematic approach to gather pertinent medical and dental information, perform necessary tests, and analyze the gathered information to develop a differential diagnosis, definitive diagnosis, and subsequent treatment plan. Most misdiagnoses can be avoided by adhering to the basic principles of diagnosis and case selection. This chapter will focus on appropriate steps to obtain information during a patient's interview regarding their medical and dental histories, clinical and radiographic signs and symptoms, and the implications of the gathered data in treatment planning.

Pulpal pain vs other pains

Several types of nonpulpal pain with or without periapical pathology simulate clinical features of pulpal and/or periapical diseases. Because of the similarities of these conditions, dentists must perform clinical tests in a systematic manner to avoid misdiagnosis and subsequent incorrect treatment. To arrive at the correct diagnosis, a provider must review all relevant patient history, clinical signs and symptoms, pulp tests, and radiographic examination. Dentists are usually the first clinicians involved in diagnosis and treatment of these conditions.[3] In order to be successful in treating these patients, it is important to have a clear understanding of the many different ways in which the patient may experience nonodontogenic versus odontogenic pain. Within the dental field, the most useful pain consultants are dentists trained in orofacial pain, endodontists, and oral and maxillofacial surgeons.[2] Pain may be acute or chronic. Acute pain arises from inflammation or injury to the pulp and periapical tissues. Chronic pain is continuous in nature and lingers long after an injury has healed or may not even be associated with an injury. Despite apparent similarities of odontogenic and nonodontogenic pain, there are some subtle but key differences in the characteristics of these conditions. Paying close attention to these differences often reduces the chance of misdiagnosis.

Characteristics of pulpal pain with or without periapical pathology

Odontogenic pain is often acute and can awaken a patient from sleep or prevent the patient from sleeping. Sleep disturbance is an important part of the differential diagnosis. It is important to ask the patient very specific questions about the impact of pain on sleep patterns.[2] Pulpal pain with or without periapical tissue pathology is easily localized initially by the patient or by the practitioner. An affected tooth is typically painful to palpation or percussion. As the pain becomes chronic, it may spread to other teeth, and it may be more difficult for the patient to identify the offending tooth or teeth. Odontogenic pain has apparent etiologic factors such as caries, leaky restorations, trauma, or fracture. Depending on the condition of the pulp, it may be very sensitive to temperature changes, or in the case of pulpal necrosis, it can have no response to thermal changes. Absence of clinical and/or radiographic signs and symptoms of pulpal or periapical disease may indicate the presence of nonodontogenic pain. Pulpal pain is usually localized and usually limited to a single tooth. This type of pain is relieved by administering local anesthetic and performing dental treatment.

Characteristics of nonpulpal pain with or without periapical pathology

Nonodontogenic pain has several accompanying features that are different from those seen in odontogenic pain.[2] Most patients who have nonodontogenic pain are extremely distressed and frequently have jumped from one provider to another as treatment failures continue to mount. A history of unsuccessful root canal treatments on a number of teeth or different procedures performed by numerous providers is a good indication for the clinician to explore the possibility of nonodontogenic pain. In contrast to odontogenic pain, patients experiencing nonodontogenic pain cannot localize the source of their discomfort and have little or no clinical or radiographic signs and symptoms of pulpal disease with or without periapical pathology. Nonodontogenic pain has no apparent etiologic factors like those for odontogenic pain. The pain does not consistently subside by administration of local anesthetic. It can be bilateral but is generally unilateral. The first group of nonodontogenic conditions that simulate odontogenic pain includes pain related to the maxillary premolars and molars adjacent to the maxillary sinuses, musculoskeletal pain, temporomandibular disorders, neuropathic pain, neurovascular pain, atypical odontalgia, neuromas, neuritis, intracranial pain, headaches, and psychologic disturbances.[2] The second group of conditions that may cause referral of pain to the teeth and simulate pulpal pain with or without periapical pathology are pain from other teeth, maxillary sinus or nasal cavities, the cervical spine, vascular structures, the heart, tumors, and other neoplasms in the head and neck.[2] The most common misdiagnosis in the first group occurs from pain in the maxillary sinus, muscles of mastication, and the temporomandibular joint (TMJ).

Patients who have maxillary sinus pain describe it as constant pressure and fullness in the region. The pain may be referred to the maxillary premolar and molar teeth. Head position or movement can often exacerbate the discomfort.[4,5] These patients usually do not have decay or restorations in the region to indicate presence of pulpal and/or periapical diseases. Consultation and referral to an ear, nose, and throat (ENT) specialist is the right course of action for these patients.

Myofascial pain is the most common muscle pain disorder of the orofacial region. The most common symptoms associated with muscle problems are pain with palpation, movement anomalies, and referred pain. These patients usually do not have decay or restorations indicating presence of pulpal or periapical disease; however, it is not uncommon to see many failed endodontic treatments as a result of misdiagnosis of this condition as pulpal and/or periapical diseases.[6] Joint disorders are identified as a major cause of nondental pain in the orofacial region and are considered a subclassification of musculoskeletal disorders.[7]

Temporomandibular joint disorders (TMDs) are one of the major causes of nonodontogenic pain. Trauma from tooth grinding or jaw clenching or trauma from external forces such as automobile accidents has been implicated as an etiology of TMD.[4,5,8] Hyperextension of temporomandibular structures during long dental procedures is another possible etiology for TMD.[2] With TMDs, palpation of the TMJ and the muscles of mastication results in pain or discomfort. During examination of the TMJ, clicking or popping in the joint can be noticed. Similar to patients with sinus pain, these patients also generally do not have decay or restorations in the region to indicate presence of pulpal and/or periapical disease. Treatment of TMD includes wearing a nightguard and taking a muscle relaxant.

Trigeminal neuralgia affects the fifth cranial nerve and can cause another common pain that can be mistaken for odontogenic pain. The etiology of trigeminal neuralgia is unknown, but demyelination, vascular malformations and the presence of pathologic cavities at the site of previous tooth extraction, periodontal lesions, and previous endodontic therapy have been implicated for this condition.[5] It is usually unilateral and involves the maxillary or mandibular branch of the fifth cranial nerve. Because of the location of the symptoms of trigeminal neuralgia relative to teeth, many of these patients are referred for root canal treatment. Patients describe their high-intensity pain as an electric-like shock with a trigger zone associated with activities such as eating, talking, or even breathing cold air.[9] The intensity of the pain is very severe and can occur for short or extended periods of time.[9] Despite the severity and intensity of pain, it usually does not awaken the patient, which helps to differentiate this type of pain from pulpal and/or periapical pain.[2]

The second group of nonodontogenic conditions that simulates odontogenic pain is referred pain. When neurons from several teeth or other structures converge on a second-order neuron that is sensitized, the potential for referred pain increases. In referred pain, the pain originating in a tooth can seem to come from another tooth or another area, even outside the mouth.[10–15] These include pain referred from one tooth to another tooth or to the ear, from the maxillary sinus to the maxillary teeth, from vascular structures to teeth, and even from cardiac muscle to teeth.

One of the most common mishaps during diagnosis is the misdiagnosis and treatment of a normal tooth instead of the offending tooth. The pain from irreversible pulpitis in a tooth can be referred to another tooth in the same quadrant or the opposite dental arch. Pain in the mandibular arch can also be referred to the ENT specialist. Careful examination of the clinical and radiographic data can prevent these mishaps.

Another common mistake is when problems in the maxillary sinuses and/or paranasal mucosa refer pain to the maxillary premolar and molar teeth. This type of pain is usually dull and increases with coughing or sneezing. In addition, lowering the head can increase pressure over the sinuses, thus exacerbating this pain.[2] Pulp testing with cold and percussion may increase the pain from the sinus. A history of upper respiratory infection, nasal congestion, or sinus problems is a good indicator of the presence of sinus problems rather than a toothache. These patients usually do not have decay or restorations in the region to indicate presence of pulpal and/or periapical diseases. Sinus radiographs, CBCT images, or a magnetic resonance imaging (MRI) can greatly help in the diagnosis of these conditions and thus prevent mishaps. Referral to an ENT specialist is indicated when these conditions are suspected.

Arteritis of the carotid or temporal arteries can present with pain in and around teeth, jaws, and related structures. Palpation of these specific anatomical locations can assist in the diagnostic process.[4,5,8] Similar to patients with sinus pain, these patients also do not have decay or restorations in the region to indicate the presence of pulpal and/or periapical diseases.

Another nonodontogenic pain that is commonly misdiagnosed is cardiac pain. Cardiac problems such as angina pectoris or acute myocardial infarction refer pain to the shoulder, to the arm, and even to the mandibular teeth, which is why these patients seek dental treatment. The dentist must be aware of the fact that this type of pain may be associated with chest pain, but occasionally they do not occur together.[2] When a toothache has a cardiac origin, it usually increases with exercise and decreases with medication such as nitroglycerin tablets. The role of the dentist in this situation is to rule out any pulpal or periapical diseases and to immediately refer the patient to a physician for treatment of the underlying cardiac problem.

Mishaps During Patient Interview

Mishaps during a patient's interview can relate to information regarding the chief complaint, health and medical history, or dental history.

Chief complaint

Recording information about why the patient is seeking care starts with their chief complaint and is the first encounter between the patient and the provider or his/her staff members. The chief complaint should be listened to very carefully and be recorded in the patient's own words. Remember, this is why the patient is seeking help. Patients usually judge the character of the provider and staff based on the outcome of treatment and how well their chief complaint was addressed. Patients want to know that your priority as a clinician is their well-being rather than the knowledge that you possess. Ignoring or not paying enough attention to the patient's chief complaint not only results in missing valuable diagnostic information, but it may also cause a lack of trust between the patient and the provider.

Health and medical history

Recording an accurate and complete medical history with vital signs is important for a thorough endodontic evaluation and subsequent diagnosis. The relationship between systemic disease and apical periodontitis has been a subject of great interest for many years.[2] This relationship is an intricate one, because both conditions share many common bioburdens and risk factors.[16–19] The common diseases that may influence endodontic pathosis, treatments, and outcomes are cardiovascular disease (CVD), diabetes, hematologic disorders, cancer, kidney disease, and neurologic disorders. Osteoresorptive agents and medications that are known to increase the risk of osteonecrosis of the jaw (bisphosphonate, denosumab, and angiogenic drugs) should be avoided when considering endodontic surgical intervention.

Cardiovascular diseases

CVDs include a group of heart and vascular systemic diseases. Some of the most common CVDs among a population might include endocarditis, myocardial infarction, hypertension, dysrhythmias, and ischemic heart disease. Systematic reviews and epidemiologic data have reported the association between endodontics and CVD, which underscores the common mechanisms and immunomodulatory effects that link these two types of diseases.[18,20] This association occurs primarily from the bacterial byproducts shared by both of these chronic diseases, resulting in inflammatory reactions, increasing C-reactive protein, interleukins, matrix metalloproteinases, and immunoglobulins, which result in NF-kB pro-inflammation gene induction.[21,22]

Endocarditis

The American Dental Association (ADA) and the American Heart Association (AHA) updated a scientific statement in 2021 to support antibiotic prophylaxis only for the highest risk patients who have recurrent episodes of native or prosthetic valve infective endocarditis.[23] The statement highlights the importance of prophylaxis for all dental procedures that involve manipulation of gingival or periapical regions.

Myocardial infarction

Nonsteroidal anti-inflammatory drugs (NSAIDs) are not recommended for patients with myocardial infarction (MI).[24] A recent MI, defined as within the past 6 months, dictates that elective dental treatment should be postponed and, if urgently needed, should be provided in consultation with the patient's physician.[25] For stress reduction, oral sedative premedication may be indicated. Vital signs should be monitored, while nitroglycerin and aspirin 81 mg should be available. An emergency container should contain additional paraphernalia. An oral and maxillofacial surgery text should be consulted for the contents of this container.

Vasoconstrictors

Epinephrine should be limited to 0.04 mg for this population. The appointment should be terminated if blood pressure readings are > 180/110. In general, vasoconstrictors are contraindicated for the following patients: recent MI, unstable angina, recent coronary artery bypass surgery (within 3 months), uncontrolled or untreated hypertension, refractory arrhythmias, uncontrolled hyperthyroidism, or uncontrolled diabetes.[25]

Nonselective beta-blockers and vasoconstrictors might result in dangerous elevation in blood pressure. Thus, it is recommended to either avoid administration of epinephrine or closely monitor blood pressure after administration of 0.017 mg epinephrine.

Anticoagulant and antiplatelet agents

Patients taking antithrombic medications may be at high risk of excessive bleeding during an endodontic surgical procedure.[26] Due to the many complications associated with Coumadin, many patients are now taking direct oral anticoagulants (DOACs). Examples of DOACs include apixaban (factor Xa inhibitor), dabigatran (factor IIa inhibitor), edoxaban (factor Xa inhibitor), and rivaroxaban (factor Xa inhibitor). Care must be taken in treating these patients, particularly when performing incision and drainage, surgical treatment, or perforation repair, because excessive bleeding may occur. Local measures to control bleeding are recommended, and discontinuation of anticoagulant medication is not advised.[26] Patients on Coumadin should not receive fluconazole or metronidazole because both drugs increase the concentration of Coumadin.

Digoxin

Patients on digoxin should not receive epinephrine, because it would increase the risk for arrhythmia.

Diabetes mellitus

Diabetes is a metabolic disorder that is caused by either a deficiency or a resistance to insulin, which results in poor circulation, healing, and outcomes.[17,27] The microangiopathies from diabetes can cause problems with eyes, kidneys, extremities, and any other area where small arteries are located. A high prevalence of periapical radiolucencies within the type 2 diabetes population has been reported.[28] The authors suggested that controlling the disease with medications (insulin, metformin, statin) was associated with lower prevalence of apical periodontitis. This indicates that when treating these patients, the astute provider should know the patient's current hemoglobin A1c status (HbA1c).

Hematologic diseases

Sickle-cell anemia

Patients with sickle cell anemia have a high prevalence of orofacial pain and pulp necrosis.[29,30]

Hemophilia

Congenital bleeding disorders should be identified and treated appropriately. NSAIDs should be avoided as these patients are at great risk of bleeding from invasive dental procedures. Patients with hemophilia and von Willebrand disease may be managed with desmopressin and aminocaproic acid. Factor VIII replacement might be required prior to the treatment for hemophilia A, and Factor IX replacement may be required prior to an invasive treatment for hemophilia B. Local hemostatic agents should be used to control bleeding.

White blood cell disorders

White blood cells (WBCs) constitute three groups: granulocytes, lymphocytes, and monocytes. Because WBCs are responsible for defense against microbial invasion, defects in WBCs can result in infection and delayed healing. Bisphosphonates and denosumab are anti-resorptive drugs that are used for treatment of myeloma.[31,32] Though similar in their anti-resorptive action, the two drugs work differently: Denosumab acts by binding to and inhibiting RANKL, and bisphosphonates inhibit osteoclasts.[33] Both of these medications and another group of drugs, angiogenesis inhibitors, have been associated with medication-related osteonecrosis of the jaw (MRONJ).[34] These drugs are also used for osteoporosis, multiple myeloma, and/or cancer therapy.[35] As such, care must be used in treating these patients when manipulating hard tissues. Denosumab belongs to a group of anti-cancer drugs called *monoclonal antibodies*. These drugs have also been associated with external cervical resorption.[36]

Chronic kidney disease

Chronic kidney disease (CKD) and end-stage renal disease (ESRD) are conditions where renal osteodystrophy can occur secondary to high levels of parathyroid hormone. A clinician must not confuse the lesions with a periapical radiolucency. These patients should not receive NSAIDs, tetracycline, high doses of acyclovir, or high doses of amoxicillin or cephalexin.[37] They may be on immunosuppressant drugs and anticoagulant agents.

Neurologic diseases

Lyme disease

Lyme disease can mimic orofacial pain. As such, a clinician must ensure that all clinical signs and symptoms come together to form an accurate and logical diagnosis.

Multiple sclerosis

Multiple sclerosis is a common autoimmune disease where demyelination of the corticospinal tract neurons takes place. It can mimic trigeminal neuralgia and should be included in a differential diagnosis. Trigeminal neuralgia can occur secondary to multiple sclerosis and can mimic orofacial pain.[38]

Cancer

Chemotherapy drugs cause immunosuppression. Additionally, antiresorptive agents—such as bisphosphonates and denosumab—and angiogenesis inhibitors may be administered to these patients.[39] These drugs are also used for osteoporosis.[40] As discussed previously, these medications may result in MRONJ. For this reason, the clinician should be completely familiar with the patient's medical history and medications and know when to request the patient's complete blood count (CBC) with differentials.

Consultation with the patient's physician is highly recommended for surgical interventions. Occasionally, antibiotics may be required for patients whose WBC count is outside of the norm (normal value may be in the range of 4,000–10,000/mL and neutrophil should be 50% cell/mL).

Patients with radiation > 60 Gy to the head or throat have an 11-fold increased risk of osteoradionecrosis.[41] Thus, surgical interventions should be avoided.

Pregnancy

According to the joint statement by the ADA and the American College of Obstetricians and Gynecologists, endodontic therapy can be safely performed without delay at any time during pregnancy.[42] Class B pregnancy drugs, which include lidocaine and prilocaine, acetaminophen, cephalosporins, clindamycin, and azithromycin, are preferred,[43] though acetaminophen should be used sparingly.[44] Caution should be exercised when using epinephrine because it contracts the uterine and vascular walls, resulting in reduced blood flow to the fetus.[45]

Smoking

Smoking is related to high prevalence of pulpal necrosis and apical periodontitis.[28,46] However, it is unknown if it would be associated with worse endodontic outcomes.[46]

Dental history

Recent visit(s) to other provider(s) might provide valuable information regarding the etiology of the patient's chief complaint. Information regarding recent trauma or restorations and previous treatment for temporomandibular dysfunction may indicate the type of treatment that would be most appropriate for a patient. When taking dental history, the clinician should ask about the presence and the nature of the pain, any swelling, broken or loose teeth, tooth discoloration, and/or a bad taste. Missing this information while recording a dental history can easily result in misdiagnosis and inappropriate treatment.

If there are two or more concurrent complaints, the history of each complaint must be obtained.[47] When pain is the chief complaint of the patient, the following questions should be asked regarding the characteristics and the nature of the existing pain: the location, onset, cause, and character of the pain (short, sharp, long lasting, dull, throbbing, continuous, occasional); if there is interference of sleep or work; if there is any worsening of the condition in the morning or evening; whether there is spontaneity (nonspontaneous or spontaneous); if any postural changes affect the pain; and if anything makes the pain better or worse (hot, cold, biting). Quantification of the amount of pain (on a Likert scale of 0 to 10) not only gives the practitioner an idea about the severity of the pain; it also allows comparison of the pain from visit to visit, particularly if there is residual pain after treatment.[47]

Mishaps During Clinical Examination

A clinical examination consists of careful observation and diagnostic testing of extraoral and intraoral tissues to compare them with other normal structures without apparent pathosis.

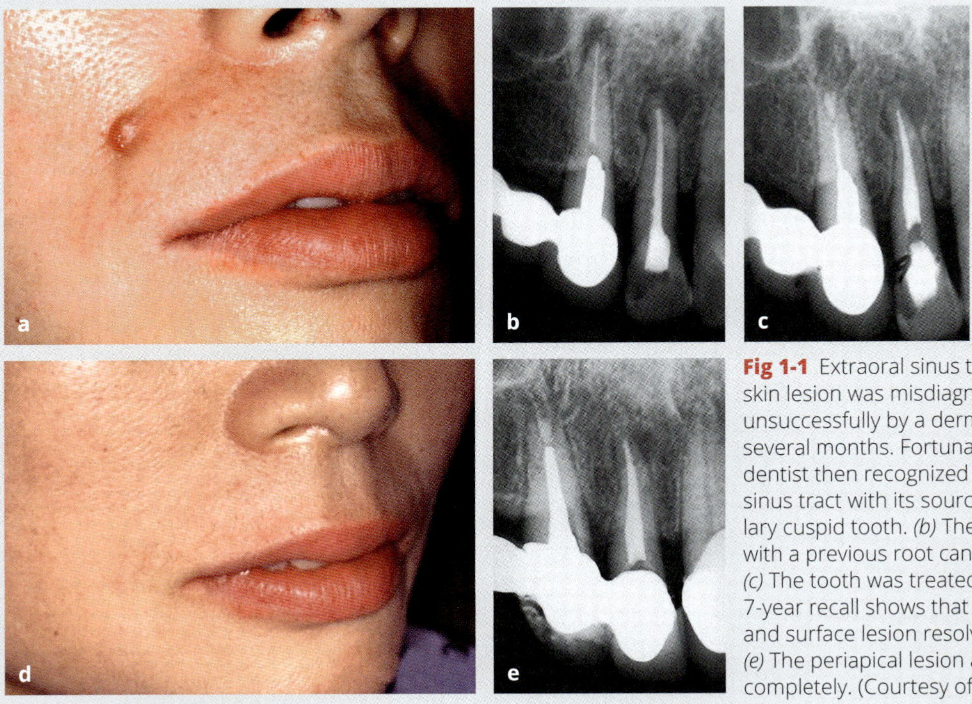

Fig 1-1 Extraoral sinus tract. *(a)* This facial skin lesion was misdiagnosed and treated unsuccessfully by a dermatologist for several months. Fortunately, the patient's dentist then recognized it to be a draining sinus tract with its source being a maxillary cuspid tooth. *(b)* The pulp was necrotic with a previous root canal treatment. *(c)* The tooth was treated surgically. *(d)* A 7-year recall shows that the sinus tract and surface lesion resolved completely. *(e)* The periapical lesion also resolved completely. (Courtesy of Dr C.J. Hong.)

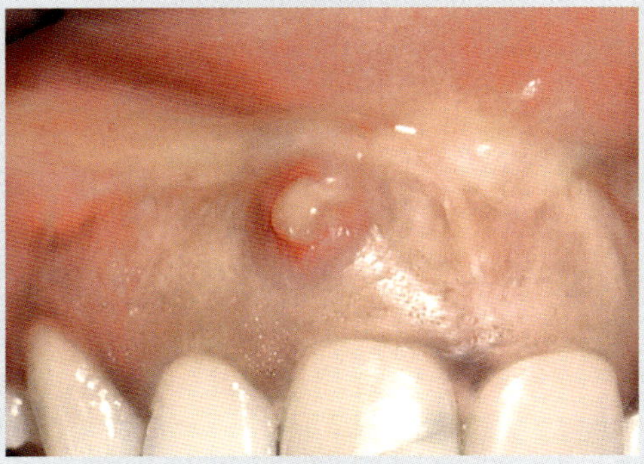

Fig 1-2 Intraoral sinus tract. Presence of a stoma usually indicates existence of a necrotic pulp and a chronic apical abscess.

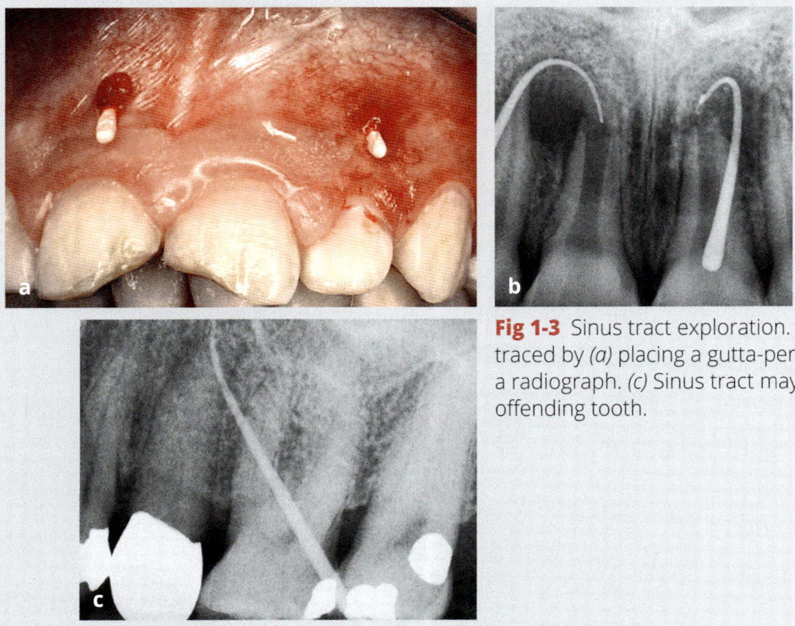

Fig 1-3 Sinus tract exploration. Sinus tracts should always be traced by *(a)* placing a gutta-percha in them and *(b)* exposing a radiograph. *(c)* Sinus tract may appear far away from the offending tooth.

Extraoral examination

During extraoral examination of a patient, the general appearance, skin tone, and facial asymmetry are evaluated. The presence or absence of swelling, discoloration, redness, extraoral scars, sinus tracts, and lymphadenopathies should also be evaluated. A careful extraoral examination can identify the cause of the patient's chief complaint and may help to reveal the cause of intraoral pathosis. A good example of this condition is the presence of an extraoral fistula related to a mandibular or maxillary tooth (Fig 1-1). A common mishap is misdiagnosis of these conditions as skin infections and subsequently treating them with medications and multiple surgeries.

Intraoral examination

Intraoral examination consists of close observation and testing of soft and hard tissues of the oral cavity. A soft tissue examination includes a careful visual evaluation and digital evaluation of the lips, oral mucosa, cheeks, tongue, periodontium, palate, and muscles of mastication. The alveolar mucosa and gingiva are examined for the presence of inflammation, ulceration, discoloration, and sinus tract formation. The presence of a stoma usually indicates a necrotic pulp, while a chronic apical abscess might indicate a periodontal abscess (Fig 1-2). Sinus tracts should always be traced by placing a gutta-percha in them and then confirming with a radiograph. A common mishap is the assumption of some clinicians that the sinus tracts appear adjacent to the offending tooth. That is not always true. A sinus tract may appear far away from the offending tooth (Fig 1-3). When swelling is present, questions must be asked regarding when the swelling began, how quickly the swelling increased in size, the nature of the swelling (fluctuant, indurated, tender), if there is drainage from the swelling, and if the swelling is associated with an excessively mobile or tender tooth.[47] Answers to these questions can determine whether the swelling is from a periapical abscess or a periodontal abscess. This information may help prevent misdiagnosis and mistreatment.

Before performing clinical tests, the teeth should be examined with a mirror and an explorer for discolorations, fractures, abrasions, erosions, caries, failing restorations, or other abnormalities.[2,47] A discolored crown is often pathognomonic of pulpal pathosis or the sequela of past root canal treatment (Fig 1-4).

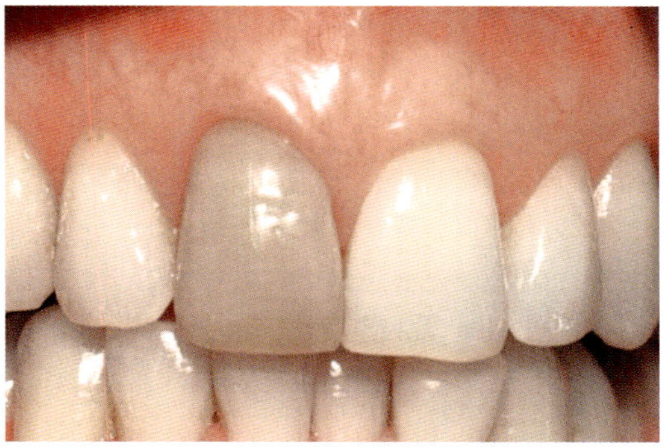

Fig 1-4 A discolored incisor may indicate the presence of a tooth with necrotic pulp, calcified pulp chamber, or inadequate previous root canal treatment.

Clinical tests

Clinical tests include several methods to determine the presence or absence of pathologic changes in the dentition. The reason for using a number of tests is that each test has its inherent limitations and must be interpreted carefully in conjunction with all other information available. In order to improve the outcome of these diagnostic tests, each test should be explained in simple terms to the patient. It is important to include a control (comparison) tooth of a similar type to the suspected tooth or teeth. A common mistake during performing clinical tests is the exclusion of control teeth for comparison, but a control tooth provides vital information for the clinician to compare the patient's baseline responses. The clinical tests used during diagnosis include percussion, palpation, probing, vitality tests, and radiographic examination.

Percussion

Percussion is performed either by using the end of a mirror handle held parallel or perpendicular to the crown or by applying gentle digital pressure on a very tender tooth to identify the offending tooth with pulpal or periapical disease. When a painful response is obtained, it only indicates the presence of inflammation somewhere in the periodontal ligament of the tooth. Repetitive strain of the periodontal ligament through clenching, presence of gross malocclusion, or traumatic injury to teeth can cause inflammation of the periodontal ligament without pulpal and/or periapical disease.[2] A common mistake during a percussion test is the assumption that the tenderness of a tooth to percussion is due to the presence of a tooth with periapical inflammation. To avoid this mistake, the presence of other etiologies should be considered, such as deep decay and/or restorations in teeth with sensitivity to percussion.

Palpation

Palpation sensitivity indicates the presence of inflammation in the periapical tissues of a tooth and is more reliable than percussion sensitivity testing. A painful response to palpation usually indicates presence of periapical inflammation in a tooth with pulpal and/or periapical disease.

Pulp sensitivity tests

Currently, there are three methods to determine pulp response: cold, hot, and electrical tests. These tests do not determine the *vitality* of the dental pulp; they only determine the level of *sensitivity* of the dental pulp to these stimuli. Selection of the appropriate test is based on the patient's chief complaint to check for reproducibility of the symptoms that simulate the patient's complaint. If a patient's chief complaint is sensitivity to cold, the results of hot or electrical tests for that patient are generally irrelevant.

The cold test is the most reliable method to determine the presence or absence of vital tissue in a tooth. After the tooth is dried and isolated with cotton rolls, a cold stimulus is applied to the buccal or lingual surface of the tooth close to the cementoenamel junction (CEJ). Presence of prolonged pain after application of cold to a tooth usually is an indication of irreversible pulpitis. However, absence of a response to cold does not necessarily mean the presence of a necrotic pulp. There are patients who present with very little or no response to thermal changes without having pulpal pathosis. A false negative response is often obtained when cold is applied to teeth with calcific metamorphosis, whereas a false positive response may result if cold contacts gingiva or is transferred to adjacent teeth with vital pulps. Gingival recession and attachment loss decrease sensitivity to cold testing.[48] Common errors for this test are lack of isolation of a test tooth, lack of a control tooth for comparison, and misunderstandings regarding the possibilities for false positive and negative responses.

An electric pulp test determines the sensitivity of the pulp to this stimulus. After the tooth is dried and isolated with cotton rolls, an electric stimulus is applied to the buccal or lingual surface of the tooth with a small amount of toothpaste on the electrode of the pulp tester as a conduction agent. False positive and false negative results can be the main problems with this test.[49] Small canals or pulp-canal obliteration may lead to false negative responses.[50] Some clinicians use the exact readings during this test as an indication of pulpal status. However, the exact number of the reading is not significant because it does not detect subtle degrees of pulpal vitality.[51] Additionally, this test does not indicate if there is partial necrosis, particularly in a multirooted tooth. The common errors for electric testing are lack of proper isolation of the test tooth, absence of control tooth for comparison, and lack of knowledge regarding the shortcomings of this test.

The heat test is the least reliable, and it should only be used in patients who complain about heat sensitivity.[52] After isolating the tooth with a rubber dam to prevent false positive responses from adjacent teeth, heat is applied to the buccal or lingual surface of the suspected tooth. As with cold, the presence of prolonged pain after application of heat to a tooth usually is an indication of the presence of irreversible pulpitis. Like cold and electric pulp testing, the common errors for this test are lack of proper isolation of the suspect tooth, the absence of a control tooth for comparison, and lack of knowledge regarding the shortcomings of this test.

Currently, a single diagnostic device capable of applying thermal and electrical stimuli and transillumination is not available. The convenience of having a single diagnostic test is overlooked because the current gold standard for testing requires different materials and techniques. Figure 1-5 shows the current devices used for pulp sensitivity tests. A single diagnostic device capable of providing cold, heat, electricity, and light in one comprehensive setting would increase diagnostic accuracy of pulp testing.

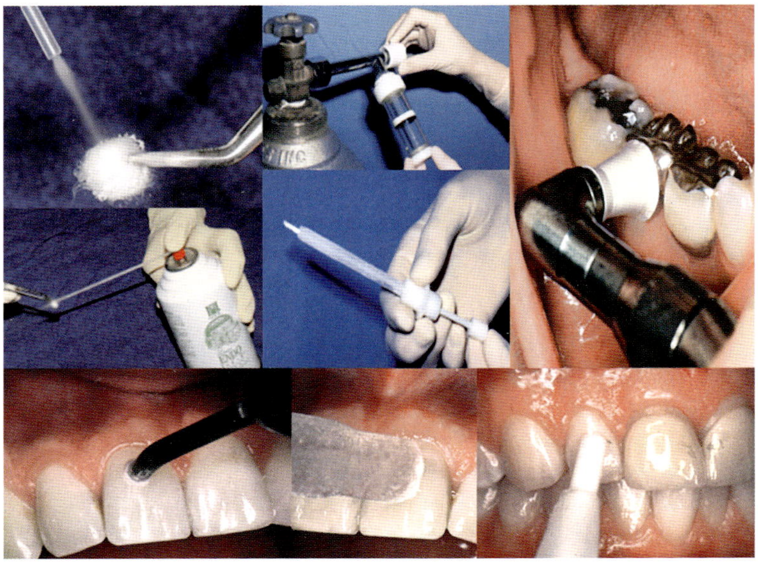

Fig 1-5 The current devices for pulp sensitity tests.

Probing

Probing is an important clinical test but, unfortunately, is the least used test for diagnosis and treatment planning. Periapical and periodontal lesions both destroy periradicular tissues and may mimic each other. Probing is a diagnostic tool that can accurately differentiate between these two problems. Periodontal defects have been classified into three major categories.[53–55] They are either of pulpal origin (endodontic), periodontal origin, or both endodontic and periodontic origin (true combined lesions).

Primary periodontal defects of endodontic origin

A periodontal defect of endodontic origin is usually associated with a tooth with pulpal necrosis (Fig 1-6a). Periodontal probing usually indicates normal sulci around the tooth except in one area with a narrow defect. This defect is not a true periodontal pocket because adequate cleaning, shaping, and obturation of the root canal system usually leads to complete resolution (Figs 1-6b and 1-6c). A common mishap is inadequate probing to determine the etiology of the periodontal pocket.

Primary periodontal defects of periodontal origin

A periodontal defect of periodontal origin is usually associated with generalized gingivitis and/or periodontitis resulting from the accumulation of plaque and/or calculus formation (Fig 1-7). Teeth with these defects respond normally to pulp sensitivity testing. When probing, the crest is within normal limits. Then, in a "step-down" fashion, the probe reaches deeper. The pocket depth decreases in a "step-up" manner and reaches the normal depth on the other side of the pocket.[53] A common mishap in this situation is a false assumption that these lesions are of pulpal origin and that the tooth or teeth will respond positively to root canal treatment.

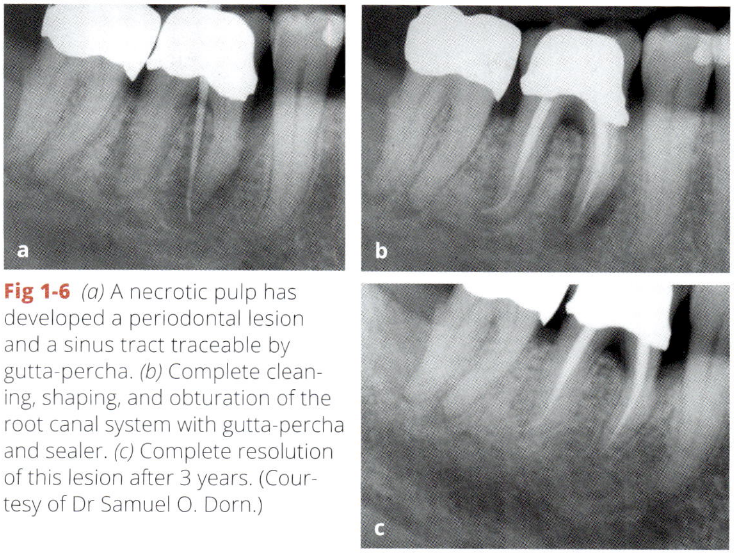

Fig 1-6 *(a)* A necrotic pulp has developed a periodontal lesion and a sinus tract traceable by gutta-percha. *(b)* Complete cleaning, shaping, and obturation of the root canal system with gutta-percha and sealer. *(c)* Complete resolution of this lesion after 3 years. (Courtesy of Dr Samuel O. Dorn.)

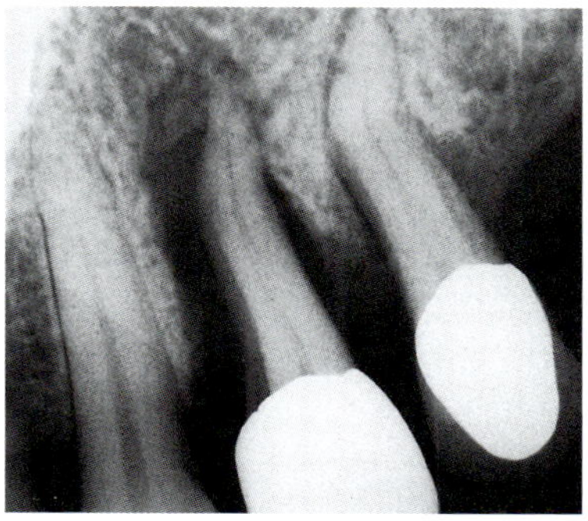

Fig 1-7 Periapical radiograph of left maxillary premolar region reveals the presence of severe periodontal lesions in this area with generalized vertical and horizontal bone loss along the root surfaces.

Primary periodontal defects of endodontic-periodontic origin (true combined lesions)

These defects have two concurrent components: a periodontal component and a periapical component (Fig 1-8a). A true combined defect is usually associated with clinical signs and symptoms of generalized gingivitis and/or periodontitis. A tooth with a true combined lesion is unresponsive to pulp vitality tests. Similar to a lesion of periodontal origin, a defect of this type is wide and V-shaped.[56] True combined lesions require endodontic and periodontal treatments (Fig 1-8b). A common mishap in this situation is a false assumption that these lesions will respond positively to exclusively endodontic or periodontal treatment.

Fig 1-8 *(a)* A true combined endodontic-periodontic lesion is observed in the second mandibular premolar. *(b)* Endodontic and periodontal treatments of this tooth have resulted in the decrease of these lesions in 6 months.

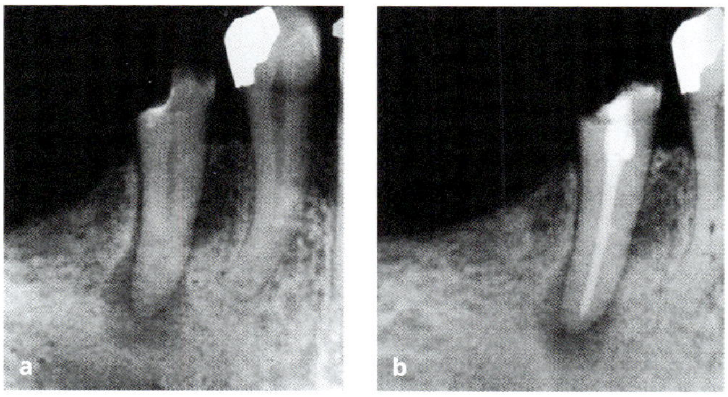

Mobility

Like periodontal probing, the mobility test is underused and overlooked in many cases, and it is often not correctly recorded.[57] The mobility test can possibly determine the etiology of the disease and its prognosis. Teeth with extreme mobility as a result of periodontal disease have little periodontal support and usually a poor prognosis. A severe periapical abscess can cause excessive mobility, which usually decreases dramatically after successful root canal treatment. A common mishap is a false assumption that all teeth with severe mobility, regardless of their etiology, have a poor prognosis and need extraction.

Mishaps During Radiographic Examination

Radiographic examinations are essential for the evaluation of hard tissues (see chapter 2). However, their value is overestimated by some clinicians who often rely more on radiographic findings than clinical findings. This attitude is a mistake and can lead to misdiagnosis and incorrect treatment. Radiographic examinations reveal the relationship between teeth and the adjacent neurovascular bundle and maxillary sinuses as well as the presence or absence of carious lesions, defective restorations, previous endodontic treatment(s), abnormal pulpal and periapical appearances, impacted teeth, and bone loss from periapical and periodontal diseases.[58] They may also reveal structural changes and bony disease unrelated to the pulp. However, radiographs are two-dimensional (2D) images and may not reveal the full picture of a clinical problem. Exposing more than one radiograph from different angles may minimize this shortcoming.

CBCT provides 3D images and dramatically aids in the diagnosis of complex cases. CBCT imaging eliminates the anatomical noise that is present in 2D imaging, particularly in areas of structural overlap such as the posterior region of the maxilla.[59] CBCT images can detect periapical pathosis in an earlier stage of disease than 2D imaging techniques.[60] CBCT was reported to have twice the odds of detecting a periapical lesion than traditional 2D periapical radiography.[61] The disadvantages of using CBCT imaging are increased radiation exposure, high cost, and lack of availability in all dental offices. Exposing CBCT images is recommended for difficult diagnoses, complex anatomy, evaluation of prior treatment complications, assessment of potential surgical cases, and evaluation of cases with traumatic injuries or resorption.[62,63]

A number of radiolucent lesions of nondental origin simulate the radiographic appearance of endodontic lesions. Because of their similarities, dentists must use their knowledge and perform clinical tests in a systematic manner to arrive at a diagnosis and avoid critical mistakes. Pulp responsive tests are the most important aids in differentiating between endodontic and non-endodontic lesions. Teeth associated with radiolucent periradicular lesions have necrotic pulps and therefore generally do not respond to pulp tests. In contrast, lesions of non-pulpal origin usually do not affect the blood or nerve supply to an adjacent tooth pulp;

therefore, their responsiveness to various stimuli remains unaffected. Unfortunately, some clinicians use only radiographs for diagnosis without taking a complete history of the signs and symptoms and performing clinical tests. To avoid mistakes, all relevant pulp tests, radiographic examinations, clinical signs and symptoms, and details of the patient history should be used for diagnosis and treatment planning. Most radiographic changes are, in fact, endodontic and arise from pathologic changes in the pulp. However, some radiographic variations, such as anatomical variations as well as benign and malignant lesions, may simulate the appearance of periradicular lesions.[2]

Anatomical entities simulating periapical lesions of pulpal origin include large marrow spaces adjacent to the apices of teeth, submandibular fossae, maxillary sinus, apical dental papillae of developing teeth, nasopalatine foramen, mental foramen (Fig 1-9), and lingual depressions in the mandible. Associated teeth respond to vitality tests and show no clinical signs or symptoms of any disease process. Additionally, changing the cone angulation, the location of these radiolucent lesions can be moved relative to their original positions and to the root apices (see Fig 1-9b).

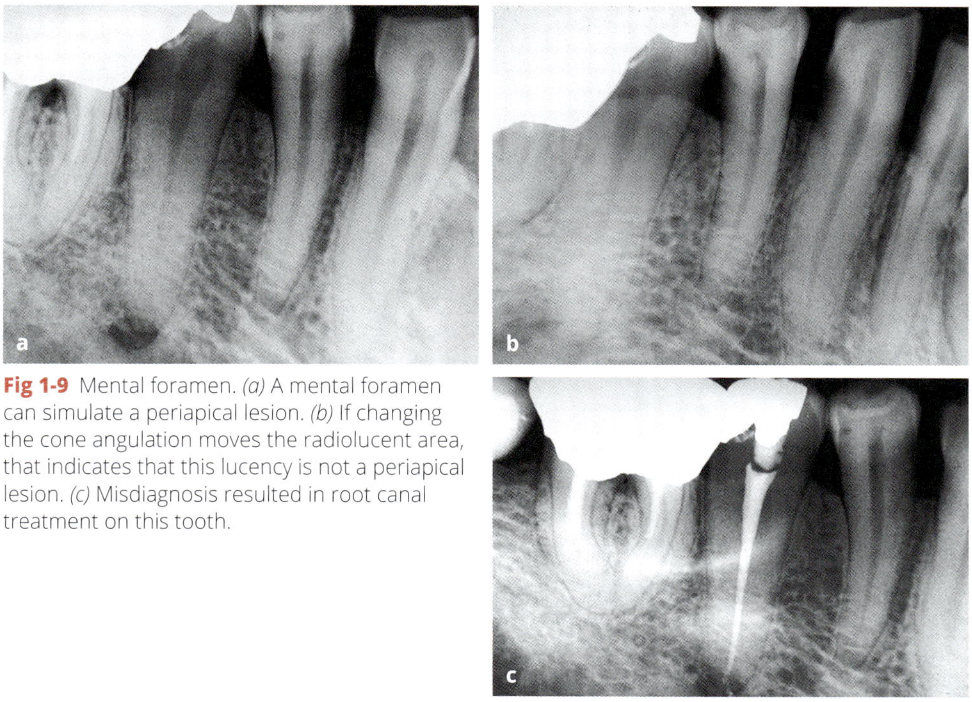

Fig 1-9 Mental foramen. *(a)* A mental foramen can simulate a periapical lesion. *(b)* If changing the cone angulation moves the radiolucent area, that indicates that this lucency is not a periapical lesion. *(c)* Misdiagnosis resulted in root canal treatment on this tooth.

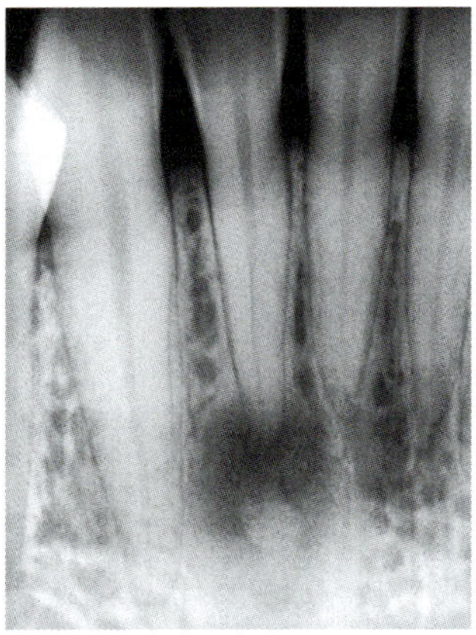

Fig 1-10 Cemental dysplasia. The initial stage of periradicular cemental dysplasia can be mistaken for a periapical lesion of pulpal origin.

Some benign lesions with radiographic appearances similar to odontogenic periradicular lesions include the initial stages of periradicular cemental dysplasia (Fig 1-10), early stages of monostotic fibrous dysplasia, ossifying fibroma, primordial cyst, lateral periodontal cyst, dentigerous cyst, nasopalatine duct cyst, solitary bone cyst, central giant cell granuloma, central hemangioma, hyperparathyroidism, myxoma, and ameloblastoma. The lamina dura around the apices of teeth associated with these lesions is usually intact, and pulp tests of these teeth respond within normal limits. To confirm the final diagnosis of these lesions, a surgical biopsy and histopathologic examination are needed.[64]

Malignant lesions that may simulate odontogenic periradicular lesions are metastatic lymphoma, squamous cell carcinoma, osteogenic sarcoma, chondrosarcoma, and multiple myeloma. Unlike endodontic lesions of pulpal origin, these lesions are usually associated with rapid and extensive hard tissue destruction (Fig 1-11). The teeth in the affected region usually remain responsive to vitality tests, but occasionally, the pulps or sensory nerves are disrupted and nonresponsive. For a more complete list as well as clinical and radiographic descriptions of these lesions, an oral and maxillofacial pathology text should be consulted.[65]

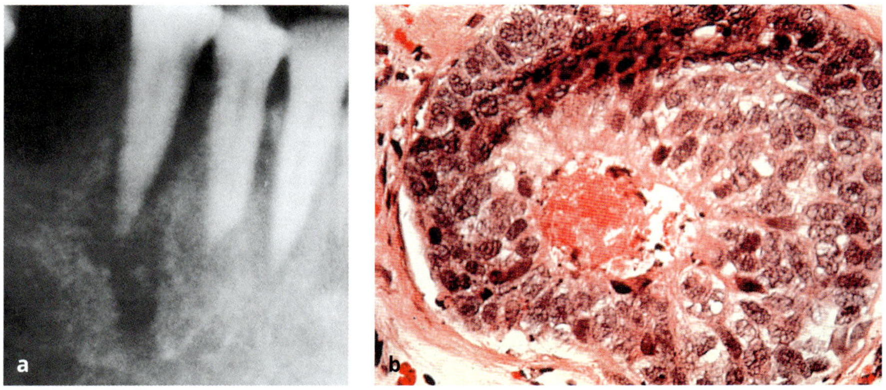

Fig 1-11 Adenocarcinoma. *(a)* Despite the presence of a lesion in the mandibular premolar, all the teeth in the region were responding within normal limits. *(b)* The lesion was fast growing, and the biopsy showed presence of an adenocarcinoma.

Mishaps During Additional Diagnostic Procedures

After systematically performing clinical and radiographic tests, it is usually possible to establish an accurate diagnosis and subsequent treatment plan. However, if the clinician is unable to make a definitive diagnosis, additional tests such as a cavity test, selective anesthesia, and transillumination might be helpful.

Test cavity

When the results of cold, heat, or electrical tests are inconclusive and the clinician cannot determine the presence of a necrotic pulp in a suspected tooth, dentin stimulation using a test cavity is the most reliable test. After careful explanation of the nature of the test to the patient, an access preparation, without anesthesia, is performed. If the pulp is vital, a pain sensation will be felt by the patient when the dentin is reached. If the pulp is necrotic, no discomfort will be felt upon entering the dentin or the pulp chamber. Unfortunately, most clinicians are not aware of the value of this test to determine the presence of a necrotic pulp in a suspected tooth. Additionally, an inadequate explanation to the patient before testing may result in a false positive response.

Selective anesthesia

Selective anesthesia is a useful test in localizing pain when the patient cannot identify the offending tooth. If a mandibular tooth is the suspect, a mandibular block could help confirm the diagnosis if the pain disappears after the injection. If a maxillary tooth is the suspect, infiltration anesthesia in an anterior to posterior fashion can help identify the suspected tooth. A common mistake in performing this test is administration of infiltration anesthetic in posterior to anterior regions. Another common mistake is the assumption that the intraligament injection identifies the offending tooth in the mandible. Intraligament injection often anesthetizes several teeth and should not be used as a diagnostic method to identify the source of pain in mandibular teeth.[66] However, using this technique for maxillary teeth is more reliable.

Bite and transillumination tests

Bite and transillumination tests are helpful methods to identify the presence or absence of cracks or fractures in teeth.[67] A common mistake in using these tests is accepting craze lines as cracks or fractures without digital examination of the involved teeth.[68]

References

1. Torabinejad M, Anderson P, Bader J, et al. Outcomes of root canal treatment and restoration, implant-supported single crowns, fixed partial dentures, and extraction without replacement: A systematic review. J Prosthet Dent 2007;98:285–311.
2. Torabinejad M, Fouad A, Shabahang S. Endodontics: Principles and Practice, ed 6. London: Elsevier, 2020.
3. Pigg M, Nixdorf DR, Law AS, et al. New International Classification of Orofacial Pain: What is in it for endodontists? J Endod 2021;47:345–357.
4. Bell WE. Orofacial Pains: Classification, Diagnosis, Management. Chicago: Year Book Medical, 1989.
5. Travell JG, Simons DG. Myofascial Pain and Dysfunction: The Trigger Point Manual. Baltimore: Williams & Wilkins, 1983.
6. Fricton J. Myofascial pain: Mechanisms to management. Oral Maxillofac Surg Clin North Am 2016;28:289–311.
7. Pertes RA, Heir GM. Chronic orofacial pain. A practical approach to differential diagnosis. Dent Clin North Am 1991;35:123–140.

8. Pertes RA, Gross SG. Clinical Management of Temporomandibular Disorders and Orofacial Pain. Chicago: Quintessence, 1995.
9. Michaelson PL, Holland GR. Is pulpitis painful? Int Endod J 2002;35:829–832.
10. Ehrmann EH. The diagnosis of referred orofacial dental pain. Aust Endod J 2002;28:75–81.
11. Reeh ES, elDeeb ME. Referred pain of muscular origin resembling endodontic involvement. Case report. Oral Surg Oral Med Oral Pathol 1991;71:223–227.
12. Silverglade D. Dental pain without dental etiology: A manifestation of referred pain from otitis media. ASDC J Dent Child 1980;47:358–359.
13. Kreiner M, Okeson JP. Toothache of cardiac origin. J Orofac Pain 1999;13:201–207.
14. Zhang S, Chiang CY, Xie YF, et al. Central sensitization in thalamic nociceptive neurons induced by mustard oil application to rat molar tooth pulp. Neuroscience 2006;142:833–842.
15. Sessle BJ. Neural mechanisms and pathways in craniofacial pain. Can J Neurol Sci 1999;26(suppl 3):S7–S11.
16. Fouad AF. Diabetes mellitus as a modulating factor of endodontic infections. J Dent Educ 2003;67:459–467.
17. Aminoshariae A, Kulild JC, Mickel A, Fouad AF. Association between systemic diseases and endodontic outcome: A systematic review. J Endod 2017;43:514–519.
18. Khalighinejad N, Aminoshariae MR, Aminoshariae A, Kulild JC, Mickel A, Fouad AF. Association between systemic diseases and apical periodontitis. J Endod 2016;42:1427–1434.
19. Gomes MS, Blattner TC, Sant'Ana Filho M, et al. Can apical periodontitis modify systemic levels of inflammatory markers? A systematic review and meta-analysis. J Endod 2013;39:1205–1217.
20. Messing M, Souza LC, Cavalla F, et al. Investigating potential correlations between endodontic pathology and cardiovascular diseases using epidemiological and genetic approaches. J Endod 2019;45:104–110.
21. Garrido M, Cardenas AM, Astorga J, et al. Elevated systemic inflammatory burden and cardiovascular risk in young adults with endodontic apical lesions. J Endod 2019;45:111–115.
22. Georgiou AC, Crielaard W, Armenis I, de Vries R, van der Waal SV. Apical periodontitis is associated with elevated concentrations of inflammatory mediators in peripheral blood: A systematic review and meta-analysis. J Endod 2019;45:1279–1295.e3.
23. Wilson WR, Gewitz M, Lockhart PB, et al. Prevention of viridans group streptococcal infective endocarditis: A scientific statement from the American Heart Association. Circulation 2021;143:e963–e978.
24. Aminoshariae A, Kulild JC, Donaldson M. Short-term use of nonsteroidal anti-inflammatory drugs and adverse effects: An updated systematic review. J Am Dent Assoc 2016;147:98–110.
25. Balakrishnan R, Ebenezer V. Contraindications of vasoconstrictors in dentistry. Biomed Pharmacol J 2013;6:409–414.
26. Aminoshariae A, Donaldson M, Horan M, Kulild JC, Baur D. Perioperative antiplatelet and anticoagulant management with endodontic microsurgical techniques. J Endod 2021;47:1557–1565.
27. Cabanillas-Balsera D, Martín-González J, Montero-Miralles P, Sánchez-Domínguez B, Jiménez-Sánchez MC, Segura-Egea JJ. Association between diabetes and nonretention of root filled teeth: A systematic review and meta-analysis. Int Endod J 2019;52:297–306.
28. Yip N, Liu C, Wu D, Fouad AF. The association of apical periodontitis and type 2 diabetes mellitus: A large hospital network cross-sectional case-controlled study. J Am Dent Assoc 2021;152:434–443.
29. Costa CPS, Thomaz É BAF, Ribeiro CCC, Souza SFC. Biological factors associating pulp necrosis and sickle cell anemia. Oral Disease 2020;26:1558–1565.
30. Costa CP, Thomaz EB, Souza Sde F. Association between sickle cell anemia and pulp necrosis. J Endod 2013;39:177–181.
31. Djulbegovic B, Wheatley K, Ross J, et al. Bisphosphonates in multiple myeloma. Cochrane Database Syst Rev 2001:CD003188.
32. Henry DH, Costa L, Goldwasser F, et al. Randomized, double-blind study of denosumab versus zoledronic acid in the treatment of bone metastases in patients with advanced cancer (excluding breast and prostate cancer) or multiple myeloma. J Clin Oncol 2011;29:1125–1132.
33. Baron R, Ferrari S, Russell RG. Denosumab and bisphosphonates: Different mechanisms of action and effects. Bone 2011;48:677–692.
34. Nicolatou-Galitis O, Schiødt M, Mendes RA, et al. Medication-related osteonecrosis of the jaw: Definition and best practice for prevention, diagnosis, and treatment. Oral Surg Oral Med Oral Pathol Oral Radiol 2019;127:117–135.
35. Khan AA, Morrison A, Hanley DA, et al. Diagnosis and management of osteonecrosis of the jaw: A systematic review and international consensus. J Bone Miner Res 2015;30:3–23.
36. Alyahya L, Myers GL. Denosumab use as a predictor variable for external cervical resorption: A case-control study. J Endod 2021;47:366–373.
37. Little JW, Miller CS, Rhodus NL. Little and Falace's Dental Management of the Medically Compromised Patient, ed 9. St Louis: Elsevier, 2018.
38. Di Stefano G, Maarbjerg S, Truini A. Trigeminal neuralgia secondary to multiple sclerosis: From the clinical picture to the treatment options. J Headache Pain 2019;20:20.

39. Beth-Tasdogan NH, Mayer B, Hussein H, Zolk O. Interventions for managing medication-related osteonecrosis of the jaw. Cochrane Database Syst Rev 2017;10:CD012432.
40. Di Fede O, Panzarella V, Mauceri R, et al. The dental management of patients at risk of medication-related osteonecrosis of the jaw: New paradigm of primary prevention. Biomed Res Int 2018; 2018:2684924.
41. Mallya SM, Tetradis S. Imaging of radiation- and medication-related osteonecrosis. Radiol Clin North Am 2018;56:77–89.
42. American Dental Association. Oral Health Topics. https://www.ada.org/en/member-center/oral-health-topics/pregnancy. Accessed 15 December 2022.
43. Ather A, Zhong S, Rosenbaum AJ, Quinonez RB, Khan AA. Pharmacotherapy during pregnancy: An endodontic perspective. J Endod 2020;46:1185–1194.
44. Aminoshariae A, Khan A. Acetaminophen: Old drug, new issues. J Endod 2015;41:588–593.
45. Lee JM, Shin TJ. Use of local anesthetics for dental treatment during pregnancy; safety for parturient. J Dent Anesth Pain Med 2017;17:81–90.
46. Aminoshariae A, Kulild J, Gutmann J. The association between smoking and periapical periodontitis: A systematic review. Clinical Oral Investig 2020;24:533–545.
47. Okeson J. Orofacial Pain Guidelines for Assessment, Diagnosis, and Management. Chicago: Quintessence, 1996.
48. Rutsatz C, Baumhardt SG, Feldens CA, Rösing CK, Grazziotin-Soares R, Barletta FB. Response of pulp sensibility test is strongly influenced by periodontal attachment loss and gingival recession. J Endod 2012;38:580–583.
49. Myers JW. Demonstration of a possible source of error with an electric pulp tester. J Endod 1998; 24:199–200.
50. Petersson K, Söderström C, Kiani-Anaraki M, Lévy G. Evaluation of the ability of thermal and electrical tests to register pulp vitality. Endod Dent Traumatol 1999;15:127–131.
51. Chen E, Abbott PV. Evaluation of accuracy, reliability, and repeatability of five dental pulp tests. J Endod 2011;37:1619–1623.
52. Rosenberg RJ. Using heat to assess pulp inflammation. J Am Dent Assoc 1991;122:77–78.
53. Harrington GW. The perio-endo question: Differential diagnosis. Dent Clin North Am 1979;23:673–690.
54. Rotstein I, Simon JH. Diagnosis, prognosis and decision-making in the treatment of combined periodontal-endodontic lesions. Periodontol 2000 2004;34:165–203.
55. Simon JH, Glick DH, Frank AL. The relationship of endodontic-periodontic lesions. J Periodontol 1972;43:202–208.
56. Bergenholtz G. Interrelationship between periodontics and endodontics. In: Lindhe J (ed). Textbook of Clinical Periodontology. Copenhagen: Munksgaard, 1983.
57. Aminoshariae A, Mackey SA, Palomo L, Kulild JC. Declassifying mobility classification. J Endod 2020; 46:1539–1544.
58. Low KM, Dula K, Bürgin W, von Arx T. Comparison of periapical radiography and limited cone-beam tomography in posterior maxillary teeth referred for apical surgery. J Endod 2008;34:557–562.
59. Patel S, Dawood A, Mannocci F, Wilson R, Pitt Ford T. Detection of periapical bone defects in human jaws using cone beam computed tomography and intraoral radiography. Int Endod J 2009;42:507–515.
60. Bhatt M, Coil J, Chehroudi B, Esteves A, Aleksejuniene J, MacDonald D. Clinical decision-making and importance of the AAE/AAOMR position statement for CBCT examination in endodontic cases. Int Endod J 2021;54:26–37.
61. Aminoshariae A, Kulild JC, Syed A. Cone-beam computed tomography compared with intraoral radiographic lesions in endodontic outcome studies: A systematic review. J Endod 2018;44:1626–1631.
62. Rodríguez G, Abella F, Durán-Sindreu F, Patel S, Roig M. Influence of cone-beam computed tomography in clinical decision making among specialists. J Endod 2017;43:194–199.
63. Viana Wanzeler AM, Montagner F, Vieira HT, Dias da Silveira HL, Arús NA, Vizzotto MB. Can cone-beam computed tomography change endodontists' level of confidence in diagnosis and treatment planning? A before and after study. J Endod 2020;46:283–288.
64. Neville BW, Damm DD, Allen CM, Chi A. Oral and Maxillofacial Pathology, ed 4. St Louis: Saunders, 2016.
65. Odell EW. Cawson's Essentials of Oral Pathology and Oral Medicine, ed 9. St Louis: Elsevier Health Sciences, 2017.
66. Smith GN, Walton RE. Periodontal ligament injection: Distribution of injected solutions. Oral Surg Oral Med Oral Pathol 1983;55:232–238.
67. Wu S, Lew HP, Chen NN. Incidence of pulpal complications after diagnosis of vital cracked teeth. J Endod 2019;45:521–525.
68. Kahler W. The cracked tooth conundrum: Terminology, classification, diagnosis, and management. Am J Dent 2008;21:275–282.

2

Radiographic Mishaps

SEYED ALIAKBAR (ALI) VAHDATI
KENNETH ABRAMOVITCH

Objectives

After reading this chapter, the reader should be able to:

1. Differentiate between the radiographic appearance of normal structures versus the appearance of abnormal or pathologic structures.
2. Understand the importance of different radiographic modalities and the possible mishaps and misdiagnoses for each modality.
3. Know how to prevent radiographic mishaps.
4. Identify technical factors contributing to an ideal radiographic image:
   - Size of x-ray emission source
   - Source-to-object distance
   - Object-to-receptor distance
   - Parallel alignment of receptor with the long axis of the tooth/teeth needing imaging
   - Perpendicular direction of x-ray beam to the tooth/teeth and the receptor long axes
5. Understand anatomical considerations that affect endodontic radiographic diagnosis and treatment:
   - Normal mandibular anatomical structures
   - Normal maxillary anatomical structures
   - Number and location of canals (SLOB rule)
6. Identify dental anomalies and radiolucent lesions of nonodontogenic origins.
7. Understand technical mishaps during endodontic radiographic diagnosis and treatment:
   - Cone cuts
   - Superimposition
   - Foreshortening
   - Elongation
8. Identify mishaps during postoperative endodontic radiographic examination.
9. Know how to use CBCT to minimize mishaps during endodontic radiographic diagnosis and treatment.

Introduction

Radiographic examinations are indispensable pillars of dental diagnosis and treatment planning. This chapter will outline the challenges of utilizing radiographic imaging for endodontic patient care and how to overcome these challenges. Constant innovation keeps x-ray imaging as one of the most progressive aspects of endodontic patient care.[1] The introduction of digital technology with the continued use of intraoral radiography as well as the progressive advances with extraoral CBCT are two examples of these innovations that will be addressed in this chapter.[2–6]

Overview of intraoral image receptors

Intraoral radiographic images can be acquired with radiographic film or digital receptors. It is important to understand that from the earliest days of photographic emulsion on glass plates until the development of plastics to support radiographic emulsion—ie, film—the term *sensors* has changed dramatically in dental imaging. Francis Mouyen introduced intraoral digital sensors in the 1980s.[2] This technology was quickly adopted by endodontists as the efficiency and completion of endodontic procedures were dramatically improved with digital sensors. Digital sensors, specifically solid-state digital sensors, are the preferred sensor type for endodontic management.

Although it has been shown that digital image quality has no major advantages over film image quality, digital sensors are by far more practical. Digital sensors are advantageous in reducing patient radiation exposure and increasing speed of image acquisition, storage, retrieval, and transmission. An additional advantage of digital sensors over film is that digital sensors omit the laborious and timely chemical film processing, which takes longer and also requires the use of a darkroom. Digital sensors have dramatically facilitated the efficiency at which endodontic procedures can be completed.[6–18]

Digital image receptors include rigid solid-state sensors and phosphor plate sensors. Intraoral digital receptors are available in sizes comparable to traditional dental film. Rigid digital receptors are typically available in sizes 1 and 2, while the phosphor plate sensors are available in variable sizes (0, 1, 2, 4). The range of available sizes depends on the specific product manufacturer. Because digital receptors cannot be sterilized, it is important to use proper infection control techniques. Sensor manufacturers provide recommendations regarding how to prepare and cover digital receptors for placement inside the patient's mouth as well as how to effectively remove barriers following completion of radiographic image acquisition.[19–21]

Rigid digital receptors are categorized as direct digital devices. These rigid receptors are usually either a complementary metal-oxide semiconductor (CMOS) sensor or a charge-coupled device (CCD) sensor, the former being the most common in contemporary use. There is also less hardware with the former, as the sensor directly connects to a computer via USB. The CCD sensor requires an analog to DC hardware connection before the signal can then connect to the computer.

These direct digital receptors convert the attenuated x-ray beam photon signal into an electronic signal. The electric energy in each pixel is then converted to a binary digital gray shade value (digitization), which is then displayed as a grayscale image on a monitor. The digital signal is also stored in the capture computer's storage media. The actual image acquisition can be displayed within 2 to 7 seconds of the exposure. The latter is dependent on the servers to which the sensors are connected. The same receptor can be used for each subsequent projection by repositioning the receptor for the next view after each exposure.[22]

Storage phosphor plates (SPP) or photostimulable phosphor (PSP) plates are known as indirect digital receptors. These plates have a europium-activated (or europium-doped) barium fluorohalide emulsion that stores the latent image as differential electric charge signals on the phosphor plate's pixels after exposure.

After the plate is exposed, the receptor is scanned with an ultraviolet laser to release light photons from the charged plate. The light intensities from the individual pixels on the phosphor plate are then assigned a numerical value for the image processing. The numerical light intensity is assigned a gray scale value that ranges from very bright to very dark, dependent on the density of the object being imaged. The different gray scale intensities are then displayed on the computer monitor, thus preserving the digital image. However, the stored electrical charges on the plates can be erased with exposure to white light so that the plates can be reused. A separate plate is needed for each projection, and the stored electrical charges on the plates must be erased with white light before reuse. There is an option for plate erasure to take place immediately after the scanning step and before exiting from the scanner.[22–27]

Software enhancement features allow the clinician to adjust the digital image in different ways. These adjustments include changes in contrast, density, zoom or magnification of particular areas of interest, image density reversal, colorization, measurement, and the application of filters for noise reduction or edge sharpening. Image enhancement tends to be subjective and is dependent on the visual preferences of the clinician interpreting the image. Using these modifications requires caution because post-processing or image enhancement/modification applications may not necessarily improve the diagnostic utility of the image and, at times, may lead to misinterpretation (Fig 2-1).[23,28–30] When used, it is only recommended to view a prior area of interest and not to view the modifications to the entire image.

Another useful tool in digital imaging is subtraction. With this process, the clinician can compare an area before and after treatment to assess the changes. The computer subtracts the two images, and the image that remains represents the difference or change in bone density between pre- and posttreatment. The challenge with digital subtraction, however, is the need to register the images prior

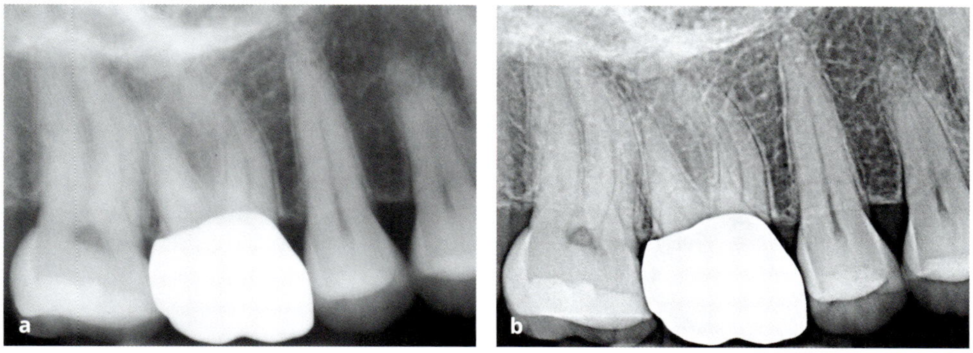

Fig 2-1 Digital periapical image *(a)* without software enhancement and *(b)* with software enhancement for sharpness. The enhanced sharpness simulates recurrent caries along the crown margin.

to subtraction. The images are rarely identical in their placement or projection geometry and must be matched structurally for the software to determine the actual changes that occurred between the two images taken at different times.

After a digital image has been obtained, it can be stored in the computer, printed, or sent electronically to referral clinicians or insurance companies, and so on. Digital radiography facilitates storage and ease of access for image viewing, printing, duplicating, and electronic transferring. Digital imaging is an integral part of a complete electronic record without the need for physical storage space and the concern that hard copy images will be physically damaged or destroyed. However, it is important to back up patient records to avoid loss of data in the event of a digital incident that may harm the originally captured digital image data. There are a variety of storage media that can be used for backup purposes. Examples include DVDs, thumb drives, external hard drives, or cloud technology. The latter two are recommended for large amounts of data storage, typically greater than 64 GB.

Digital imaging like film radiography uses x-ray beam collimators to reduce the area of exposure at the skin surface with a preference for rectangular collimation and receptor holding devices to reduce retakes. Rectangular collimation reduces both primary and scatter radiation. This not only benefits the patient by reducing exposure; the reduction in scatter also improves image quality. Because digital receptors are more sensitive to scatter radiation than film, rectangular collimation is recommended for use with digital imaging systems. There are a number of commercially available devices that can be used by clinicians to achieve rectangular collimation and reduce exposure. Current digital receptors offer equal or greater dose reduction than F-speed film with comparable diagnostic utility.

The majority of technique and exposure errors that occur with film exposures can also occur with digital receptors. The greatest advantage of digital imaging is the elimination of processing errors, which are the most common causes of retakes in film-based radiography. In addition, digital imaging eliminates the need for a darkroom and chemical processing equipment. The requirements for storage space, physical handling, and cost of processing chemicals are also eliminated. The chemical processing steps for film, the lengthy processing times, and the use of equipment require additional time and effort to perform properly.

Although digital imaging facilitates the retake and storage of dental images, it is essential that clinicians follow all the necessary recommendations to comply with the ALARA (as low as reasonably achievable) principle, thus further reducing patient radiation exposure.[19–31]

Clinical versus radiographic examinations

Radiographic images demonstrate findings beyond the scope of the clinical examination; however, it is essential to understand that these images are complementary to the clinical examination and should not replace thorough intra- and extraoral clinical evaluations. However, some clinicians often rely more on radiographic images than clinical findings. This approach is really below the standard of patient dental care and can lead to misdiagnosis, incorrect treatment, and unfavorable outcomes (see chapter 1).

Radiographic examinations assist the clinical examination in revealing the presence or absence of carious lesions and defective restorations. The radiographs are even more definitive for identifying previous endodontic treatment(s), abnormal pulpal and periapical appearances, impacted teeth, the relationship between teeth and the adjacent neurovascular bundle and maxillary sinuses, and bone loss from periapical and/or periodontal diseases.[1–3] Radiographic examinations may also reveal structural changes and bony disease unrelated to the dental pulp (see chapter 1).

Different radiographic imaging modalities

The most common dental radiographs used for endodontic purposes are periapical and bitewing images. These radiographs are two-dimensional (2D) images and will not demonstrate details of the disease process in all anatomical planes. Exposing more than one radiograph from different horizontal projection angles is typically indicated to minimize this shortcoming.

Since its inception, extraoral panoramic imaging has become very popular because of the wide-angle view of the jaws in a single exposure. However, the extraoral panoramic imaging technique lacks the resolution to show the details and intricacies within root canal systems. Therefore, endodontic patient care did not benefit from extraoral imaging until the introduction of CBCT. CBCT is a digital extraoral imaging modality that has significantly changed endodontic diagnosis and care.

CBCT provides 3D imaging and dramatically aids in the diagnosis of complex cases. 3D imaging refers to the ability of the software to generate an infinite number of multiple angle and multiple anatomical plane views of a region of interest. This potential then permits a 3D evaluation of the region of interest.

CBCT imaging overcomes the limitation of anatomical structural superimposition (eg, superimposition of the zygomatic process on maxillary molar roots; superimposition of the mental foramen on premolar apices, etc). CBCT imaging can also detect periapical pathosis at earlier stages of disease than the 2D imaging techniques. CBCT was reported to have twice the odds of detecting a periapical lesion than 2D periapical radiography. The disadvantages of using CBCT imaging are increased radiation exposure, financial cost, and lack of availability in all dental offices. CBCT scans are recommended for difficult diagnoses, complex dentoalveolar anatomy, and evaluation of cases with traumatic injuries or resorption. Further CBCT indications include evaluating prior treatment complications and assessing potential surgical cases.[32–36] The American Association of Endodontists/American Academy of Oral and Maxillofacial Radiology (AAE/AAOMR) position statement outlines the more thorough indications for CBCT in endodontic patient care.[37]

It should also be mentioned that in the modern era, imaging no longer relies solely on the use of x-rays. Other imaging modalities that benefit dental care include optical scan imaging, magnetic resonance imaging (MRI), and on the frontier, ultrasound imaging.[38,39] These modalities remain in the preliminary stages of application for endodontics, but they show potential for future benefits to endodontic care.

Potential imaging artifact and misdiagnosis in each modality

A number of artifacts, mainly object distortion, can occur during image capture that may adversely affect the radiographic interpretation in the course of endodontic treatment. An artifact is any distortion or error in the image that is unrelated to the subject being studied.

Cone cuts in the captured image, superimposition with other teeth and anatomical structures, and tooth foreshortening or elongation are the main technical problems that may arise. Anatomical challenges, on the other hand, may include superimposition over normal structures that may resemble endodontic lesions of pulpal origin. These misinterpretations may lead to misdiagnosis (see chapter 1). Therefore, to avoid critical mistakes, clinicians should systematically rely on their anatomical knowledge and clinical tests to arrive at a diagnosis. It is also crucial to have an accurate understanding of a tooth's internal anatomy. Awareness of the possible number of canals in each tooth and each root in multirooted teeth plays an important role in the outcome of endodontic treatment. Missing canal(s) in the radiographic interpretation might lead to untreated canal(s) and eventually failure of the endodontic treatment.

Identifying dental anomalies and/or variations of normal anatomical structures also plays an important role in accurate diagnosis and treatment planning. Dens evaginatus, dens invaginatus, radix entomolaris and paramolaris, and C-shaped canals are the most common anatomical variations noted in endodontic patient

2

care.[40] Clinicians also should be able to differentiate the radiographic presentation of internal, external, and cervical root resorptions. Improper recognition of these different resorption patterns can potentially lead to mistreatment and an unfavorable prognosis.

CBCT is also subject to image artifacts which are classified as either inherent, procedure-related, introduced, or patient motion. Inherent artifacts arise from limitations in the physical processes involved in the acquisition of CBCT data. Beam hardening and scattering are the two most common inherent artifacts (Fig 2-2).

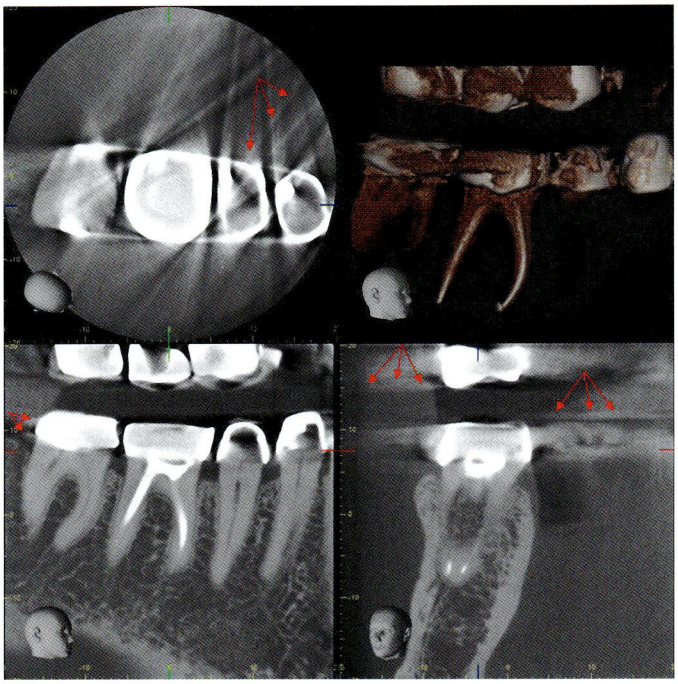

Fig 2-2 Scattering on CBCT multiplanar reconstructions. The *arrows* point to some of the areas with scatter artifacts.

As an x-ray beam passes through an object, lower energy photons are absorbed in greater numbers than higher energy photons. Consequently, a greater number of higher energy photons interact with the digital receptor. The reconstruction algorithms used to generate image displays are complex. Adding to the complexities are compromises in the image processing to account for convenience and speed (ie, time efficiency) of the image acquisition and display. These compromises actually misinterpret the degree of attenuation and assume oversaturation of the beam energy adjacent to metallic structures. This results in an image display with a dark area otherwise known as *extinct pixel display values*. This phenomenon, called *beam hardening*, results in two types of CBCT image artifacts: *(1)* distortion of metallic structures as a result of differential absorption, and *(2)* streaks and dark bands, which present adjacent dense (metallic) objects (Fig 2-3).

Scatter artifact results from x-ray photons that are diffracted from their original path after interaction with dense areas of an object. In the reconstruction algorithm, the diffracted photons create signal gain and signal loss in areas of the image display where they should not be present. The scatter causes streak artifacts that can be either light or dark bands that "streak" across the reconstructed image.

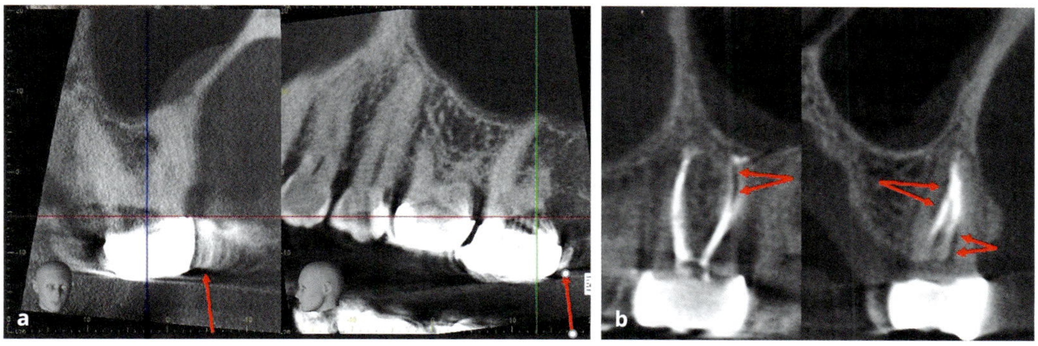

Fig 2-3 *(a)* Patient movement artifact. Note the *arrows* showing multiple edges of the metal crown. *(b)* Beam hardening artifact. The *arrows* show the dark areas that simulate voids in the root canal filling.

In clinical practice, it is advised to reduce the field size, modify patient position, or separate the dental arches to minimize scanning regions susceptible to beam hardening or streaking (eg, metallic restorations, dental implants). It is also important to remove metallic objects such as jewelry before scanning to reduce peripheral beam hardening effects superimposed on the region of interest (ROI).

Misalignment of the x-ray source to the detector creates a double contour artifact, similar to that created by patient motion. Therefore, periodic source-detector realignment may be necessary to prevent procedural artifacts.

Patient positioning and stability also play an important role in image capture. Patient motion can cause misregistration of data, which appears as double contours in the reconstructed image (see Fig 2-3a). Evaluation and consideration regarding how much the movement artifact prevents the visualization of the ROI should occur prior to rescanning. Head straps and chin cups are used to avoid motion artifact during the acquisition phase. As a general rule, using the shortest scan time possible can minimize motion artifact and also reduce the radiation dose associated with CBCT imaging.[41–43] However, this is less of an option for the high-resolution scans used for endodontic diagnosis. The high-resolution scans need longer exposure times to generate an adequate x-ray signal for the greater number of smaller pixels used in this scanning protocol. These scans also need the maximum number of basis images to obtain higher resolution.

Technical Factors Affecting Ideal Diagnostic and Working Periapical Radiographs

In order to prevent radiographic errors, it is helpful to first have an ideal reference. To simplify this understanding, a radiograph can be considered as a picture of the projected image of the teeth and surrounding structures, similar to a photograph.

The purpose of the receptor is to capture an image of the projected area of interest. The principles of diagnostic image projection for optimizing image quality are summarized below.

Size of x-ray emission source

X-ray photons should be emitted from the smallest source of radiation possible. Within the x-ray tube head, the source of x-ray photons is the focal spot on the anode of the x-ray tube. As electrons strike the focal spot during an exposure, x-rays are emitted. The smaller the focal spot, the better the image resolution. The size of the focal spot is a fixed option set by the manufacturer prior to the purchase of the x-ray unit. Over the last few decades, manufacturers have been able to decrease focal spot sizes from 1.2 mm^2 to as small as 0.5 mm^2. This is due to improvements in the inherent x-ray tube cooling systems. Some x-ray units used for other medical disciplines have different x-ray tubes with cooling systems where the focal spots are as small as 0.1 mm^2. Resolution test devices used in quality assurance programs can determine if there is age-related deterioration of the focal spot size and indicate when an x-ray head may need to be replaced. Focal spot testing is usually done in conjunction with periodic state-mandated x-ray machine inspections.[44]

Source-to-object distance

The x-ray source-to-object distance should be as long as possible. The distance between the focal spot and the object to be imaged is called the *source-to-object distance*. Machines with longer open-ended position-indicating devices (PID or cone) will enable the x-ray photons in the x-ray beam to emerge in a straighter line with less beam divergence. The resulting images will then have sharper object outlines and demonstrate less image magnification.[44]

Object-to-receptor distance

The object-to-receptor distance should be as short as possible. Placing the receptor closer to the tooth or anatomical structures being radiographed (ie, the object) also reduces magnification and improves image sharpness. In the bisecting angle technique, there is a shorter object-to-receptor distance than with the paralleling technique. However, the bisecting angle technique does not conform to the other principles of accurate image projection. As a result, it is more prone to dimensional and shape distortion and is not recommended as the primary imaging technique. *Shape distortion* is defined as deviation from the true shape or dimension of the object. The bisecting angle technique is considered a secondary method but may be necessary when parallel alignment of the receptor (ie, sensor) to the vertical axis of the teeth is not possible.[44]

Parallel alignment of receptor with the long axis of the tooth

The receptor and long axis of the tooth should be parallel to each other. When the receptor and the long axis of the tooth are parallel to each other (ie, paralleling technique), the geometric shape distortion of the radiographic image is decreased. This improves anatomical accuracy.[44]

Perpendicular direction of x-ray beam to the tooth and to the receptor

The x-ray beam should be perpendicular to the vertical axes of the tooth and receptor. The x-ray beam should ideally be perpendicular, or at a right angle, to the long axis of the tooth, which ideally would also be perpendicular to the receptor. When this principle is not followed, an error in vertical length of the object (teeth) is seen, and the resultant image will appear either foreshortened (shorter than the actual object) or elongated (longer than the actual object). A perpendicular direction of the x-ray beam improves anatomical accuracy and reduces the geometric shape distortion.[44] Table 2-1 summarizes these principles and their impact on radiographic imaging.

Table 2-1 Summary of principles and their impact on radiographic imaging

PRINCIPLES	OUTCOMES
X-rays should be emitted from the smallest source of radiation possible	Improves image sharpness
X-ray source-to-object distance should be as long as possible	Improves image sharpness Reduces magnification
Object-to-receptor distance should be as short as possible	Improves image sharpness Reduces magnification
Receptor and long axis of the tooth should be parallel to each other	Improves anatomical accuracy Reduces shape distortion
X-ray beam should be perpendicular to the tooth and the receptor	Improves anatomical accuracy Reduces shape distortion

The "perfect" radiographic technique would simultaneously incorporate all five principles of accurate image projection listed in Table 2-1. Unfortunately, an ideal technique that meets all the requirements for accurate image projection has not been identified. The paralleling technique, which typically utilizes receptor-holding devices, is the preferred intraoral technique because it follows four of the five principles of accurate image projection listed in Table 2-1 (Fig 2-4). However, shallow palatal vaults and more superior mylohyoid and genial tubercle locations make parallel placement of the receptors difficult to attain consistently.

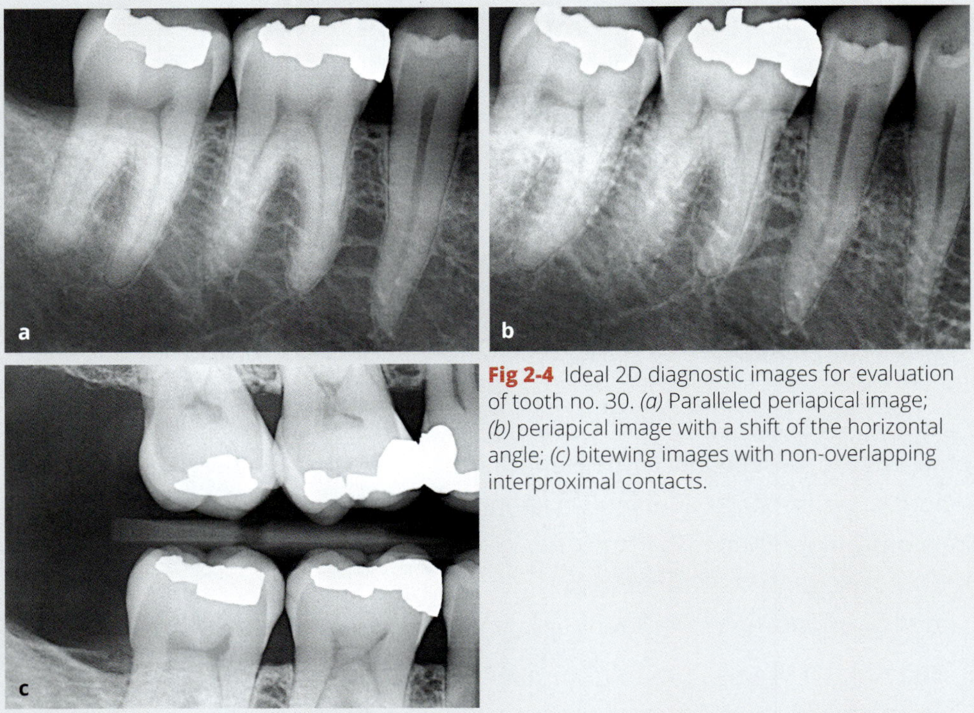

Fig 2-4 Ideal 2D diagnostic images for evaluation of tooth no. 30. *(a)* Paralleled periapical image; *(b)* periapical image with a shift of the horizontal angle; *(c)* bitewing images with non-overlapping interproximal contacts.

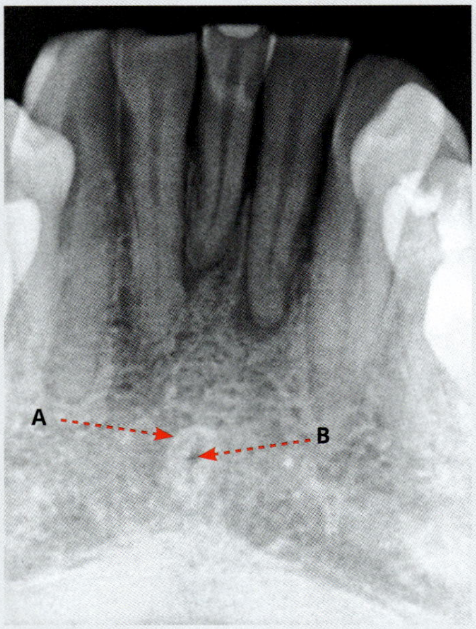

Fig 2-5 Genial tubercle and lingual foramen. The radiopaque doughnut shape (A) is the genial tubercle and the radiolucent dot in the middle (B) is the lingual foramen.

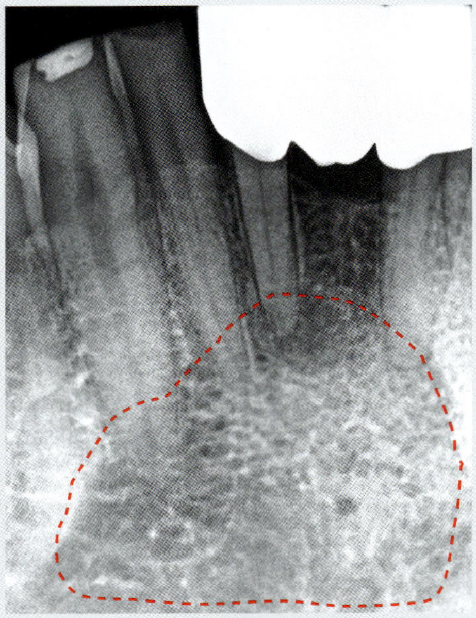

Fig 2-6 Mental fossa *(outlined dotted area)*.

Anatomical Structures That Present on Endodontic Diagnostic and Treatment Radiographs

Radiographic interpretation is based on recognizing normal anatomical landmarks and when a disease process has altered the normal anatomical patterns. Knowledge of anatomical structures is therefore essential to differentiating between normal structures, variations of normal structures (abnormalities), and disease.[17,18,44–47] There are a number of radiolucent and radiopaque anatomical structures in both the maxilla and the mandible of which the clinician should be aware. Lack of identifying normal anatomical landmarks might lead to misdiagnosis and mistreatment (see chapter 1). In addition, dental anomalies need to be identified during radiographic examination so that they are not treated as disease entities.

Normal anatomical structures presenting on mandibular images

Genial tubercle

The genial tubercle is a spiny protuberance or prominence of bone located in the midline on the lingual aspect of the mandible below the roots of the incisor teeth. This structure serves as the locus of attachment for the genioglossus and geniohyoid muscles. Although variable in appearance, the tubercle often produces a ring-like or doughnut-shaped radiopacity on mandibular incisor periapical images. The genial tubercle is also referred to as the *mental spine*[48] (Fig 2-5A).

Lingual foramen

The lingual foramen is an opening centered within the genial tubercle on the lingual aspect of the anterior mandible along the midline below the apices of the central incisor teeth. The lingual artery exits this foramen. The lingual foramen is seen on mandibular incisor periapical radiographs[48] (Fig 2-5B).

Mental fossa

The mental fossa is a concave depression on the labial aspect of the mandible. It has a diffuse radiolucent appearance above the mental ridge. The mental fossa varies in its prominence depending on the degree of concavity, thickness, and trabeculation density of the anterior mandible[48] (Fig 2-6).

Mental ridge

The mental ridge is a prominence of bone on the labial surface of the anterior mandible. This structure presents as an inverted V-shaped radiopaque ridge that extends from the premolar to canine area on each side, meeting at the midline. The mental ridge varies in its presentation, with some individuals displaying very distinct ridge anatomy while others display little or no evidence of its presence. This mandibular landmark can be recorded on incisor and partially on the lateral aspect of canine periapical radiographs[48] (Fig 2-7).

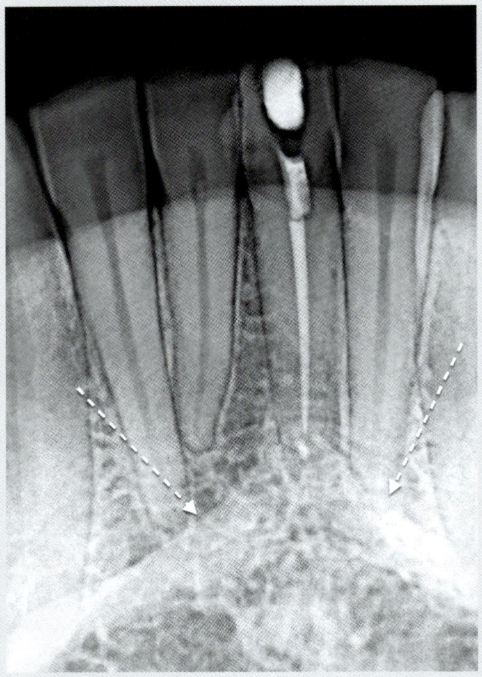

Fig 2-7 Mental ridge.

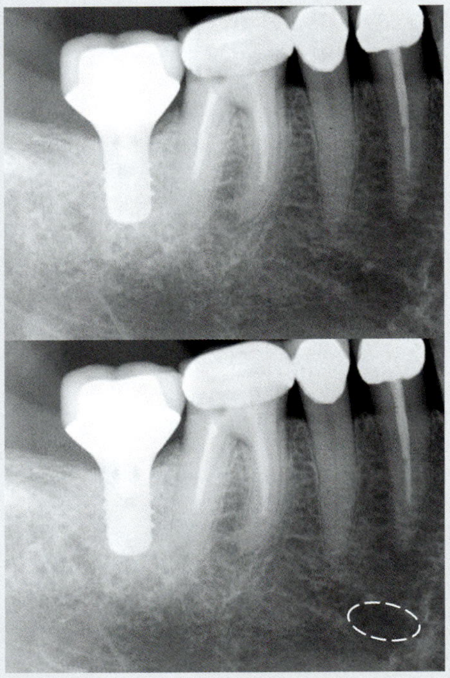

Fig 2-8 Mental foramen.

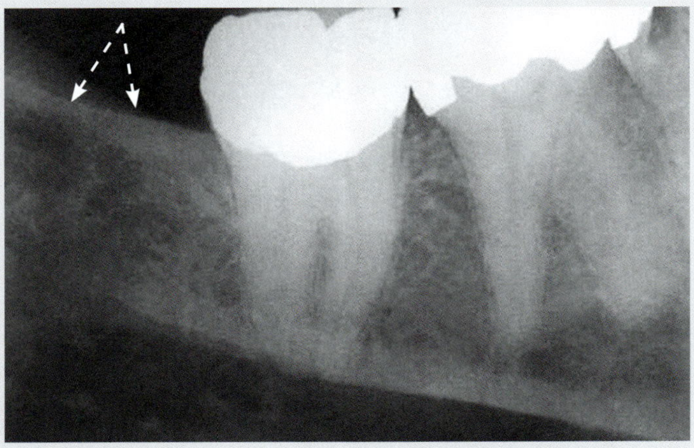

Fig 2-9 External oblique ridge.

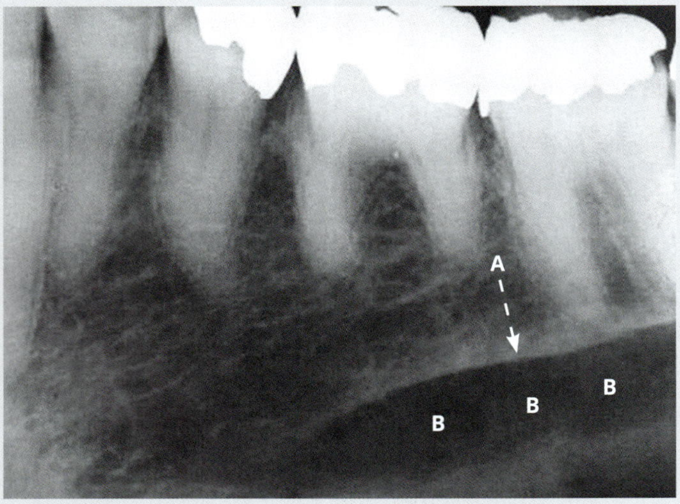

Fig 2-10 Internal oblique ridge (A); submandibular fossa (B).

Mental foramen

The mental foramen is a circular to ovoid radiolucent structure located below the roots of the mandibular premolar teeth. This structure is the opening for passage of the mental nerve and vasculature. It can be observed on mandibular molar, premolar, and lateral aspect of canine periapical radiographs. This bilateral radiolucency can be misinterpreted as a periapical lesion. However, it is easily differentiated upon closer examination of healthy adjacent teeth and their supporting structures[48] (Fig 2-8).

External oblique ridge

The external oblique ridge or line is the bony anterior border of the ramus located on the outer lateral aspect of the mandible. This ridge has an inferior-anterior diagonal course and is seen on most mandibular molar periapical and molar bitewing radiographs[48] (Fig 2-9).

Internal oblique ridge

The internal oblique ridge is the bony ridge found bilaterally on the lingual aspect of the posterior mandible. This radiopaque ridge is variable in its appearance, ranging from highly defined to barely visible. When recorded on molar periapical radiographs, it runs parallel and inferior to the external oblique ridge. The latter is more prominent and appears more frequently than the internal oblique ridge. The internal oblique ridge is also referred to as the *mylohyoid line*[48] because the mylohyoid muscle originates here (Fig 2-10A).

Submandibular fossa

The submandibular fossa is an anatomical depression on the lingual aspect of the posterior mandible. The fossa is located bilaterally and is inferior to the internal oblique ridge. This concavity is where the lateral aspect of the submandibular salivary gland rests. The submandibular fossa presents as a diffuse bilateral radiolucency, typically with few trabeculae. Due to this trace presence of trabeculae, it can appear as a much darker radiolucency, enticing the novice clinician to interpret that a pathologic lesion is present. The submandibular fossa is recorded on premolar and molar periapical images. This structure is also referred to as the *submandibular gland fossa* or *mandibular fossa*[48] (Fig 2-10B).

Mandibular canal

The mandibular canal is the pathway in bone where the inferior alveolar nerve and blood vessels course through the mandible. The canal extends from the mandibular foramen in the mid ramus and extends anteriorly to the mental foramen. This tubular bilateral radiolucency often demonstrates fine radiopaque boundaries. The mandibular canal is recorded on mandibular premolar and molar periapical radiographs. It is also referred to as the *inferior alveolar canal*[48] (Fig 2-11A).

2

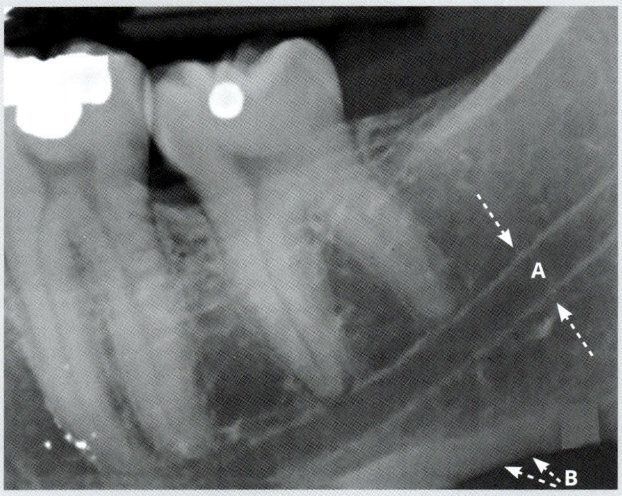

Fig 2-11 Mandibular canal (A) and mandibular lower border (B).

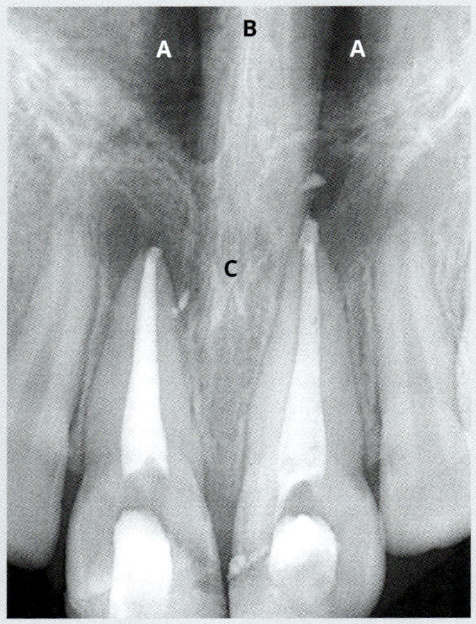

Fig 2-12 Nasal fossa (A); nasal septum (B); anterior nasal spine (C).

Table 2-2 Mandibular anatomical radiographic landmarks

LANDMARK	BRIEF DESCRIPTION	RADIOLUCENT/ RADIOPAQUE	PERIAPICAL	BILATERAL OR MIDLINE	ALTERNATE NAME(S)
External oblique ridge	Diagonal line	Radiopaque	Molar	Bilateral	External oblique line
Genial tubercle	Doughnut shape	Radiopaque	Central incisor	Midline	Mental spine
Inferior border of mandible	Horizontal band	Radiopaque	Any mandibular	Bilateral	Lower border
Internal oblique ridge	Diagonal line	Radiopaque	Molar	Bilateral	Mylohyoid line
Lingual foramen	Pinpoint dot	Radiolucent	Central incisor	Midline	
Mandibular canal	Tubular	Radiolucent	Premolar, molar	Bilateral	Inferior alveolar nerve canal
Mental foramen	Circular, ovoid	Radiolucent	Premolar, canine	Bilateral	
Mental fossa	Diffuse	Radiolucent	Central incisor	Midline	
Mental ridge	Inverted V	Radiopaque	Central incisor, lateral incisor, canine	Bilateral	
Submandibular fossa	Diffuse	Radiolucent	Premolar, molar	Bilateral	Submandibular gland fossa, mandibular fossa

Lower border of the mandible

The lower or inferior border of the mandible appears as a radiopaque band of dense cortical or lamellar bone demarcating the inferior aspect of the mandible. This structure can be observed on any mandibular periapical radiograph where the x-ray beam's vertical angulation is excessive[48] (Fig 2-11B).

Table 2-2 summarizes the mandibular anatomical radiographic landmarks.

Normal anatomical structures presenting on maxillary images

Nasal fossae

The nasal fossae (plural; singular: fossa) are the nasal air spaces located above the maxillary anterior teeth on either side of the maxillary midline. A midline partition made up of the vomer and septal cartilage separates the left nasal fossa from the right. These air spaces appear on maxillary central incisor periapical views and partially on lateral incisor and canine periapical radiographs[48] (Fig 2-12A).

Nasal septum

The nasal septum is a midline bony radiopaque structure that divides the nasal cavity into right and left chambers. It is a radiopaque landmark visible on maxillary central incisor periapical radiographs[48] (Figs 2-12B and 2-13A).

Anterior nasal spine

The anterior nasal spine (ANS) is a bony projection at the anterior midline extent of the nasal fossa. The right and left processes fuse to form a pointy anterior spine. Radiographically, the ANS appears as a V-shaped or triangular pointed radiopacity. This structure is recorded on maxillary central incisor periapical radiographs[48] (Fig 2-12C).

Inferior nasal concha

The inferior nasal concha or inferior turbinate bone projects into the inferior aspect of the nasal fossae from the lateral walls of the nasal cavity. These bilateral mildly radiopaque structures are sometimes visible on central and lateral incisor periapical radiographs[48] (Fig 2-13B).

Mid-palatine suture

The mid-palatine suture is the interface of the two halves of the maxilla where they join at the midline. The mid-palatine suture is also referred to as the *median palatal suture*. It courses from the alveolar crest along the midline to the posterior aspect of the hard palate. It is a very thin suture line, so it may not always project on radiographs. If it is notable, it appears as a thin "jagged" midline linear radiolucency on maxillary central incisor periapical radiographs[48] (Fig 2-14A).

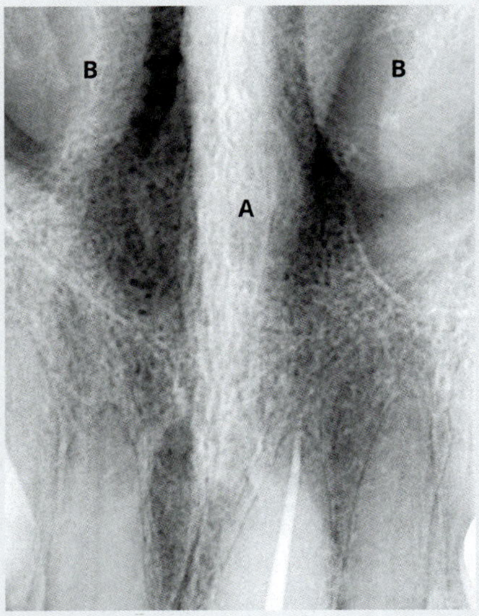

Fig 2-13 Nasal septum (A); inferior nasal concha (B).

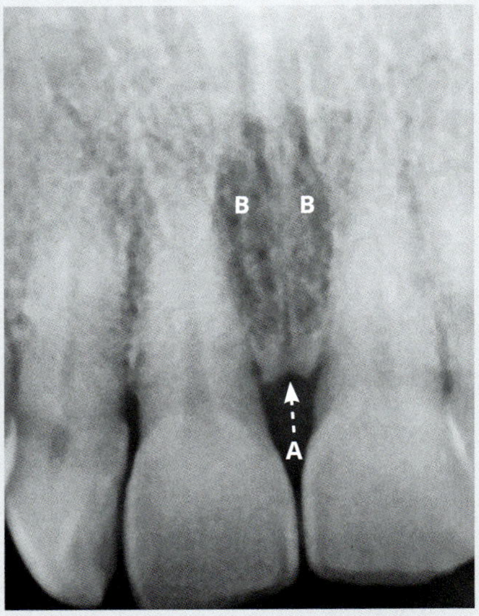

Fig 2-14 Mid-palatine suture (A); incisive foramen (B).

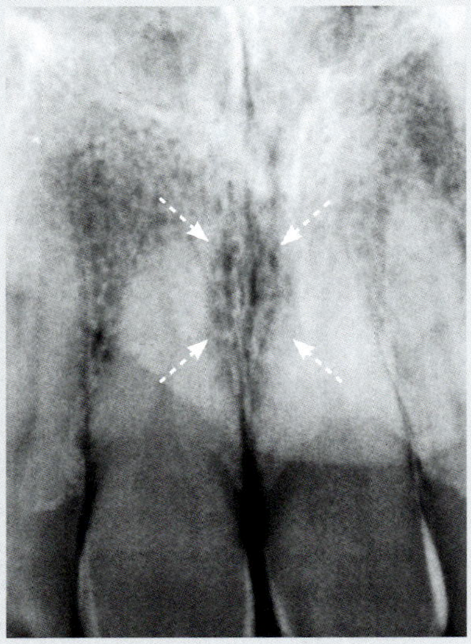

Fig 2-15 Incisive foramen.

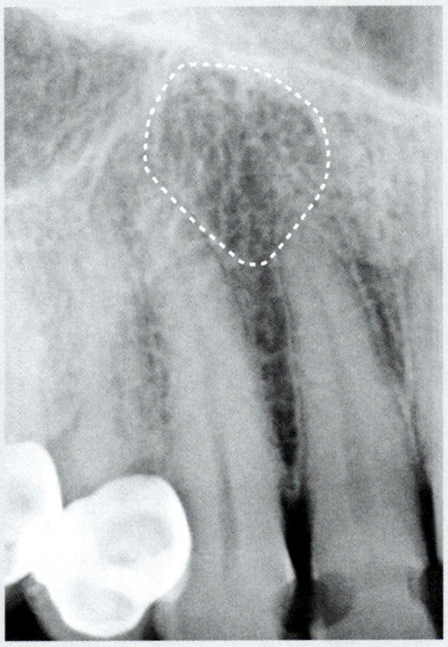

Fig 2-16 Lateral fossa.

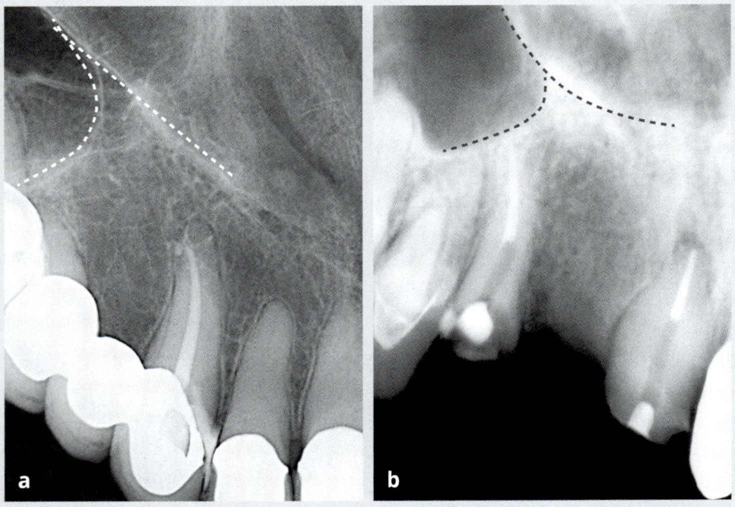

Fig 2-17 *(a and b)* Inverted Y.

Incisive foramen

The incisive or nasopalatine foramen is a maxillary midline structure on the lingual aspect of the hard palate between or just apical to the central incisor roots. The foramen is the termination of the nasopalatine canal. Radiographically, it appears between the roots of the central incisor teeth as a round to oval radiolucency less than one centimeter in greatest dimensions. It has a range of sizes and shapes, so variation is not unusual. This structure is recorded on maxillary central incisor periapical radiographs[48] (Figs 2-14B and 2-15).

Lateral fossa

The lateral fossa is a slight concavity or depression on the labial aspect of the maxilla medial to the canine eminence and in the vicinity of the lateral incisor root. This diffuse radiolucency appears bilaterally and is recorded on lateral incisor and canine periapical radiographs. It is sometimes referred to as the *canine fossa*[48] (Fig 2-16).

Inverted Y (or X)

The inverted Y is a radiographic landmark that depicts where the nasal fossa borders with the maxillary sinus. The boundary between them is shaped like an upside-down letter Y or an X, hence its name. The inverted Y is a classic radiographic landmark of the right and left anterior maxilla. The fossa is positioned toward the midline while the sinus extends toward the posterior aspect of the maxilla. Typically, the vertex of the inverted Y is apical to the maxillary canine root apex. However, based on the horizontal projection angle, the position relative to the canine apex may vary. The more tangent the horizontal angle of the x-ray beam is to the junction of these two airspaces, the more this structure looks like an inverted Y. If the horizontal angle is not tangent to this partition, then it will look more like an X[48] (Fig 2-17).

Nasal soft tissue

The soft tissue of the nose, including the tip and ala (lateral aspect of nares), often can be seen superimposed over the roots of the cuspids and incisors. The nasal soft tissues have a faint radiopaque appearance[48] (Fig 2-18).

Maxillary sinus

The maxillary sinus is the most inferior of the paired paranasal sinuses. These prominent radiolucent air-filled cavities are located above the posterior teeth on the right and left sides of the maxilla. The sinus cavities are horizontally oblong bilateral structures with fine corticated radiopaque borders. The maxillary sinus may contain septa that appear as radiopaque lines within the body of the sinus cavity. The size of the maxillary sinus can be quite variable and sometimes encroaches inferiorly into the alveolar process and rests adjacent to the superior and lateral surfaces of posterior roots. If posterior teeth are extracted, there is also

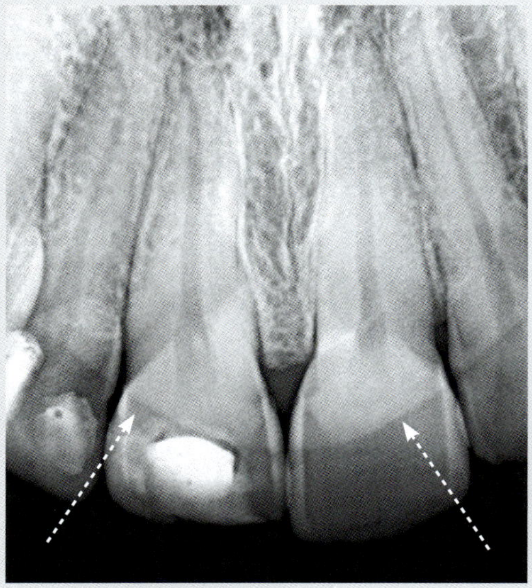

Fig 2-18 Nasal soft tissue.

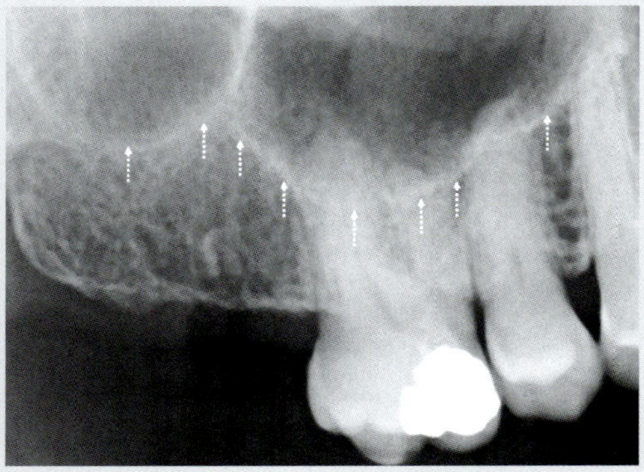

Fig 2-19 Maxillary sinus.

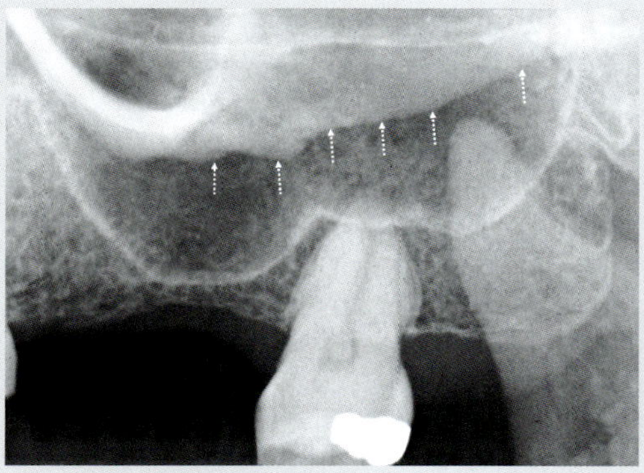

Fig 2-20 Zygomatic bone.

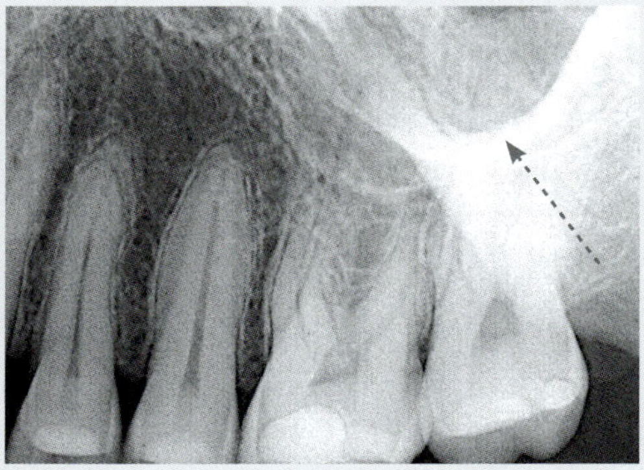

Fig 2-21 Zygomatic process.

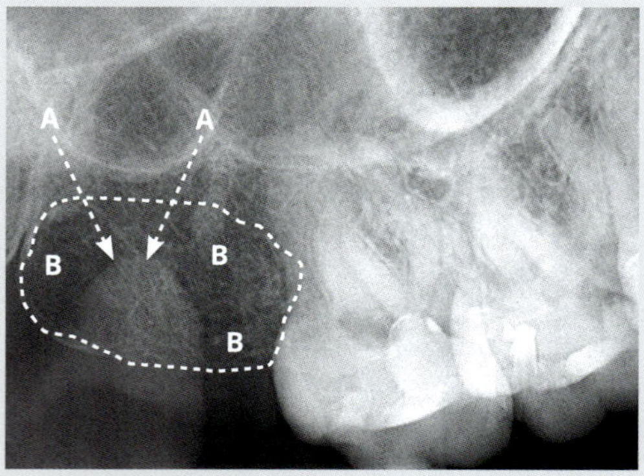

Fig 2-22 Coronoid process (A); maxillary tuberosity (B).

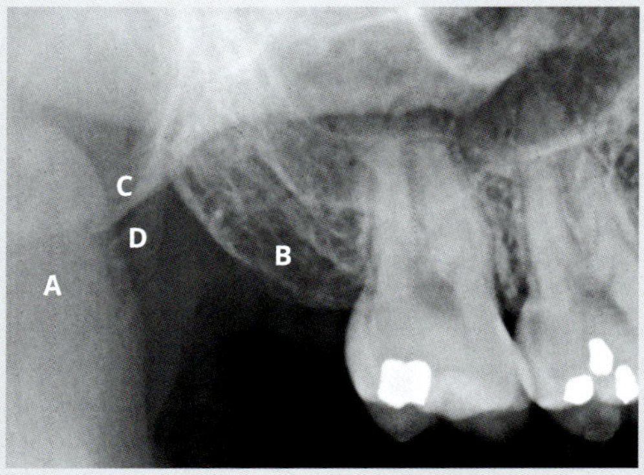

Fig 2-23 Coronoid process (A); maxillary tuberosity (B); pterygoid plate (C); hamular process (D).

a tendency after healing for the maxillary sinus spaces to get larger and extend inferiorly into edentulous alveolar arch space. Typically, the sinus cavities appear uniform right to left. The maxillary sinus is sometimes referred to as the *maxillary antrum* and can be observed on both maxillary premolar and molar periapical radiographs and partially on lateral-canine periapical radiographs[48] (Fig 2-19).

Zygomatic bone

The zygomatic bone attaches to the right and left sides of the posterior maxilla. It is quadrangular in shape and broadens as it extends posteriorly. This bilateral radiopaque structure has several synonymous terms, including the *malar bone*, *zygoma*, and *cheek bone*. The zygomatic bone can be seen on maxillary premolar and molar periapical radiographs[48] (Fig 2-20).

Zygomatic process of the maxilla

The zygomatic process is the radiopaque U-shaped structure representing where the most anterior part of the zygomatic bone attaches to the maxilla. This process is positioned anterior and medial to the zygoma. The zygoma then extends posteriorly. This structure is sometimes referred to as the *malar process* and can be seen on maxillary premolar and molar periapical radiographs[48] (Fig 2-21).

Coronoid process

The coronoid process of the mandible is the bilateral triangular bony portion of the anterosuperior aspect of the mandibular ramus. This mandibular structure can be recorded on maxillary molar periapical radiographs as the mandible moves forward when the patient's mouth is open. It appears as a bilateral triangular or thumb-like radiopacity on posterior maxillary images. The triangular portion projects anteriorly. The coronoid process is the only mandibular structure recorded on maxillary periapical radiographs[48] (Figs 2-22A and 2-23A).

Maxillary tuberosity

The maxillary tuberosity is the rounded terminal part of the maxillary alveolar process. This radiopaque structure appears bilaterally on maxillary molar periapical radiographs and often on maxillary molar periapical and molar bitewing radiographs. The tuberosity curves superiorly at the end of the maxillary alveolar process[48] (Figs 2-22B and 2-23B).

Pterygoid plates

The lateral and medial pterygoid plates are located posterior to the maxillary tuberosity. They project a single image configured like a thin wing of bone extending posteriorly from the tuberosity. This bilateral radiopacity is occasionally recorded on maxillary molar periapical images when the receptor is positioned posterior to the maxillary tuberosity. However, in most cases, the receptor does

2

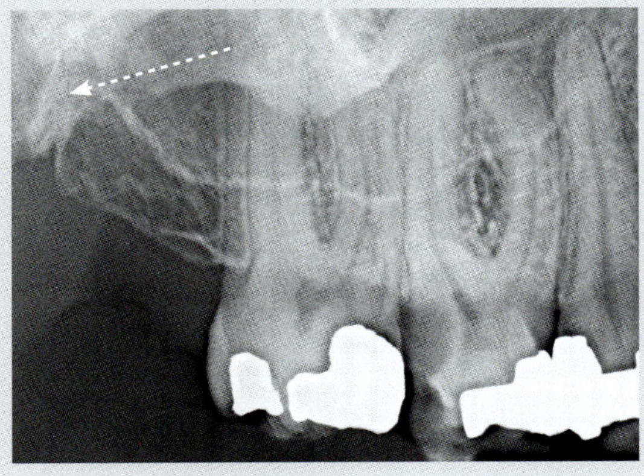

Fig 2-24 Pterygoid plate.

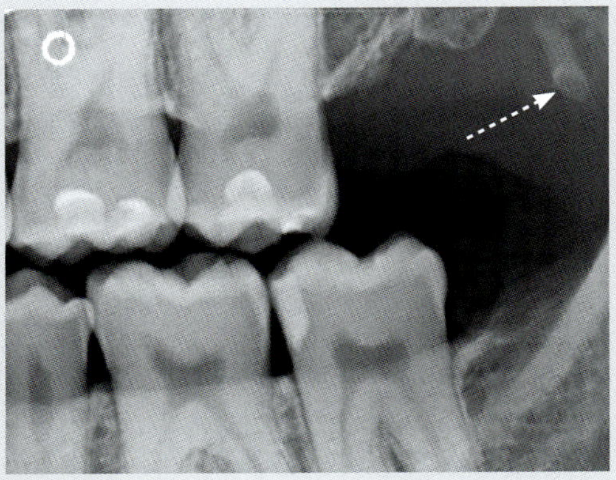

Fig 2-25 Hamular process.

Table 2-3 Maxillary anatomical radiographic landmarks

LANDMARK	BRIEF DESCRIPTION	RADIOLUCENT/ RADIOPAQUE	JAW REGION	BILATERAL OR MIDLINE	ALTERNATE NAME
Anterior nasal spine	Triangular point	Radiopaque	Central incisor	Midline	
Coronoid process	Triangular	Radiopaque	Molar	Bilateral	
Hamular process	Finger-like	Radiopaque	Molar	Bilateral	Pterygoid hamulus
Incisive foramen	Round/oval	Radiolucent	Central incisor	Midline	Nasopalatine foramen
Inferior nasal concha	Round/oval	Radiopaque	Central incisor	Bilateral	Inferior nasal turbinate
Inverted Y	Upside-down Y	Radiopaque	Lateral incisor, canine	Bilateral	
Lateral fossa	Diffuse	Radiolucent	Lateral incisor	Bilateral	Canine fossa
Maxillary sinus	Horizontally oblong	Radiolucent	Premolar/ molar	Bilateral	Maxillary antrum
Maxillary tuberosity	Rounded	Radiopaque	Molar	Bilateral	
Midpalatine suture	Vertical line	Radiolucent	Central incisor	Midline	Median palatal suture
Nasal fossa	Vertically oblong	Radiolucent	Central incisor, lateral incisor, canine	Bilateral	Nasal cavity
Nasal septum	Vertical band	Radiopaque	Central incisor	Midline	
Pterygoid plates	Wing of bone	Radiopaque	Molar	Bilateral	
Zygomatic bone	Quadrangle shape	Radiopaque	Premolar/ molar	Bilateral	Malar bone
Zygomatic process	U-shaped	Radiopaque	Premolar/ molar	Bilateral	Malar process

not reach this far posteriorly, as the patient may not tolerate receptor positioning this far posterior in the oral cavity[48] (Figs 2-23C and 2-24).

Hamular process

The hamular process, or pterygoid hamulus, is a tiny finger or hook-like inferior projection of bone from the medial pterygoid plate. This bilateral radiopacity occasionally appears on maxillary molar periapical radiographs and molar bitewings when the receptor is positioned sufficiently posteriorly to record it[48] (Figs 2-23D and 2-25).

Table 2-3 summarizes maxillary anatomical radiographic landmarks.

It is also paramount to know that anatomical entities simulating periapical lesions of pulpal origin include large marrow spaces adjacent to the apices of teeth, submandibular fossae, maxillary sinus, apical dental papillae of developing teeth (Fig 2-26), nasopalatine foramen, mental foramen, and lingual depressions in the mandible. Associated teeth may respond to vitality tests and show no clinical signs and symptoms of any disease process. Additionally, by using the tube shift technique, the location of these radiolucent "lesions" can be moved relative to their original positions and to the root apices. True periapical lesions do not shift when other alternate tube shift images are taken.

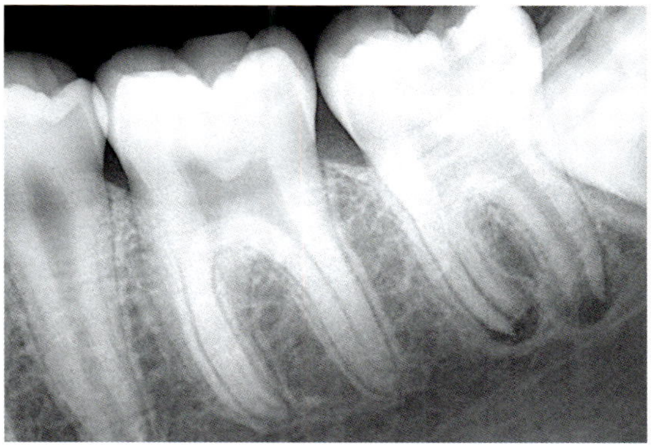

Fig 2-26 Apical dental papilla of developing tooth no. 18.

Number and location of canals (SLOB rule)

One other anatomical challenge is due to a fundamental limitation of intraoral radiographs. Standard intraoral periapical and bitewing images offer only 2D anterior-posterior and superior-inferior perspectives. This limitation automatically results in superimposition and can cause misinterpretation and mistreatment of root canals.

Localization of foreign objects and impacted teeth as well as differentiating a buccal versus lingual canal in a single root require a buccolingual perspective. To overcome these 2D imaging challenges, extraoral CBCT imaging is a more efficient option and will be discussed in detail at the end of this chapter.

However, in the absence of access to CBCT, an alternative intraoral technique for object localization is the tube-shift method. This technique is known by different terms, including Clark's rule, the buccal object rule, and most commonly, the SLOB rule. "SLOB" is an acronym for "same-lingual, opposite-buccal." This technique was first described by Clark in 1910.[45] The principal of the tube shift technique is capturing two different angle projections of the intraoral object by shifting the horizontal angulation of the x-ray tube. The first image acts as a reference image. The comparison of positional changes of the object between the first image and the second image taken after the horizontal shift of the tube determines whether the object is located more toward the buccal or the lingual aspect. For example, if the tube is horizontally shifted mesially compared to the first image and the object in question appears to move distally (in the opposite direction to the tube), the object of interest is positioned on the buccal side. If the object of interest moves in the same direction as the tube, then the object is positioned toward the lingual side. In contrast, if the tube is horizontally shifted distally compared to the first image and the object moves mesially, the object of interest is positioned on the buccal. This technique is crucial for identifying the number and location of root canals in roots with more than one canal or if there is difficulty identifying a buccal from a lingual root. Missed canals are one of the major reasons for the failure of initial nonsurgical root canal treatments (NSRCTs)[46–50] (Fig 2-27).

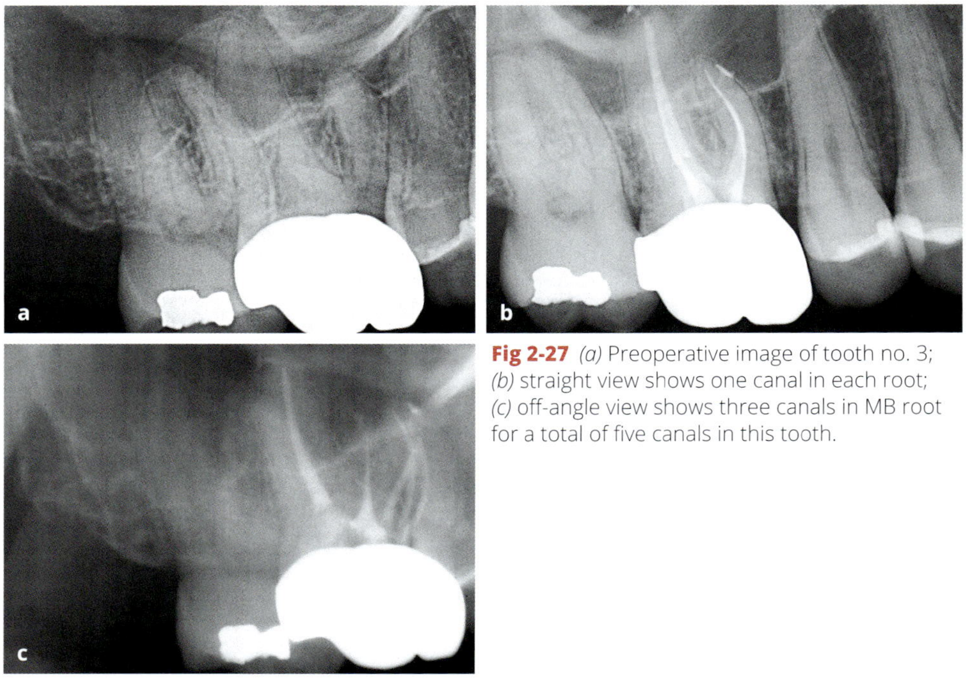

Fig 2-27 *(a)* Preoperative image of tooth no. 3; *(b)* straight view shows one canal in each root; *(c)* off-angle view shows three canals in MB root for a total of five canals in this tooth.

Dental Anomalies

Another essential area of radiographic interpretation is identifying dental anomalies. Anomalies are not disease processes. They are variations of the normal anatomical presentation. Often, they do not require treatment but do require a proper diagnosis that would rule out a disease entity. Some anomalies are more predisposed to disease processes like caries, periodontal disease, and pulpal infection. The number and scope of possible dental anomalies that present in the jaws are beyond the scope of this chapter; however, the anomalies presented here are those that may be more predisposed to endodontic interventions or are often misdiagnosed leading to unnecessary or improper treatment.

Microdontia

Microdontia is a term used to describe one or more primary or permanent teeth that appear normal in every respect, except for their small size. They can be found in any tooth-bearing area of the jaws and in individuals of all ages. Permanent maxillary lateral incisors and permanent maxillary third molars have a higher prevalence of microdontia. In addition, they are often associated with osteogenesis imperfecta, Ehler-Danlos syndrome, and Down syndrome.[51] Another microdont, the peg lateral incisor, is a manifestation of the agenesis of the maxillary lateral incisor nonsyndromic genetically inherited trait[52] (Fig 2-28).

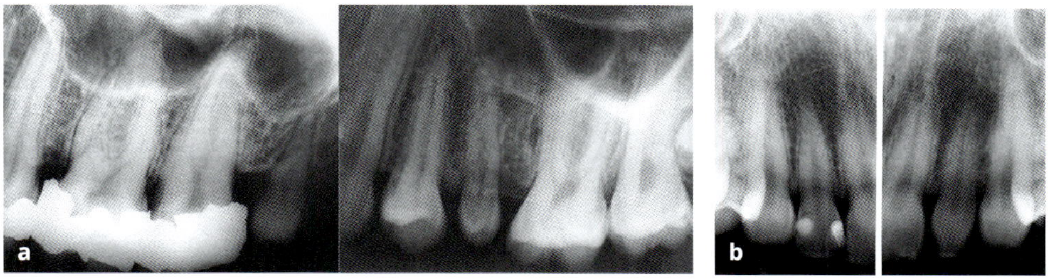

Fig 2-28 Microdontia. *(a)* Note that the maxillary third molar and the maxillary premolar are appreciably smaller than the adjacent molar and premolar, respectively. *(b)* Note the size of the no. 10 peg lateral incisor crown in comparison to the contralateral no. 7 lateral incisor.

Dens invaginatus

Dens invaginatus, also known as *dens in dente*, is a developmental anomaly believed to result from invagination of the marginal ridges on the lingual surface of maxillary incisors. The maxillary lateral incisors are most frequently affected. Dens invaginatus is recognized on radiographs as an inverted "pear-shaped" radiolucency formed by the invagination of the marginal ridges at the cingulum area. This invagination forms a thin layer of enamel and dentin that projects over the pulp. Plaque collecting in the anatomical constriction of the cingulum area is difficult to remove with oral hygiene procedures, leading to a high risk of a carious pulp exposure. There is no predilection based on sex, age, or race. If there is a carious pulp exposure, the patient often presents with pain and/or a periapical radiolucency[51] (Fig 2-29). Prophylactic restoration with a composite resin closes the constriction at the cingulum and minimizes the risk of caries and pulp exposure.

Denticle

Also known as *pulp stone* or *endolith*, a denticle is a round or oval-shaped calcified entity inside the pulp chamber of either a permanent or primary tooth. The denticle appears as a uniform, dense, radiopaque mass with well-defined borders. Its size can vary from 1 mm in diameter to total obliteration of the pulp chamber. Clinically, there is no predilection based on age or race, and it is usually asymptomatic[53] (Fig 2-30).

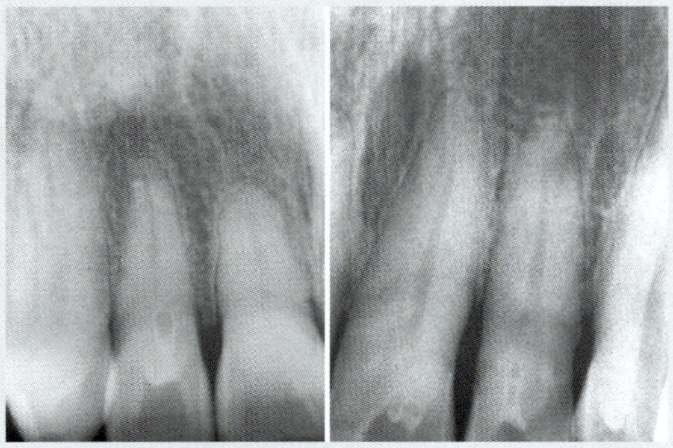

Fig 2-29 Periapical images of dens invaginatus. Note the radiolucent pattern with the radiopaque enamel outline apical to the cingulum of the lateral incisors.

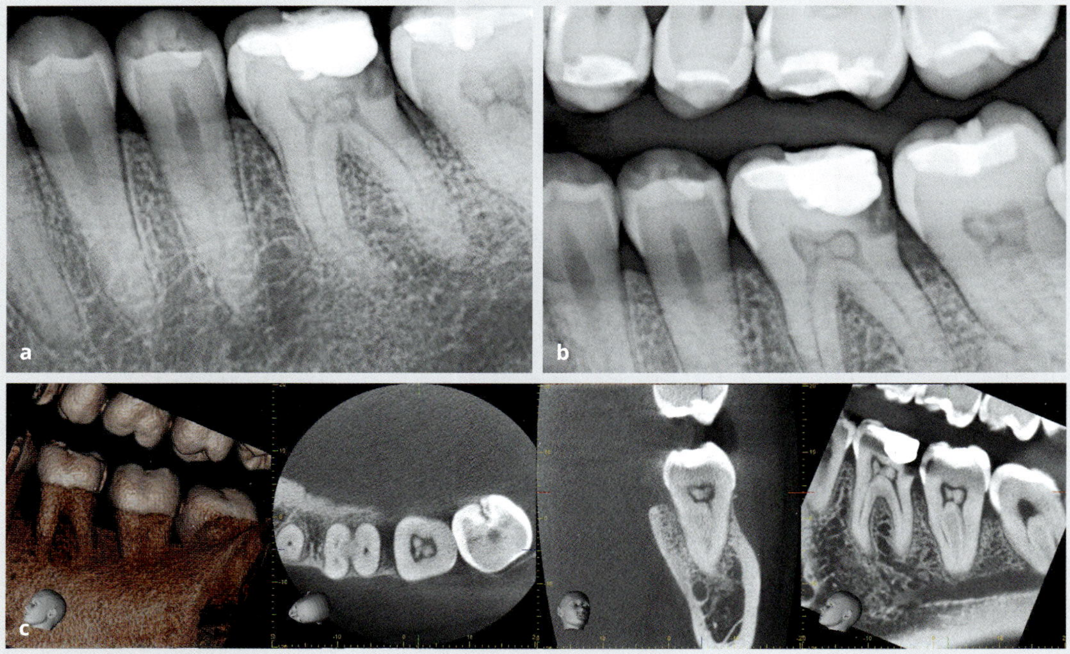

Fig 2-30 *(a)* Periapical image, *(b)* bitewing image, and *(c)* CBCT reconstruction of a denticle or pulp stone in teeth nos. 18 and 19.

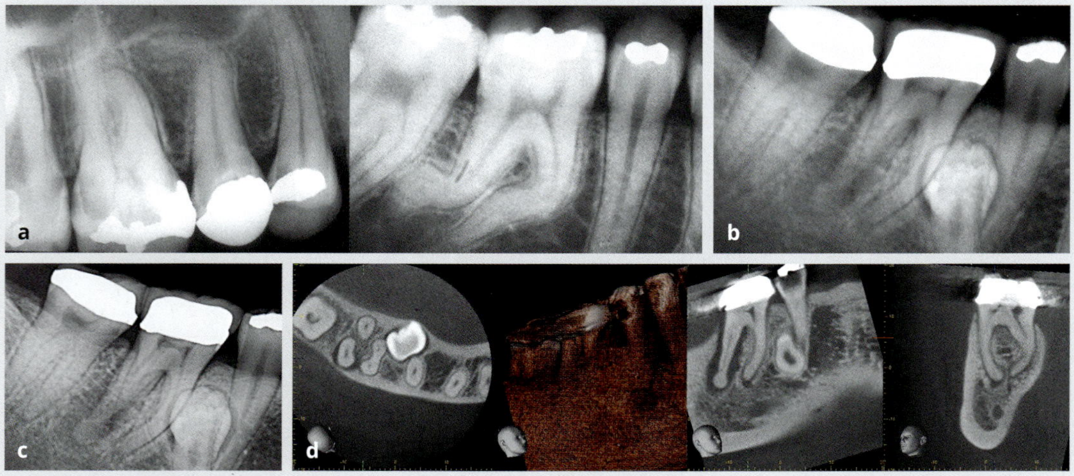

Fig 2-31 *(a)* Molars (teeth nos. 3 and 30) and premolar (no. 4) with sharp dilacerations. *(b)* Straight view periapical image of tooth no. 30 with radix entomolaris and hypercementosis at the distal root apex. An impacted supernumerary premolar is also present. *(c)* Off-angle periapical image. *(d)* CBCT multiplanar reconstructions.

Dilaceration

An abnormal distortion in the root of a tooth or at a junction of the crown and root of a tooth is called a *dilaceration*. Trauma during tooth development is believed to be the etiology of this distortion. It may occur in either the permanent or the primary dentition, with the former being more frequent. There is no predilection based on sex or race, and it may be diagnosed in any age group. Aside from the bent or excess curvature of a root's morphology, the tooth appears normal. Clinically, dilaceration is asymptomatic.[51] It is only of significance if the tooth requires extraction or needs root canal treatment, as the dilaceration adds a measure of complexity to these treatment procedures (Fig 2-31).

Hypercementosis

Hypercementosis, also known as *cementum hyperplasia*, is a change in the shape of a permanent tooth root due to the deposition of excessive amounts of secondary cementum. It is often described as "club-shaped," a bulbous root morphology, or the shape of a flame on a matchstick. Regardless of the shape of the altered root, it usually maintains the normal width of the periradicular periodontal ligament. Secondary cementum may form over the entire root surface or be limited to one area. Because cementum is less radiopaque than dentin, the border between the two is distinguishable. Hypercementosis mainly affects the premolar and molar teeth. There is a higher incidence of occurrence in the mandible. There is no predilection based on race or sex, and it is rarely diagnosed in individuals younger than 6 years old. Clinically, the affected tooth is vital and asymptomatic in most cases. Hypercementosis is often associated with systemic disorders, such as acromegaly and osteitis deformans (Paget disease)[51] (Fig 2-32; see also Figs 2-31b to 2-31d).

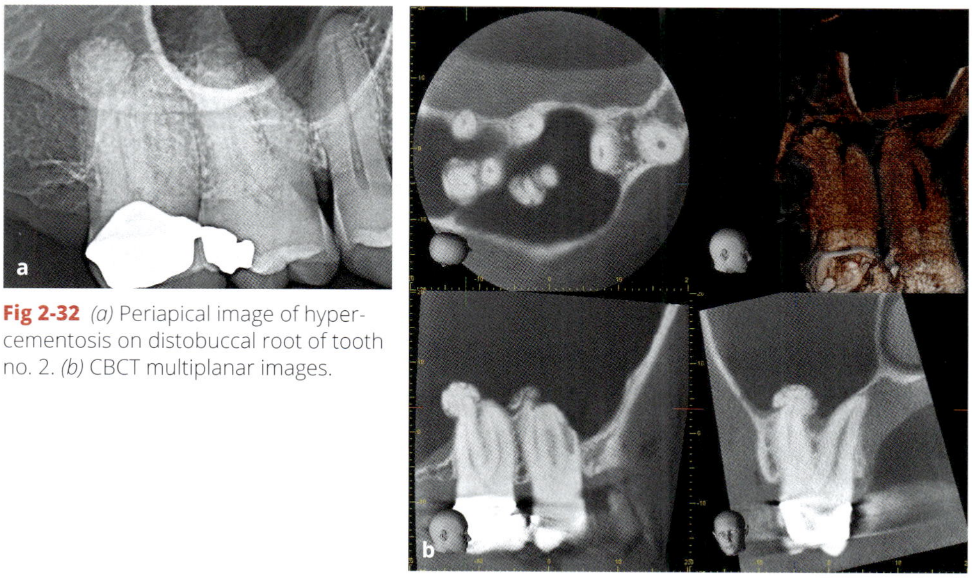

Fig 2-32 *(a)* Periapical image of hypercementosis on distobuccal root of tooth no. 2. *(b)* CBCT multiplanar images.

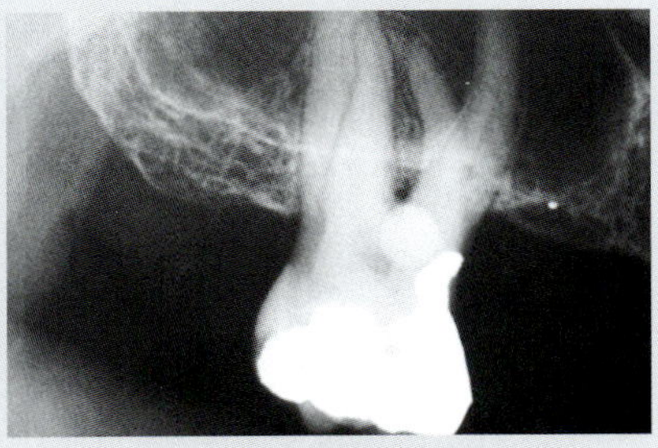

Fig 2-33 Enamel pearl. (Case courtesy of Dr Dwight D. Rice.)

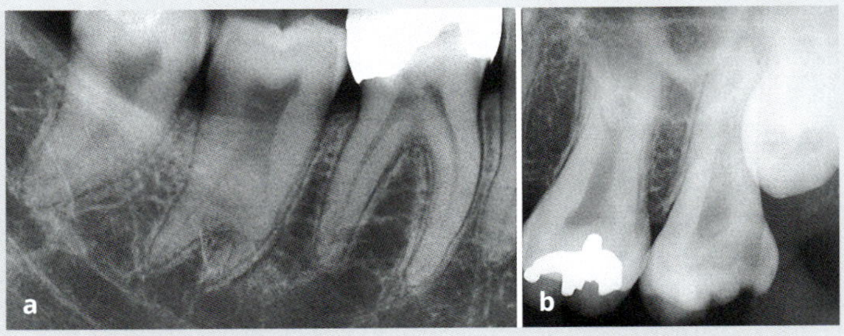

Fig 2-34 Taurodontia in a *(a)* mandibular and *(b)* maxillary molar.

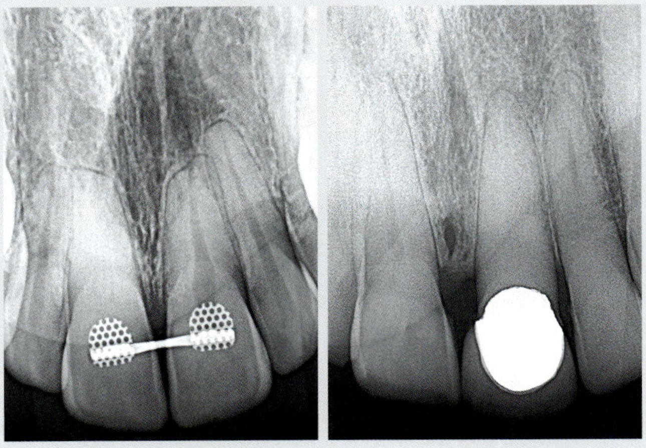

Fig 2-35 Pulpal obliteration.

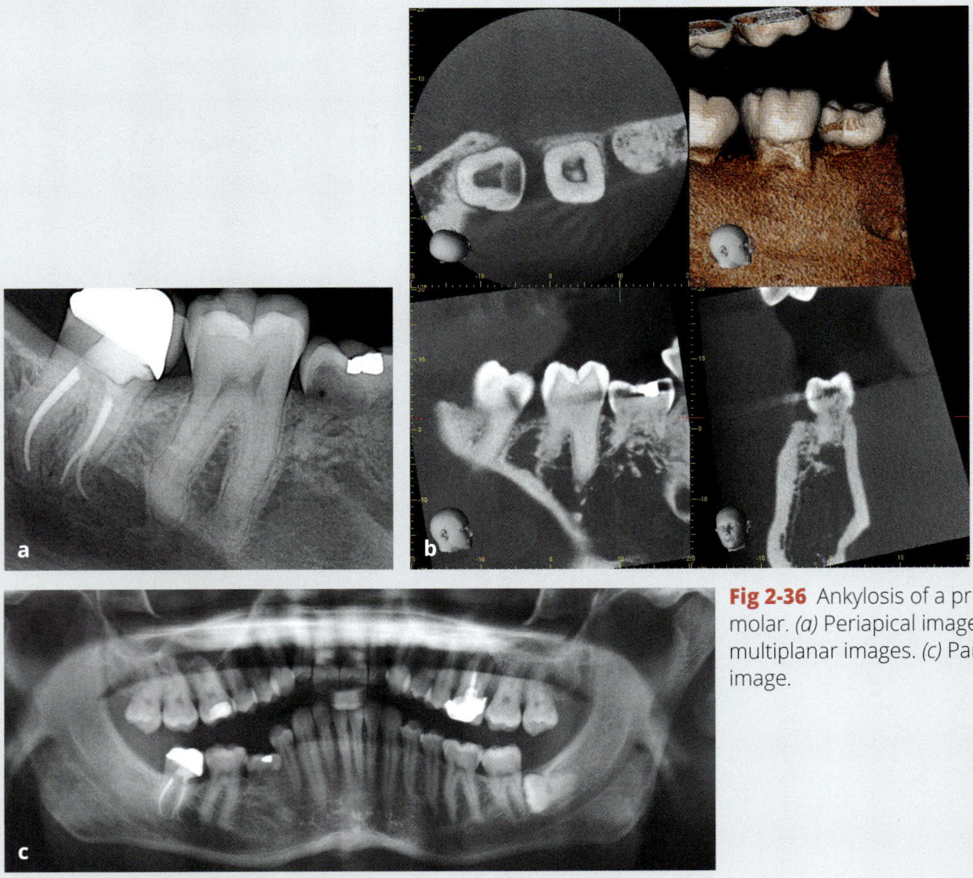

Fig 2-36 Ankylosis of a primary molar. *(a)* Periapical image. *(b)* CBCT multiplanar images. *(c)* Panoramic image.

Enamel pearl

An enamel pearl is a small semicircular bulk of enamel attached to the surface of a permanent tooth. Typically, it is a single spherical mass found at the cementoenamel junction in or near the bifurcation or trifurcation of the multirooted teeth, particularly the maxillary first molar. There is no gender predilection. The enamel pearl appears as a well-defined, round or ovoid, dense radiopacity with or without a normal lamina dura or a periodontal ligament-like space present. The diameter or long axis of an ovoid enamel pearl ranges from 1 to 5 mm. Clinically, it is usually asymptomatic[51] (Fig 2-33).

Taurodont

Taurodont, or "bull-like tooth," describes any tooth that congenitally develops a large body and pulp chamber with very little root formation. The size and length of the taurodont is usually within normal limits. It is rarely noted in children under 6 years old. Taurodonts do not pose any significant clinical problems unless a taurdont needs endodontic treatment or extraction. The larger, vertically deeper pulp chamber makes it more difficult to access molar root canals. The smaller roots are also more likely to fracture during exodontia[40,51,54] (Fig 2-34).

Pulpal obliteration

Partial or total constriction of the pulp chamber and/or root canal of a tooth, often referred to as *pulpal sclerosing*, can lead to the loss of the pulp space or pulpal obliteration. A various number of permanent or deciduous teeth may be affected. There is no predilection based on tooth type, age, sex, or race for pulpal obliteration. It appears as a generalized blockage of the pulp. Although pulpal obliteration is often associated with pulpitis from dental caries or trauma, or developmental disorders such as dentinogenesis imperfecta, the patient is often asymptomatic[51] (Fig 2-35).

Ankylosis

Ankylosis of a tooth is often described as the proliferation of bone between the cementum or dentin of a root and the alveolar bone, with elimination of any intervening soft tissue. Although the etiology is uncertain, there is often a history of blunt trauma or a dental infection. There is no age, race, or sex predilection. Primary molars are most commonly affected, but ankylosis may affect any of the primary or permanent dentition. On radiographic images, the radiolucent periodontal ligament space is replaced with a radiopaque region confluent with the surrounding bone. In some cases, the root may have a moth-eaten appearance with an irregular peripheral outline. Consequently, there may also be a reduction in the overall size of the tooth. Clinically, the affected tooth is generally asymptomatic[51] (Fig 2-36).

Abrasion

Abrasion is defined as pathologic wearing of coronal tooth structure by mechanical means. The extent of wear is variable, ranging from under 1 mm to total destruction of the coronal tooth structure. Radiographically, the abrasion area appears more radiolucent than the remainder of the crown, and it often has irregular borders. Abrasion can affect the primary or permanent dentition, and there is no age, sex, or race predilection. Improper tooth brushing technique, abrasive dentifrice, ill-fitting partial dentures, personal habits, and occupational hazards are some of the etiologies of abrasion. The patient is often asymptomatic[51] (Fig 2-37).

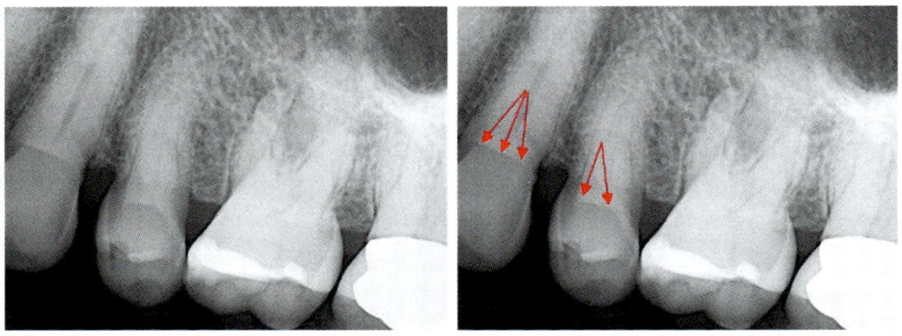

Fig 2-37 Abrasion on the cuspid and premolar from excessive tooth brushing (ie, toothbrush abrasion).

Erosion

Erosion is defined as pathologic wearing down of coronal tooth structure by chemical means. Similar to dental abrasion, the extent of wear is also variable, ranging from under 1 mm to total destruction of the coronal tooth structure. The erosion area appears more radiolucent than the remainder of the crown, and it often has well-defined borders. Similar to abrasion, erosion can also occur with the primary or permanent dentition, and there is no age, sex, or race predilection. It is notable that the mesial and distal surfaces of teeth are rarely affected. Clinically, tooth surfaces affected by erosion often appear as either a smoothly polished, disc-shaped cavity or as a pitted tooth surface. Occupational hazards, diet, medications, and low salivary pH value are some of the etiologic factors of erosion[51] (Fig 2-38).

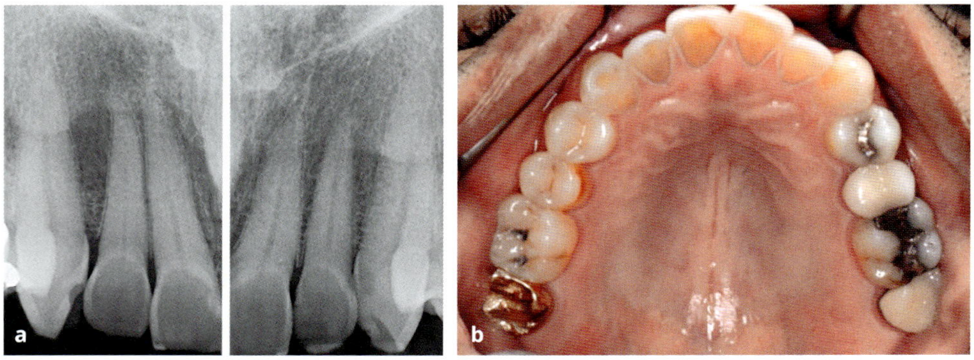

Fig 2-38 *(a)* Erosion of tooth structure noted on the lingual surfaces of the maxillary incisors by the thinning of the enamel on the marginal ridges and cingulum areas. *(b)* Clinical image of the lingual surface erosion due to bulimia.

Attrition

Attrition is defined as age-related loss of tooth structure from tooth-to-tooth contact. The extent of tooth reduction is variable, ranging from under 1 mm to total wear of the coronal tooth structure. In cases of excess parafunction or factitial injury, the rate of attrition can be more excessive. Usually, the pattern of wear is irregular. In addition to the reduction in tooth size, pulpal and root canal obliteration may also occur. Attrition may be associated with any primary or permanent teeth, and there is no age, sex, or race predilection. Occupational hazards, especially with jobs where a patient is exposed to abrasive airborne materials, malpositioned teeth, or a coarse diet, are some of the etiologies where more excessive or pathologic attrition is noted. The patient is often asymptomatic unless the wear is rapid enough to cause symptoms of pulpitis[51] (Fig 2-39).

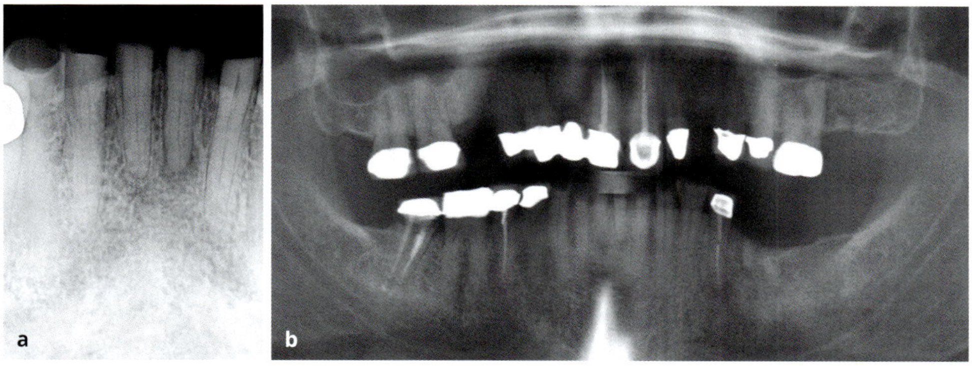

Fig 2-39 Attrition of mandibular anterior dentition. *(a)* Periapical image. *(b)* Panoramic image.

External resorption

External resorption, or *external resorptive defect*, is the loss of coronal or root structure in a primary or permanent tooth initiating at the outer surface and continuing inward (or axially) toward the pulp. Generally, the pulp walls are not affected. This results in either a smooth or irregular periphery. The loss of tooth structure can vary from a linear dimension of 1 mm to total destruction of the tooth. Although the etiology is not fully clear, normal physiologic resorption, previous orthodontic treatment, trauma, or congenital defects are believed to be some of the most common etiologic factors. Again, there is no age, sex, or race predilection[51] (Fig 2-40).

Internal resorption or internal resorptive defect

Contrary to external resorption, internal resorption is the loss of dentin originating from the pulp chamber and continuing outward toward the root surface. Although it may affect either the primary or permanent dentition, internal resorption is mostly found in permanent teeth. Internal resorption generally results in a well-defined round or oval radiolucent area in the central portion of a tooth, associated with the pulp chamber and occasionally extending to the external

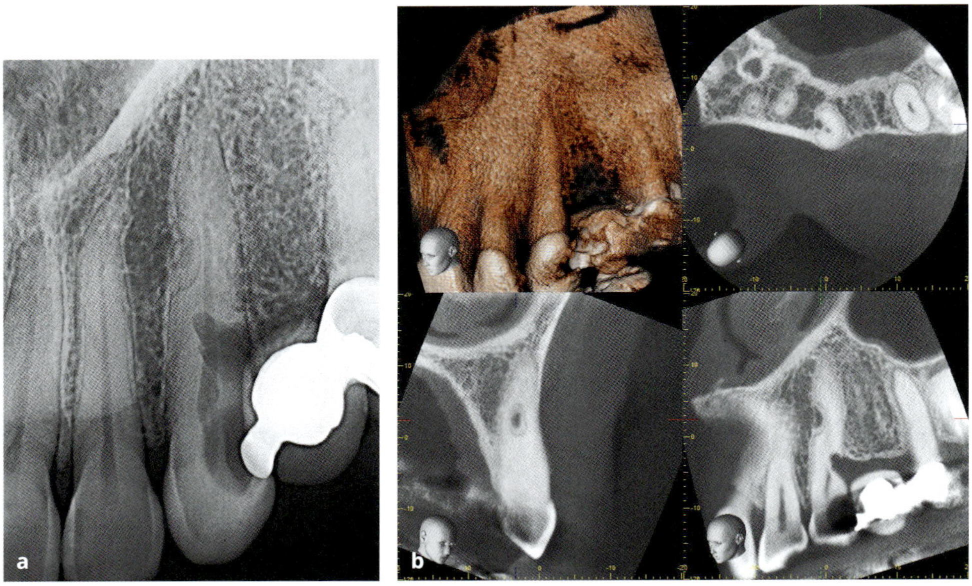

Fig 2-40 External root resorption on tooth no. 11. The cervical radiolucency seems to be iatrogenic (accidental during preparation for fixed partial denture rest), but the distal mid-root resorption is external root resorption. *(a)* Periapical image. *(b)* CBCT image.

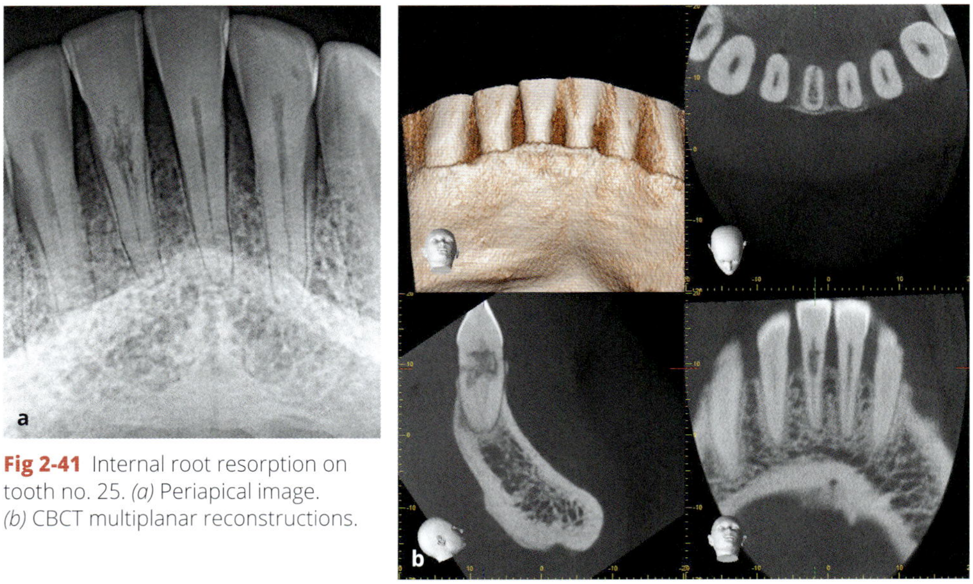

Fig 2-41 Internal root resorption on tooth no. 25. *(a)* Periapical image. *(b)* CBCT multiplanar reconstructions.

surface of the root. However, the resorbed area may also assume any shape, and its linear size may vary on radiographs from less than 1 mm to total destruction of the tooth. Similar to other forms of tooth structure loss, there is no age, sex, or race predilection. In many cases, there is a history of a pulpotomy or another trauma to the affected tooth. Clinically, there may be a pink color to the coronal tooth structure that is characteristic of internal resorption[51] (Fig 2-41).

Table 2-4 summarizes the dental anomalies presented in this chapter.

TABLE 2-4 Summary of dental anomalies

DENTAL ANOMALY	BRIEF DESCRIPTION	RADIOLUCENT/ RADIOPAQUE	COMMON TEETH AFFECTED	SYMPTOMS	ALTERNATE NAME
Microdontia	Teeth that are smaller in size and stature	N/A	Maxillary lateral incisors and maxillary third molars	Asymptomatic	Dwarf teeth and peg laterals
Dens invaginatus	Infolding of margical ridges at the cingulum, which gives the appearance of a tooth within a tooth	Mixed	Maxillary lateral incisor	Pain and/or periapical radiolucency	Dens in dente
Denticle	Calcified, uniform, dense body within a pulp chamber	Radiopaque	Any permanent or primary	Asymptomatic	Pulp stone, endolith
Dilaceration	Shape of the root has a sharp bend or a twisted course	N/A	Any permanent	Asymptomatic	
Enamel pearl	Globular mass at the cementoenamel junction	Radiopaque	Maxillary first molar	Asymptomatic	
Hypercementosis	Deposition of excessive amounts of secondary cementum	Radiopaque	Permanent mandibular premolar and molar	Asymptomatic	Cementum hyperplasia
Taurodont	Large body and pulp chamber, with very little root formation	N/A	Molar	Asymptomatic	Bull-like tooth
Pulpal obliteration	Partial or total constriction of the pulp chamber and/or root canal	Radiopaque	Any permanent or primary	Asymptomatic	
Ankylosis	Partial or complete elimination of PDL	N/A	Any permanent or primary	Asymptomatic	
Abrasion	Mechanical wear of tooth structure	Radiolucent	Any permanent or primary	Asymptomatic	
Erosion	Chemical wear of tooth structure	Radiolucent	Any permanent or primary	Asymptomatic	
Attrition	Wearing down of tooth structure by tooth-to-tooth contact	N/A	Any permanent or primary	Asymptomatic	
External resorption	Resorption that starts from the root surface and moves toward the pulp	Radiolucent	Any permanent or primary	Asymptomatic	
Internal resorption	Resorption that starts in the pulp and moves outward	Radiolucent	Any permanent or primary	Asymptomatic	

Radiolucent Lesions of Nonodontogenic Origin

There are several radiolucent lesions of nonpulpal origin that mimic the radiographic appearance of endodontic lesions of pulpal origin. Due to these similarities, clinicians should systematically perform clinical tests to assist with a diagnosis and avoid critical mistakes (see chapter 1). Pulp responsive tests are the most important aids in differentiating between endodontic and non-endodontic lesions. Teeth with necrotic pulps and radiolucent periradicular lesions generally do not respond to pulp tests. However, the neurovasculature to teeth adjacent to lesions of nonpulpal origin is not usually affected, and the response of these teeth to various pulpal stimuli remains unaffected. Unfortunately, some clinicians use only radiographs to establish a diagnosis without taking a complete history of the signs and symptoms and performing clinical tests. Therefore, in addition to the radiographic examination, all relevant pulp tests, clinical signs and symptoms, and patient history details should be used for diagnosis and treatment planning to be as accurate as possible.

Even though most radiographic changes are of endodontic origin and arise from pathologic changes in the pulp, other radiographic variations, such as anatomical variations, anomalies, and benign and malignant lesions, may simulate the appearance of periradicular endodontic lesions.[55]

The following benign odontogenic lesions may have radiographic appearances similar to endodontic periradicular lesions: initial stages of periradicular cemental dysplasia, lateral periodontal cysts, dentigerous cysts, odontogenic keratocysts, odontogenic myxomas, and ameloblastomas. Nonodontogenic lesions that may have radiographic appearances similar to endodontic periradicular lesions include early stages of monostotic fibrous dysplasia, early stage ossifying fibromas, nasopalatine duct cysts, solitary bone cysts, central giant cell granulomas, and central hemangiomas (see chapter 1). The pulp tests of teeth adjacent to these lesions respond within normal limits, and the lamina dura around the apices of teeth associated with these lesions is often not affected. Surgical biopsy and histopathologic examination are needed to establish a diagnosis for these lesions.[56]

Malignant lesions that may simulate odontogenic periradicular lesions include metastatic lymphoma, squamous cell carcinoma, osteosarcoma, chondrosarcoma, and multiple myeloma. In most of these malignant lesions, rapid and extensive hard tissue destruction is a common finding, which is in contrast to endodontic lesions of pulpal origin. Although the teeth in the affected region can remain responsive to vitality tests, in some cases, the dental pulps or sensory nerves are disrupted and nonresponsive. More details on the clinical and radiographic description of these lesions can be found in established textbooks[44,57,58] (see chapter 1).

Technical Mishaps During Endodontic Radiographic Diagnosis and Treatment

Correctly exposing intraoral receptors incorporates four basic steps: receptor placement, vertical angulation alignment of the position indicating device (PID), horizontal angulation alignment of the PID (cone), and x-ray beam centering. Technical errors can occur if any of these steps are performed inadequately.

Receptor placement errors

Inadequate coverage/missing apices

A very common receptor placement error is inadequate coverage of the area to be examined radiographically. This error typically occurs in molar images due to patient discomfort maintaining or tolerating proper receptor placement. Each periapical and bitewing in a complete radiographic examination has well-established placement criteria. These criteria describe the structures of interest that should be recorded on each image. Consistent application of these criteria is essential to minimize receptor placement errors.

Improper receptor placement can cause missing apices. Placing the receptor more lingual to the teeth, where the palate and floor are deeper, will make positioning easier and more comfortable for the patient. Placement of the bite block and receptor in the correct position first and then having the patient slowly bite to maintain the placement is the preferred and most effective approach. In addition, when using receptor holders, the bite block should be placed on the teeth to be imaged and not on the opposing teeth. If the bite block is placed on the opposing teeth and the patient is required to bite the receptor into place, a placement error is likely to result[48] (Fig 2-42).

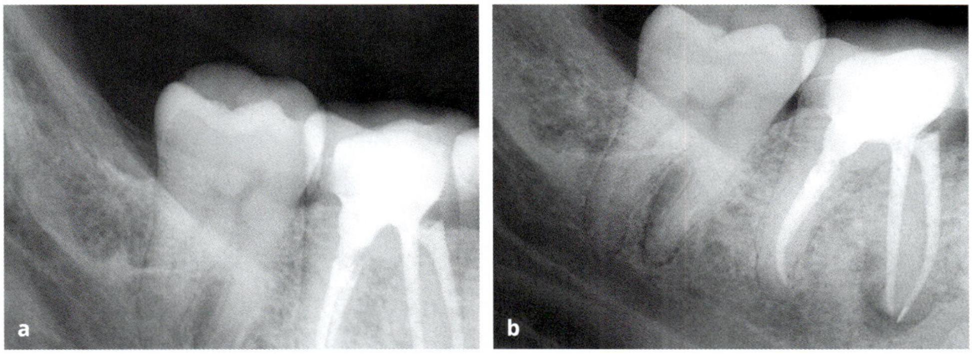

Fig 2-42 *(a)* Inadequate periapical coverage. *(b)* Corrected periapical coverage.

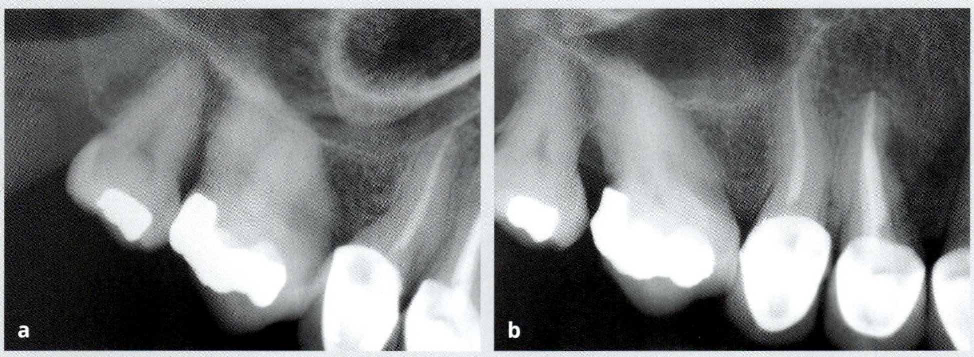

Fig 2-43 *(a)* Tilted occlusal plane. *(b)* Corrected periapical image with the bite block closer to or contacting the occlusal surfaces.

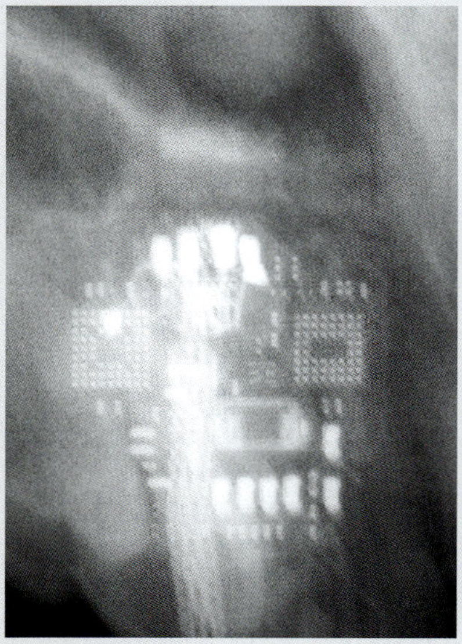

Fig 2-44 Backward placement of solid-state intraoral receptor.

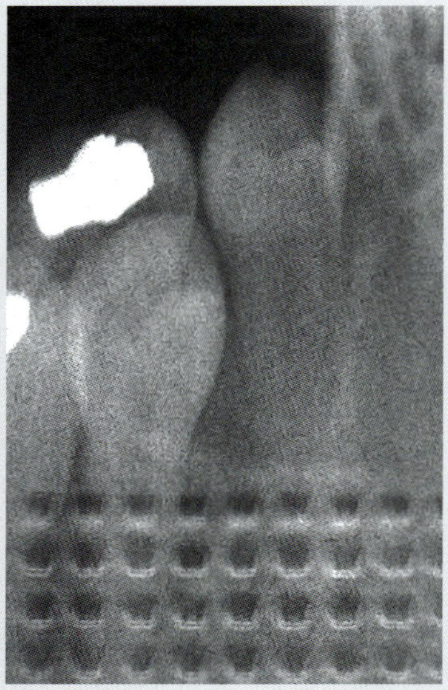

Fig 2-45 Backward placement of PA film.

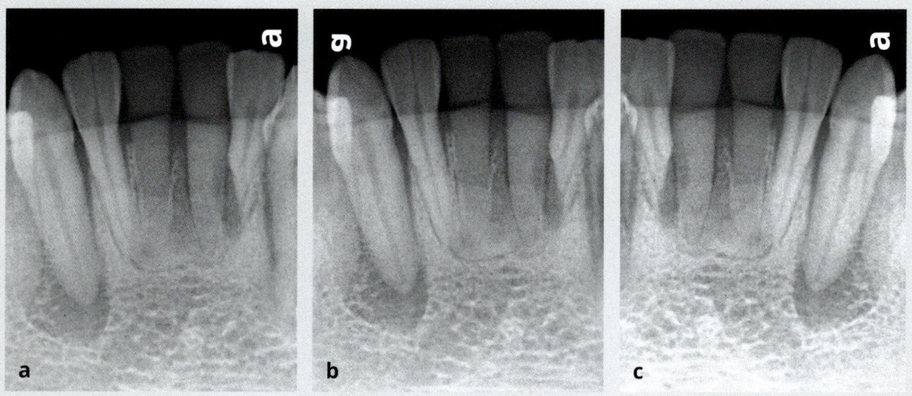

Fig 2-46 Example of the confusion created by exposing a PSP backward. This case shows images taken on a model. *(a)* The proper orientation of the anterior right mandible. Note the letter "a" orientation marker in the top right. *(b)* Periapical radiograph of the same area with the plate positioned back to front. Note the letter "a" orientation marker in the top left is also back to front. *(c)* The same image as part *b*, but the image is flipped showing the letter "a" oriented to read correctly. However, when this is done, the image presents incorrectly as a periapical image of the anterior left mandible. This type of error causes confusion and can lead to errors in anatomical identification, diagnosis, and treatment, and can possibly even lead to medicolegal problems.

Tilted occlusal plane

The occlusal plane will appear slanted or diagonal on the recorded image when the occlusal edge of the receptor is not placed parallel to the occlusal plane. When exposing bitewing radiographs, the edges of the receptor may come in contact with the curvature of the palate or the lingual aspect of the mandible. When this occurs, the occlusal plane will appear slanted. To avoid this error, the capture surface of the receptor must be placed perpendicular to the occlusal plane and farther away from the teeth toward the sagittal midline where there is more vertical depth in the oral cavity for the receptor to fit and therefore be more comfortable for the patient. For periapical radiographs, the bite block must be in contact with the occlusal or incisal surfaces of the teeth being imaged (Fig 2-43).

Placement on the opposing teeth or too close to the teeth will cause the receptor to displace when it contacts bony anatomy. The PSP receptor orientation dot or plate marker should be placed toward the crowns of the teeth for periapical images and toward the mandible for bitewing images to reduce interference with viewing the structures of interest on the recorded image.[48]

Back-to-front sensor placement

In order to produce an acceptable image, the exposure side of any receptor must be facing the x-ray source. Backward placement is rather improbable with the rigid solid-state digital receptors because of the wire attachment on the nonexposure side of the sensor. However, if this happens, instead of an image of the teeth, the electronic circuit board is in the image (Fig 2-44).

The back-to-front placement of a film in the mouth causes the lead foil inside the packet to face the radiation source instead of the film directly. As a result, the lead foil decreases the x-ray beam intensity before the x-ray photons reach the film. This error causes the imprinted pattern on the foil, a diamond effect, or a herringbone pattern on the processed film. This error also results in a lighter image and reversal of the image (Fig 2-45).

The backward placement of the receptor may also occur with phosphor plate receptors. This problem can lead to confusion about the correct anatomical area recorded when the images are sequenced (mounted) in a template (Fig 2-46). Attention to the orientation of the receptor inside the mouth is critical for correct anatomical orientation and avoidance of diagnostic errors.[48]

Receptor artifacts

With phosphor plate receptors, bending may occur due to space compromises and contact with the curvature of the mandibular lingual or palatal cortex and/or by mishandling the receptors. These receptors can be arched but should never be completely bent to a degree that will create a crease mark. It is best to use the smallest receptor size that will adequately cover the teeth in need without producing excessive discomfort to the patient. If a plate is scratched, crimped, or folded, the embedded emulsion will become damaged, compromising the image quality (Figs 2-47a to 2-47c). Smaller receptors, correct placement, and careful handling will minimize receptor bending and other receptor distortions that produce image artifacts.

Although rigid digital receptors cannot be bent, they can be accidentally dropped on the floor, and the wires that attach them to the computer can be damaged or projected onto the image (Fig 2-47d). Excess pressure on the receptor from dropping or biting can damage the sensor and create "dead" or nonreactive pixels on

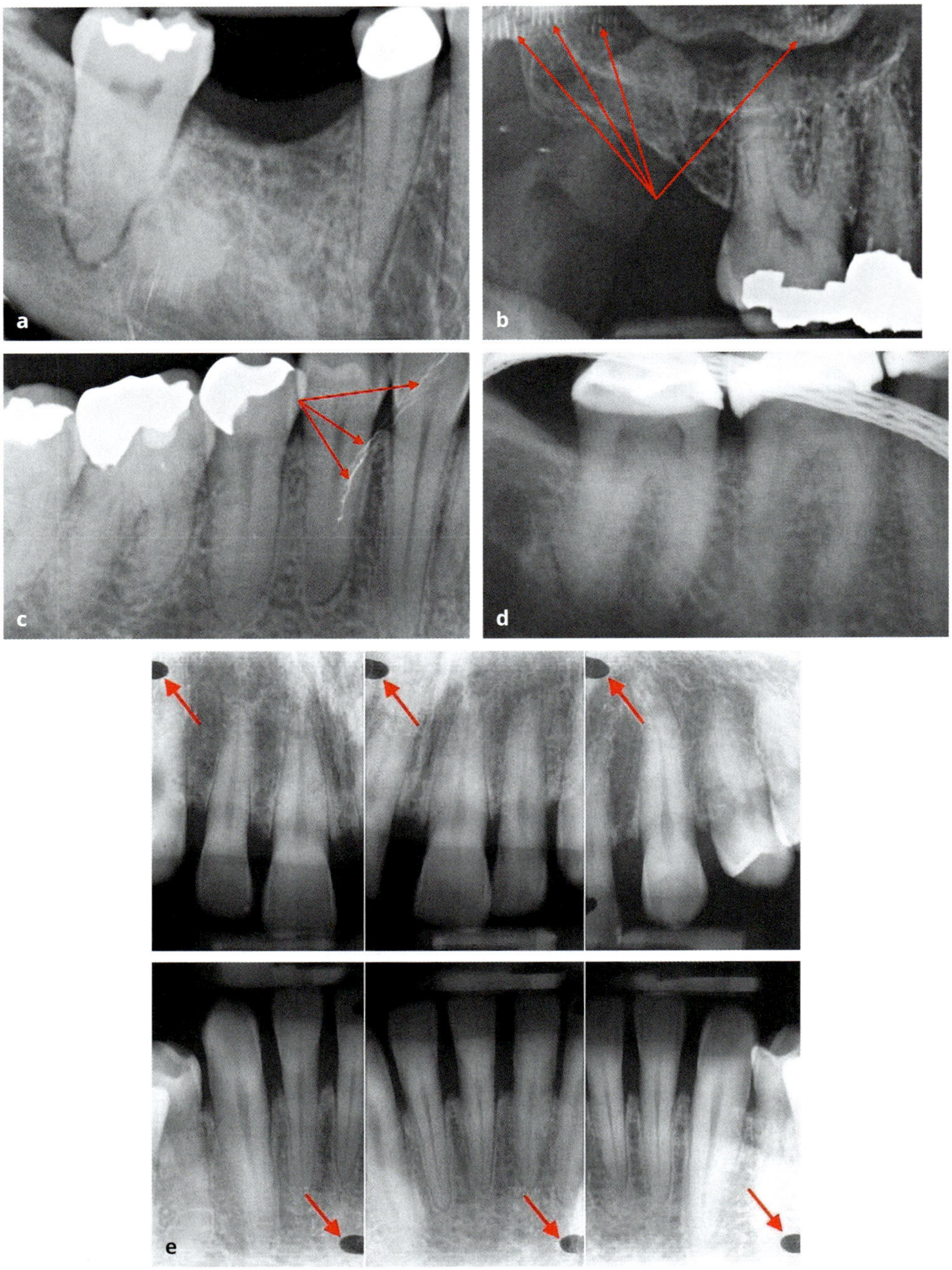

Fig 2-47 Receptor artifacts. *(a)* Scratches on PSP plate in no. 31 PA region. *(b)* Hemostat damage to the PSP emulsion. *(c)* Damage to the PSP emulsion from a permanent crease caused by bending. *(d)* Solid-state wire artifact. *(e)* Dead zone from compression/biting damage to pixels.

the receptor surface (Fig 2-47e). These incidents can result in permanent damage to the silicone plates, which degrades image quality.[48]

Vertical alignment errors

The length of the teeth on the recorded image is controlled by vertical angulation. When applying the paralleling technique and using receptor holders, the vertical angulation is dictated by the holding device to help align the x-ray beam perpendicular to both the receptor and the teeth. Therefore, in order to ensure proper vertical angulation, it is important that the clinician place the receptor parallel to the vertical axis of the teeth. Vertical alignment errors occur more often with the bisecting angle technique, resulting in either elongation or foreshortening of the length of the teeth. In the bisecting angle technique, the beam is perpendicular to the plane that bisects or divides the angle formed by the vertical axes of the teeth and the receptor. With this bisecting angle technique, the margin for error in vertical linear dimension is very small, so elongated or foreshortened images are more common.

It is important to determine the cause of an image distortion in order to correct it if a retake radiograph is necessary.[48]

Elongation

Elongation, or lengthening of the images of the teeth and surrounding structures, happens due to under-angulation of the x-ray beam (ie, inadequate vertical angle). In other words, when elongation occurs using the paralleling technique, the angle of the x-ray beam is less than the angle of the long-axis plane of the teeth. In order to correct this error, the clinician must increase the vertical angulation (Fig 2-48a). For the maxillary arch, the positive vertical angulation must be increased (PID pointing down); for the mandibular arch, the negative vertical angulation must be increased (PID pointing up).

As mentioned earlier, this error can also occur when using the bisecting angle technique. However, the error is often caused by the x-ray beam being perpendicular to the long axis of the teeth rather than perpendicular to the plane that bisects the angle between the teeth and the receptor.[48]

Foreshortening

Foreshortening, or shortening of images of the teeth and the surrounding structures, can also result from improper vertical angulation due to over-angulation of the x-ray beam (ie, excessive vertical angle). While using the paralleling technique, foreshortening can occur when the angle of the x-ray beam is greater than the vertical angle needed to be perpendicular to the long axis plane of the teeth. In order to correct foreshortening when using the paralleling technique, the clinician should decrease the positive vertical angulation for maxillary projections and decrease the negative vertical angulation for mandibular projections[48] (Figs 2-48b and 2-48c).

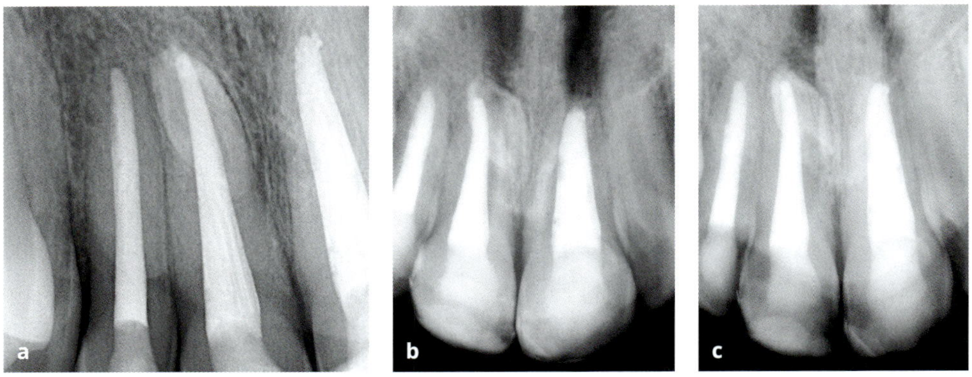

Fig 2-48 *(a)* Elongation and cone cut periapical image; *(b)* same area with foreshortening and *(c)* adequate image of the same area. Incidentally, a mesiodens is superimposing the apical one-fourth of tooth no. 8.

Horizontal alignment errors—Superimposition/overlap of anatomical structures

With proper horizontal alignment of the x-ray beam, the interproximal contacts of the teeth will be open and not overlapped on the image. This will facilitate a thorough radiographic caries evaluation and assessment of alveolar bone levels, both important components of a thorough clinical and radiographic examination. In order to open the interproximal surfaces, the x-ray beam should be aimed directly between the targeted teeth. Horizontal alignment errors cause the image to shift anteriorly or posteriorly, resulting in the overlap of the contact areas of proximal surfaces (Fig 2-49).

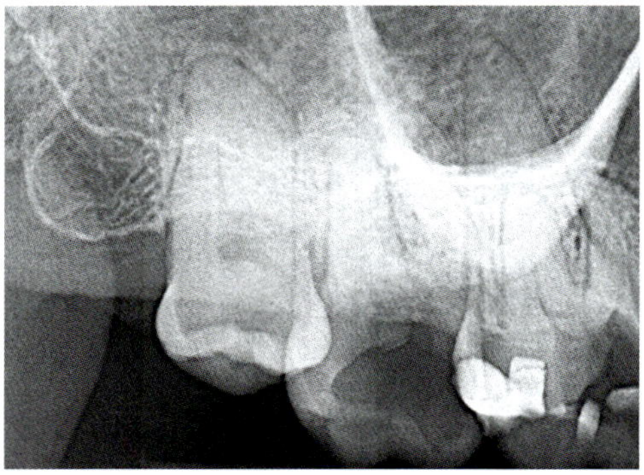

Fig 2-49 Superimposition.

To determine if the horizontal angulation is incorrect, the clinician should evaluate the extent of the overlap. The buccal object rule can be used to determine the movement of the buccal and lingual cusps when trying to understand the error. Buccal objects move in the opposite direction compared to the direction of the x-ray tube head, while lingual objects move in the same direction as the movement of the x-ray tube head. Application of the buccal object rule to determine the cause of interproximal overlapping requires evaluation of the position of the x-ray tube head and the direction of the overlapping on the bitewing image. For example, if the x-ray head is placed too posteriorly, the buccal cusps will shift in an anterior direction relative to the lingual cusps, and the interproximal surfaces will overlap.

In contrast, if the x-ray head is too anterior in position, the buccal cusps will shift to the posterior direction relative to the lingual cusp, and again, the interproximal surfaces will overlap. To avoid this error, the central ray must pass through the proximal surfaces of the teeth so the contacts are open and do not overlap. To aid in determining the correct horizontal angle, the clinician can place the end of a cotton-tip applicator into the contact zone. This method will help visualize the direction of the x-rays to open the interproximal teeth contacts.

When using receptor-holding devices, horizontal errors can occur from improper horizontal alignment of the receptor. These errors can be avoided by placing the receptor in the same horizontal plane as the buccal and lingual surfaces of the teeth so that the x-ray beam travels directly through the contact areas. This will position the receptor parallel to the buccal plane of the teeth as well as parallel to the instrument indicator ring.[48]

Beam centering errors—Cone cuts

The central ray should be aligned over the receptor's center, with the x-ray beam directed perpendicular to the receptor; otherwise, a cone cut occurs. Cone cuts appear as a radiopaque or clear zone on the radiographic image. The shape of the cone cut depends on the type of collimator used, round or rectangular, when exposing the receptor[48] (Fig 2-50).

Table 2-5 summarizes technical errors.

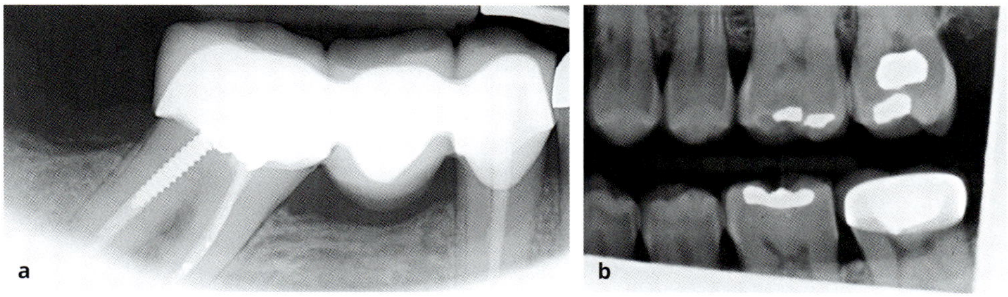

Fig 2-50 Cone cut with *(a)* round collimator and *(b)* rectangular collimator.

TABLE 2-5 Technical error summary

ERROR	CAUSE	CORRECTION
Receptor placement	Improper receptor positioning	Place receptor in correct location
Backward placement	Non-exposure side toward x-rays	Place exposure side toward x-rays
Receptor artifacts	Bending, curving, marring	Select proper size; handle gently
Elongation	Inadequate vertical angulation	Increase the vertical angulation
Foreshortening	Excessive vertical angulation	Decrease the vertical angulation
Overlapping	Incorrect horizontal angulation	Direct x-ray through the contacts
Cone cut	X-ray beam not centered	Center x-ray beam over receptor

Post-Endodontic Radiographic Examination Mishaps

Root canal therapy results in the elimination or reduction of bacteria; thereafter, the healing may begin. Inflammatory cytokines and mediators within the lesion transition from a pro-inflammatory, destructive phase to an anti-inflammatory and proliferative nature. Osteoprogenitor cells undergo differentiation into osteoblasts, which secrete bony matrix to replace bone destroyed from apical periodontitis.[59] Since 1956, the benchmarks for successful endodontic therapy have been assessed according to Strindberg's criteria. These criteria include complete radiographic healing of the periapical lesion.[60]

Healing determination

Periapical radiography has been the main modality to evaluate the healing of apical periodontitis, specifically by monitoring the resolution of the radiolucency at the apex of the tooth.[61] Preoperative periapical radiographs aid in the diagnosis of apical periodontitis and serve as the baseline to evaluate the resolution of the lesion after treatment is initiated. A decrease in size of the radiolucency suggests healing is taking place. Conversely, an increase in the size of the periapical lesion suggests the lesion is not healing and that the disease is still aggressive. However, if the size of the lesion is consistent or unchanged, it is more difficult to discern the situation and, subsequently, how to proceed with treatment.[62–64]

Because periapical radiography is only two-dimensional, the amount of information provided is limited. For instance, the buccolingual dimensions cannot be assessed in periapical radiographs. In addition, superimposition of adjacent anatomical structures such as the maxillary sinus may interfere with appropriate interpretation. Studies have shown that in some instances, bone must be demineralized by 30% to 50% in order to visualize these lesions radiographically.[65] It has been suggested that periapical lesions are not detected by periapical radiographs if confined only to cancellous bone or if less than 12.5% of bone loss exists in the area.[66] Many other authors have confirmed that perforation of the cortical bone is necessary for radiographic detection of lesions.[67–70] These reasons explain why the healing of periapical lesions may not be detected by periapical radiography for many years after treatment.

In contrast, CBCT aids in the visualization of periapical lesions not seen otherwise due to small size or being confined in cancellous bone.[71,72] Additionally, CBCT allows assessing and measuring of periapical lesions in three orthogonal planes. Disadvantages of CBCT include higher radiation exposure, high levels of scatter artifact on the images (metal posts), and increased costs to the patient.[73,74]

In addition, many believe CBCT is overestimating the frequency of periapical lesions[56] and, in return, leading to possible overtreatment of otherwise asymptomatic radiolucencies. A recent study showed that 20% of teeth with successful root canal treatment based on conventional periapical imaging had CBCT radiolucencies measuring greater than 1 mm of apical PDL width.[75,76] If one cannot determine the histologic diagnosis of the periradicular radiolucency, the study states that despite the presence of a lesion using CBCT, no further treatment is warranted if the patient is asymptomatic. These radiolucencies may not be pathologic changes, and therefore clinical decision-making must not be solely based on radiographic interpretation.[76]

CBCT has a higher probability of detecting the presence of a periapical lesion, and a periapical radiograph has a higher probability of missing a periapical lesion. Even though healing may be present, it is a very dynamic process and may be affected by many factors. Therefore, a combination of clinical and radiographic examination should be used to prevent misdiagnosis and over/mistreatment in a postoperative evaluation; in addition, despite the advantages of CBCT, clinicians must still consider the higher costs and potentially higher radiation dose to the patient. When CBCT is indicated as the radiographic modality of choice, the clinician should use a CBCT with a limited field of view (FOV) of 50 mm × 50 mm or less. The limited FOV exposes a smaller area of the jaws and is programmed with smaller voxel sizes, which offer higher resolution and lower radiation dose to the patient.[76,77]

Use of CBCT to Minimize Mishaps for Endodontic Radiographic Diagnosis, Treatment, and Postoperative Evaluation

CBCT technology was developed at the end of the last millennium,[78,79] and it has very quickly made a huge impact on the field of endodontics. CBCT has been shown to overcome many of the limitations attributed to periapical radiography.[80-83] This imaging modality aids in the visualization of periapical lesions not seen otherwise due to small early-stage sizes or limitations of 2D imaging in cancellous bone.[71,72] In addition, CBCT allows the opportunity to assess and measure the periapical lesion in multiple dimensions.[73]

A joint position paper released by the American Association of Endodontists and the American Academy of Oral and Maxillofacial Radiology provides evidence-based guidance to clinicians for using CBCT in the field of endodontics.[37] In general, the use of CBCT should be limited to the assessment and treatment of complex endodontic conditions.

Recommendations

The following are the recommendations from the AAOMR /AAE joint position statement[37] on the use of CBCT in endodontic diagnosis and treatment planning:

1. Intraoral radiographs should be considered the imaging modality of choice in the evaluation of the endodontic patient.

2. Limited FOV CBCT should be considered the imaging modality of choice for diagnosis in patients who present with contradictory or nonspecific clinical signs and symptoms associated with untreated or previously endodontically treated teeth. (CBCT imaging has the ability to detect periapical pathosis before it is apparent on 2D radiographs.)
3. Limited FOV CBCT should be considered the imaging modality of choice for initial treatment of teeth with the potential for extra canals and suspected complex morphology, such as mandibular anterior teeth and maxillary and mandibular premolars and molars, and dental anomalies.
4. If a preoperative CBCT has not been taken, limited FOV CBCT should be considered the imaging modality of choice for intra-appointment identification and localization of calcified canals.
5. Intraoral radiographs should be considered the imaging modality of choice for immediate postoperative imaging.
6. Limited FOV CBCT should be considered the imaging modality of choice if clinical examination and 2D intraoral radiographs are inconclusive in the detection of vertical root fracture (VRF).
7. Limited FOV CBCT should be the imaging modality of choice when evaluating the nonhealing of previous endodontic treatment to help determine the need for further treatment, such as nonsurgical, surgical, or extraction.
8. Limited FOV CBCT should be considered the imaging modality of choice for nonsurgical retreatment to assess endodontic treatment complications, such as overextended root canal obturation material, separated endodontic instruments, and localization of perforations.
9. Limited FOV CBCT should be considered the imaging modality of choice for presurgical treatment planning to localize root apex/apices and to evaluate the proximity to adjacent anatomical structures.
10. Limited FOV CBCT should be considered the imaging modality of choice for surgical placement of implants.
11. Limited FOV CBCT should be considered the imaging modality of choice for diagnosis and management of limited dentoalveolar trauma, root fractures, luxation and/or displacement of teeth, and localized alveolar fractures in the absence of other maxillofacial or soft tissue injury that may require other advanced imaging modalities.
12. Limited FOV CBCT should be considered the imaging modality of choice in the localization and differentiation of external and internal resorptive defects and the determination of appropriate treatment and prognosis.

Conclusion

Intraoral radiographic imaging is an invaluable tool, providing critical information for the diagnosis and treatment of dental disease and other oral conditions. These cost-effective, high-resolution images continue to be the primary method for dental imaging. To ensure the production of high-quality diagnostic images, the clinician must attend to the principles of optimal image projection. In addition, the clinician must be able to manage the patient effectively during radiographic procedures and be well versed in the identification and correction of errors when they occur. The clinician is also responsible for eliminating unnecessary retakes and minimizing radiation exposure to the patients under their care.

There are many specific situations where the 3D image reconstructions produced by CBCT facilitate diagnosis and influence treatment. Therefore, in order to prevent radiographic mishaps, misdiagnoses, and mistreatments, clinicians should consider using CBCT scans whenever indicated, as outlined by the AAE/AAOMR joint statement on CBCT imaging for endodontic diagnosis and treatment. In addition, general dentists and other specialty disciplines should consider an endodontist as part of the dental team when the diagnosis and treatment complexities call for their clinical expertise.

References

1. Gittinger JW. Inside out: Early investigations of x-ray by two Harvard-educated physicians revealed the technology's benefits—and dangers. Harvard Med Alum Bull 2008.
2. Mouyen F, Benz C, Sonnabend E, Lodter JP. Presentation and physical evaluation of RadioVisioGraphy. Oral Surg Oral Med Oral Pathol. 1989;68:238–242.
3. Ong EY, Pitt Ford TR. Comparison of radiovisiography with radiographic film in root length determination. Int Endod J 1995;28:25–29.
4. Low KMT, Dula K, Bürgin W, von Arx T. Comparison of periapical radiography and limited cone-beam tomography in posterior maxillary teeth referred for apical surgery. J Endod 2008;34:557–562.
5. Patel S, Dawood A, Mannocci F, Wilson R, Pitt Ford T. Detection of periapical bone defects in human jaws using cone beam computed tomography and intraoral radiography. Int Endod J 2009;42:507–515.
6. Akdeniz BG, Soğur E. An ex vivo comparison of conventional and digital radiography for perceived image quality of root fillings. Int Endod J 2005;38:397.
7. Bhaskaran V, Qualtrough AJE, Rushton VE, Worthington HV, Horner K. A laboratory comparison of three imaging systems for image quality and radiation exposure characteristics. Int Endod J 2005;38:645.
8. Kositbowornchai S, Hanwachirapong D, Somsopon R, Pirmsinthavee S, Sooksuntisakoonchai N. Ex vivo comparison of digital images with conventional radiographs for detection of simulated voids in root canal filling material. Int Endod J 2006;30:287.
9. Burger CL, Mork TO, Hutter JW, Nicoll B. Direct digital radiography versus conventional radiography for estimation of canal length in curved canals. J Endod 1999;25:260.
10. Holtzmann DJ, Johnson WT, Southard TE, Khademi JA, Chang PJ, Rivera EM. Storage-phosphor computed radiography versus film radiography in the detection of pathologic periradicular bone loss in cadavers. Oral Surg Oral Med Oral Pathol 1998;86:90.
11. Sullivan JE Jr, Di Fiore PM, Koerber A. Radiovisiography in the detection of periapical lesions. J Endod 2000;26:32–35.
12. Al-Rawi W, Teich S. Evaluation of physical properties of different digital intraoral sensors. Compend Contin Educ Dent 2013;34:e76–e83.
13. Christensen GC. Digital radiography sensors. Which is best? Clinicians Report 2011;4(9):1–3.
14. Iannucci JM, Howerton LJ. Dental Radiography: Principles and Techniques, ed 5. St Louis: Elsevier, 2017:72–103.

15. Thomson EM, Johnson ON. Essentials of Dental Radiography for Dental Assistants and Hygienists, ed 10. New York: Pearson, 2018:78–105.
16. Mallya SM, Lam EWN. White and Pharoah's Oral Radiology: Principles and Interpretation, ed 8. St Louis: Elsevier, 2018:89–118.
17. Iannucci JM, Howerton LJ. Dental Radiography: Principles and Techniques, ed 5. St Louis: Elsevier, 2017:152–196.
18. Thomson EM, Johnson ON. Essentials of Dental Radiography for Dental Assistants and Hygienists, ed 10. New York: Pearson, 2018:158–194.
19. Bedard A, Davis TD, Angelopoulos C. Storage phosphor plates: How durable are they as a digital dental radiographic system? J Contemp Dent Pract 2004;5:57–69.
20. White SC, Pharoah MJ. Oral Radiology: Principles and Interpretation, ed 7. St Louis: Elsevier, 2014.
21. Parks ET, Williamson GF. Digital radiography: An overview. J Contemp Dent Pract 2002;3:23–39.
22. Gormez O, Yilmaz HH. Image post-processing in dental practice. Eur J Dent 2009;3:343–347.
23. Brettle D, Carmichael F. The impact of digital image processing artefacts mimicking pathological features associated with restorations. Br Dent J 2011;211:167–170.
24. Gray BM, Mol A, Zandona A, Tyndall D. The effect of image enhancements and dual observers on proximal caries detection. Oral Surg Oral Med Oral Pathol Oral Radiol 2017;123:e133–e139.
25. Costa ED, Brasil DM, Gaêta-Araujo H, Oliveira-Santos C, Freitas DQ. Do image enhancement filters in complementary metal oxide semiconductor and photostimulable phosphor imaging systems improve the detection of fractured endodontic instruments in periapical radiography? Oral Surg Oral Med Oral Pathol Oral Radiol 2021;131:247–255.
26. Zhang W, Abramovitch K, Thames W, Leon IL, Colosi DC, Goren AD. Comparison of the efficacy and technical accuracy of different rectangular collimators for intraoral radiography. Oral Surg Oral Med Oral Pathol Oral Radiol Endod 2009;108:e22–e28.
27. Versteeg CH, Sanderink GC, van Ginkel FC, van der Stelt PF. An evaluation of periapical radiography with a charge-coupled device. Dentomaxillofac Radiol 1998;27:97–101.
28. Clark JL, Wadhwani CP, Abramovitch K, Rice DD, Kattadiyil MT. Effect of sharpening on radiographic image quality. J Prosthet Dent 2018;120:927–933.
29. Schweitzer DM, Berg RW. A digital radiographic artifact: A clinical report. J Prosthet Dent 2010;103:326–329.
30. Liedke GS, Spin-Neto R. Vizzotto MB, Da Silveira PF, Dias Silveira HE, Wenzel A. Diagnostic accuracy of conventional and digital radiography for detecting misfit between the tooth and restoration in metal-restored teeth. J Prosthet Dent 2015;113:39–47.
31. American Dental Association Council on Scientific Affairs, US Department of Health and Human Services, Public Health Service, Food and Drug Administration. Dental Radiographic Examinations: Recommendations for Patient Selection and Limiting Radiation Exposure. Revised 2012. https://www.fda.gov/media/84818/download. Accessed 4 Nov 2022.
32. Patel S, Dawood A, Mannocci F, Wilson R, Pitt Ford T. Detection of periapical bone defects in human jaws using cone beam computed tomography and intraoral radiography. Int Endod J 2009;42:507–515.
33. Bhatt M, Coil J, Chehroudi B, Esteves A, Aleksejuniene J, MacDonald D. Clinical decision-making and importance of the AAE/AAOMR position statement for CBCT examination in endodontic cases. Int Endod J 2021;54:26–37.
34. Aminoshariae A, Kulild JC, Syed A. Cone-beam computed tomography compared with intraoral radiographic lesions in endodontic outcome studies: A systematic review. J Endod 2018;44:1626–1631.
35. Rodríguez G, Abella F, Durán-Sindreu F, Patel S, Roig M. Influence of cone-beam computed tomography in clinical decision making among specialists. J Endod 2017;43:194–199.
36. Viana Wanzeler AM, Montagner F, Vieira HT, Dias da Silveira HL, Arús NA, Vizzotto MB. Can cone-beam computed tomography change endodontists' level of confidence in diagnosis and treatment planning? A before and after study. J Endod 2020;46:283–288.
37. AAE and AAOMR joint position statement: Use of Cone Beam Computed Tomography in Endodontics 2015 Update. Oral Surg Oral Med Oral Pathol Oral Radiol 2015;120:508–512.
38. Cotti E, Esposito SA, Musu D, Campisi G, Shemesh H. Ultrasound examination with color power Doppler to assess the early response of apical periodontitis to the endodontic treatment. Clin Oral Investig 2018;22:131–140
39. Reda R, Zanza A, Cicconetti A, et al. Ultrasound imaging in dentistry: A literature overview. J Imaging 2021;7:238.
40. Ahmed HMA, Dummer PMH. A new system for classifying tooth, root and canal anomalies. Int Endod J 2018;51:389–404.
41. Mora MA, Mol A, Tyndall DA, Rivera EM. In vitro assessment of local tomography for the detection of longitudinal tooth fractures. Oral Surg Oral Med Oral Path Oral Radiol Endod 2007;103:825–829.
42. Katsumata A, Hirukawa A, Noujeim M, et al. Image artifact in dental cone beam CT. Oral Surg Oral Med Oral Path Oral Radiol Endod 2006;101:652–657.

43. Barrett JF, Keat N. Artifacts in CT: Recognition and avoidance. Radiographics 2004;24:1679–1691.
44. Mallya SM, Lam EWN. White and Pharoah's Oral Radiology: Principles and Interpretation, ed 8. St Louis: Elsevier, 2018.
45. Clark CA. A method of ascertaining the relative position of unerupted teeth by means of film radiographs. Proc R Soc Med 1910;3:87–90.
46. Walton R. Endodontic radiographic techniques. Dent Radiogr Photogr 1973;46:51.
47. Tamse A, Kaffe I, Fishel D. Zygomatic arch interference with correct radiographic diagnosis in maxillary molar endodontics. Oral Surg Oral Med Oral Pathol 1980;50:563–566.
48. Miles DA, Van Dis ML, Williamson GF, Jensen CW. Radiographic Imaging for the Dental Team, ed 4. St Louis: Elsevier, 2008.
49. Richards AG. The buccal object rule. Dent Radiogr Photogr 1980;53:37–56.
50. Klein RM, Blake SA, Nattress BR, Hirschmann PN. Evaluation of x-ray beam angulation for successful twin canal identification in mandibular incisors. Int Endod J 1997;30:58–63.
51. Hubar JS. Fundamentals of Oral and Maxillofacial Radiology. Hoboken, NJ: Wiley-Blackwell, 2017: 149–169.
52. Letra A, Chiquet B, Hansen-Kiss E, et al. Nonsyndromic tooth agenesis overview. In: GeneReviews. Seattle: University of Washington, 1993.
53. Syryńska M, Durka-Zajac M, Janiszewska-Olszowska J. Prevalence and location of denticles on panoramic radiographs. Ann Acad Med Stetin 2010;56:55–57.
54. Jafarzadeh H, Azarpazhooh A, Mayhall JT. Taurodontism: A review of the condition and endodontic treatment challenges. Int Endod J 2008;41:375–388.
55. Eli B, Said-Al-Naief N, Torabinejad M. Differential diagnosis of pains and radiolucencies of nonpulpal origin. In: Torabinejad M, Fouad A, Shabahang S (eds). Endodontics: Principles and Practice. St Louis: Elsevier, 2020.
56. Neville BW, Damm DD, Allen CM, Chi AC. Oral and Maxillofacial Pathology, ed 4. St Louis: Elsevier, 2016:453–459.
57. Odell EW, Cawson RA. Cawson's Essentials of Oral Pathology and Oral Medicine. St Louis: Elsevier, 2017.
58. Neville BW, Damm DD, Allen CA, Chi AC. Oral and Maxillofacial Pathology, ed 4. St Louis: Elsevier, 2016:400.
59. Ricucci D, Siqueira JF Jr. Endodontology: An Integrated Biological and Clinical View. Chicago: Quintessence, 2013.
60. Strindberg LZ. The dependence of the results of pulp therapy on certain factors; An analytic study based on radiographic and clinical follow-up examinations. [Tr. from the Swedish manuscript. Stockholm, 1956.
61. Patel S, Durack C, Abella F, Shemesh H, Roig M, Lemberg K. Cone beam computed tomography in endodontics—A review. Int Endod J 2015;48:3–15.
62. Orstavik D. Time-course and risk analyses of the development and healing of chronic apical periodontitis in man. Int Endod J 1996;29:150–155.
63. Eriksen HM, Orstavik D, Kerekes K. Healing of apical periodontitis after endodontic treatment using 3 different root-canal sealers. Endod Dent Traumatol 1988;4:114–117.
64. Murphy WK, Kaugars GE, Collett WK, Dodds RN. Healing of periapical radiolucencies after nonsurgical endodontic therapy. Oral Surg Oral Med Oral Pathol Oral Radiol Endod 1991;71:620–624.
65. Bender IB. Factors influencing the radiographic appearance of bony lesions. J Endod 1997;23:5–14.
66. Bender IB, Seltzer S. Roentgenographic and direct observation of experimental lesions in bone: I. 1961. J Endod 2003;29:702–706.
67. Shoha RR, Dowson J, Richards AG. Radiographic interpretation of experimentally produced bony lesions. Oral Surg Oral Med Oral Pathol Oral Radiol Endod 1974;38:294–303.
68. Lee SJ, Messer HH. Radiographic appearance of artificially prepared periapical lesions confined to cancellous bone. Int Endod J 1986;19:64–72.
69. Paurazas SB, Geist JR, Pink FE, Hoen MM, Steiman HR. Comparison of diagnostic accuracy of digital imaging by using CCD and CMOS-APS sensors with E-speed film in the detection of periapical bony lesions. Oral Surg Oral Med Oral Pathol Oral Radiol Endod 2000;89:356–362.
70. Tsai P, Torabinejad M, Rice D, Azevedo B. Accuracy of cone-beam computed tomography and periapical radiography in detecting small periapical lesions. J Endod 2012;38:965–970.
71. Lofthag-Hansen S, Huumonen S, Gröndahl K, Gröndahl HG. Limited cone-beam CT and intraoral radiography for the diagnosis of periapical pathology. Oral Surg Oral Med Oral Pathol Oral Radiol Endod 2007;103:114–119.
72. Ahlowalia MS, Patel S, Anwar HMS, et al. Accuracy of CBCT for volumetric measurement of simulated periapical lesions. Int Endod J 2013;46:538–546.
73. Aminoshariae A, Kulild JC, Syed A. Cone-beam computed tomography compared with intraoral radiographic lesions in endodontic outcome studies: A systematic review. J Endod 2018;44:1626–1631.

74. Petersson A, Axelsson S, Davidson T, et al. Radiological diagnosis of periapical bone tissue lesions in endodontics: A systematic review. Int Endod J 2012;45:783–801.
75. Torabinejad M, Rice DD, Maktabi O, Udochukwu O, Abramovitch K. Prevalence and size of periapical radiolucencies using cone-beam computed tomography in teeth without apparent intraoral radiographic lesions: A new periapical index with a clinical recommendation. J Endod 2018;44:389–394.
76. Cotton TP, Geisler TM, Holden DT, Schwartz SA, Schindler WG. Endodontic applications of cone-beam volumetric tomography. J Endod 2007;33:1121–1132.
77. Goldman M, Perason AH, Darzenta N. Endodontic success—Who's reading the radiograph. Oral Surg Oral Med Oral Pathol Oral Radiol Endod 1972;33:432–437.
78. Mozzo P, Procacci C, Tacconi A, Martini PT, Andreis IA. A new volumetric CT machine for dental imaging based on the cone-beam technique: Preliminary results. Eur Radiol 1998;8:1558–1564.
79. Arai Y, Tammisalo E, Iwai K, Hashimoto K, Shinoda K. Development of a compact computed tomographic apparatus for dental use. Dentomaxillofac Radiol 1999;28:245–248.
80. Velvart P, Hecker H, Tillinger G. Detection of the apical lesion and the mandibular canal in conventional radiography and computed tomography. Oral Surg Oral Med Oral Pathol Oral Radiol Endod 2001;92:682–688.
81. Liang Y-H, Jiang L, Gao X-J, Shemesh H, Wesselink PR, Wu MK. Detection and measurement of artificial periapical lesions by cone-beam computed tomography. Int Endod J 2014;47:332–338.
82. Garcia de Paula-Silva FW, Wu MK, Leonardo MR, Bezerra da Silva LA, Wesselink PR. Accuracy of periapical radiography and cone-beam computed tomography scans in diagnosing apical periodontitis using histopathological findings as a gold standard. J Endod 2009;35:1009–1012.
83. Bender IB, Seltzer S. Roentgenographic and direct observation of experimental lesions in bone: II. 1961. J Endod 2003;29:707–712.

3

Management of Challenges and Mishaps Associated with the Treatment of Teeth with Necrotic Pulps, Open Apices, and Apical Periodontitis

JOSEPH A. PETRINO
MAHMOUD TORABINEJAD

Objectives

After reading this chapter, the reader should be able to:

1. Discuss the etiology of pulpal necrosis in teeth with open apices.
2. Elaborate treatment options for teeth with necrotic pulp and open apices.
3. State the type of tissues found in the root canals after regenerative endodontics.
4. Enumerate the challenges and mishaps during diagnosis and treatment planning.
5. Discuss the challenges and mishaps during regenerative endodontic procedures.
6. State the challenges after performing regenerative endodontic procedures.

Teeth with necrotic pulps, open apices, and apical periodontitis present a significant challenge to clinicians. At the present time, we have two treatment options: mineral trioxide aggregate (MTA) apexification and regenerative endodontic procedures. The purpose of this chapter is to discuss the challenges, pitfalls, and management of these teeth.

The primary objective of endodontic treatment has always been the preservation of the patient's natural dentition.[1] The endodontic literature reveals that endodontic treatment has a high success and survival rate.[1] However, the immature tooth with necrotic pulp and apical periodontitis is one of the most challenging situations to treat. The presence of the incompletely developed open apices makes it difficult to use the conventional and accepted protocols for adequate cleaning and shaping as well as obtaining a three-dimensional obturation. Furthermore, the use of intracanal medicaments and the thin root walls associated with these teeth can make these teeth susceptible to root fractures.[2-4] Cvek reported that immature teeth have a higher frequency of cervical root fracture compared to mature teeth.[5]

The Immature Tooth with Pulpal Necrosis and Apical Periodontitis

Etiology

Prior to discussing treatment options for teeth with necrotic pulps and open apices, it is important to describe some common etiologies for these teeth. It is well established that pulpal necrosis occurs because of bacterial infection from caries.[6] Traumatic luxation or avulsion injuries can result in severance of the blood supply and subsequent pulpal ischemia, which leads to pulpal necrosis and often a secondary infection with bacteria.[7] Unlike a fully mature tooth, the consequence of pulpal necrosis in teeth with open apices is the cessation of root development, thus making endodontic treatment with conventional techniques and materials difficult and sometimes impossible. Figure 3-1 represents a typical immature tooth with necrotic pulp and an open apex. Immature teeth have open and often divergent apices that are not suitable for complete cleaning and obturation with conventional materials and methods. In addition, because of their thin walls, these teeth are susceptible to fracture after treatment.[4] Furthermore, the use of medicaments in the treatment of these teeth can also increase the likelihood of root fracture.[2,3]

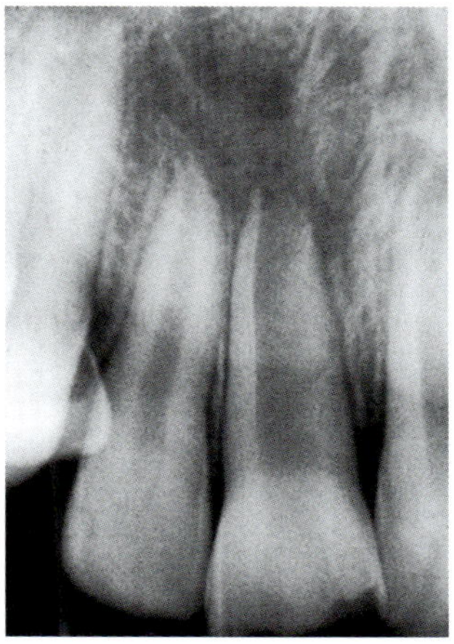

Fig 3-1 Typical presentation of an immature tooth with a necrotic pulp and apical periodontitis. Note the thin root walls and blunderbuss apex, which make disinfection and obturation via conventional means difficult.

Traumatic injuries

Traumatic injuries represent a common etiology for teeth with necrotic pulps, open apices, and apical periodontitis. The overall incidence of dental trauma in patients of all ages is 5%. That figure increases to 17% in patients ages 0 to 6 years.[8] The incidence of dental trauma is higher in boys than girls. Additionally, anterior maxillary teeth are most commonly affected,[9,10] whereas maxillary central incisors are more affected than lateral incisors (66% versus 17%, respectively). Traumatic injuries are more common in permanent teeth.[11,12] Uncomplicated crown fractures (without pulp exposure) are the most common traumatic injuries (41% to 68%).[13–15] The incidence of pulp necrosis after uncomplicated crown fractures is low (2% to 5%), but when there is a concomitant injury such as a luxation, the chance of necrosis increases, especially in teeth with closed apices (55% to 65%) as compared to those with open apices (3.5% to 11%). The traumatized dental pulps in teeth with open apices have greater chances to heal and survive compared to those with closed apices.[16–18] If an immature permanent tooth is avulsed and replanted, the risk of pulp necrosis is as high as 77%.[19]

Dental anomalies

Less frequent etiologic factors that can cause pulpal necrosis following trauma are dental anomalies such as dens evaginatus, dens invaginatus, or radicular lingual or palatogingival groove. In these conditions, bacteria have direct access to the pulp through the malformations. Dens evaginatus, which is an occlusal tubercle formed during development by folding of inner enamel epithelium into the stellate reticulum, is most commonly found in mandibular second premolars.[20] Dens evaginatus has been reported to be prevalent in 1% to 4% of Asian populations and in up to 15% of Alaskan Yupik and Iñupiat people and North American Indian populations.[20–22] Dens invaginatus, on the other hand, is formed from in-folding of the inner enamel epithelium and odontoblast layer into the pulp. Dens invaginatus has an overall prevalence of 1% to 10% and is observed most commonly in maxillary lateral incisors. If the pulp is exposed, as in the most severe cases of dens invaginatus, the communication passes directly to the apical papilla, communicating with the apical third of the canal and giving a direct entrance for bacterial penetration. The radicular lingual groove in dens invaginatus cases is mostly found in maxillary lateral incisors and is less common in central incisors.[23–25]

Treatment Options

MTA apical plug (MAP)

As stated earlier, teeth with necrotic pulps, open apices, and apical periodontitis present many challenges to the clinician. Historically, clinicians treated these teeth over several visits, often spanning several months, using calcium hydroxide ($Ca(OH)_2$) to induce a hard tissue barrier to prevent over extrusion of obturation materials.[26] While this treatment had a high success rate, the drawbacks included the long treatment time, lack of patient compliance, and potential weakening of the root due to long-term use of $Ca(OH)_2$ during treatment.[2,3] Fortunately, clinicians now can perform single visit apexification, known as MTA apexification or MTA apical plug (MAP), which is carried out by placement of an apical barrier. This significantly reduces the number of visits and time to complete treatment.[27–29]

The clinical protocol for one-step treatment varies from clinician to clinician. After obtaining profound local anesthesia, access is made, and root canal(s) are debrided with hand instrumentation. Disinfection is accomplished by passive irrigation of root canals with 1.5% to 5.25% NaOCl while performing the canal instrumentation. For patients who present with soft tissue swelling around the buccal gingiva or with draining sinus tract, intracanal medicament using $Ca(OH)_2$ is necessary with temporization with cotton pellet and temporary restoration. Subsequently, after confirming the resolution of the soft tissue lesions, placement of MTA into the root canal apex may proceed by drying the canals using extra-coarse paper points (Video). In certain cases, a collagen membrane (eg, CollaPlug or CollaTape, Zimmer Biomet) can be placed in contact with the periradicular tissues at the apex to serve as an internal matrix to prevent or minimize the extrusion of MTA into the periradicular tissues. Apical condensation of MTA using large pluggers, the back end of paper points, or gutta-percha points may be necessary to ensure the material adaptation to the most apical extent of the divergent root canal apices. Radiographs should be taken to confirm the adequate placement of the apical MTA plug and assess the density and thickness of the apical plug. After placing at least 5 mm of MAP and ensuring adequate apical seal, the coronal root canal space may be filled with either MTA or flowable gutta-percha, depending on the clinical needs and restorative plan for the tooth. Coronal restoration may be finalized using bonded composite material.

VIDEO

Radiographic follow-up examination should be scheduled to assess resolution of apical periodontitis and absence of complications after both 6 and 12 months postoperatively. Figure 3-2 represents a successful case completed with MAP. Most importantly, one-step apexification has been shown to have high rates of success compared to traditional $Ca(OH)_2$ apexification.[30] However, the main limitation of apexification, whether via $Ca(OH)_2$ or otherwise, is that these treatment modalities do not allow for further root development in most cases. Following treatment, the teeth still possess a large open apex and underdeveloped root structures with thin and short root canal walls. Not surprisingly, there is increased probability of root fracture in teeth treated by apexification. Figure 3-3 represents a cervical fracture following apexification treatment.

Regenerative endodontic procedures

There are many different regenerative endodontic procedure (REP) protocols that lead to successful treatment outcomes. Despite calling these procedures "regenerative," it is important to realize that these procedures do not predictably cause pulpal regeneration. Several terms have been proposed to describe these

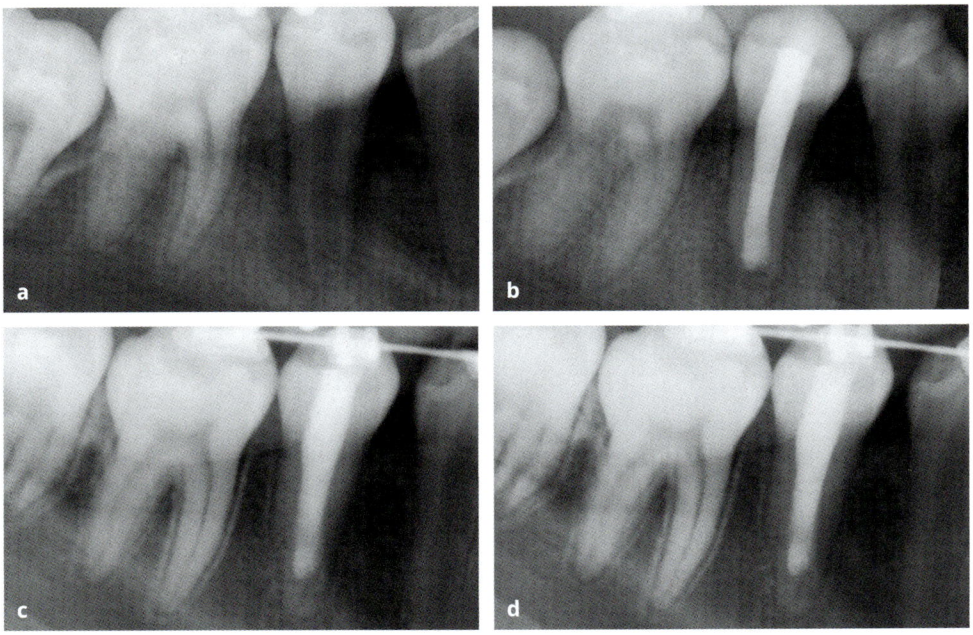

Fig 3-2 *(a)* Tooth no. 29 presented with immature apex, necrotic pulp, and apical periodontitis. *(b)* Completion of MTA apexification (MAP). *(c)* The 1-year recall showing healing of the apical periodontitis. *(d)* The 2-year recall displaying healing. Note that this tooth now displays further root development.

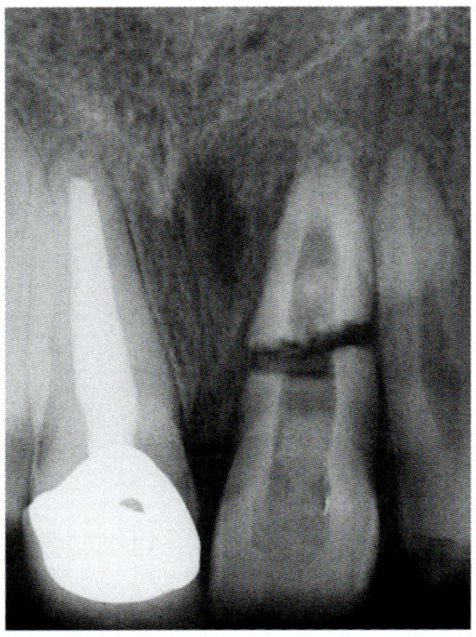

Fig 3-3 Cervical root fracture of tooth no. 9 following treatment by apexification. The thin dentin in immature teeth makes the cervical area prone to fracture.

types of procedures, including *revitalization*, *revascularization*, or *maturogenesis*. Like "regenerative," none of these terms is entirely correct. That being said, the term *regenerative endodontic procedures* (REPs) will be used to describe all the procedures intended to restore a functional pulp dentin complex. The American Association of Endodontists (AAE) has developed a resource, AAE Clinical Considerations for a Regenerative Procedure,[31] which outlines detailed protocols for REP. In addition, these treatment recommendations closely resemble those of the European Society of Endodontology (ESE).[32] In essence, the cases that would benefit from REP include those teeth with necrotic pulps and open apices that have adequate coronal tooth structure to be restored with direct restoration and without the need for a post. Debridement of the root canal space may proceed with minimal instrumentation and irrigation with low concentration of 1.5%

NaOCl, followed by placement of intracanal $Ca(OH)_2$ or triple antibiotic paste (TAP) dressing to disinfect the root canal system and resolve periradicular pathosis. These teeth are then temporarily restored until the second appointment.

After confirming the absence of severe periradicular inflammation, such as soft tissue swelling or draining sinus tract, the tooth is ready for the second phase of REP. The patient is anesthetized again with a local anesthetic without vasoconstrictor (eg, 3% mepivacaine), and the tooth is isolated with rubber dam. After intracanal irrigation with 17% ethylenediaminetetraacetic acid (EDTA) and visual confirmation of the absence of draining exudate or necrotic debris, bleeding is induced into the root canal space by agitation of periapical tissues beyond the root apex using a small file to allow the blood clot formation to the level of the cementoenamel junction (CEJ). Collagen matrix (eg, CollaPlug or CollaTape) may be placed over the blood clot to provide a barrier onto which MTA or other tricalcium silicate cements can be placed as coronal capping material.

For the final visit, the patient should be recalled for a 1-week postoperative check to confirm the absence of periradicular infection and the resolution of their symptoms. The tooth can then be restored with direct restoration (eg, composite resin over MTA or other tricalcium silicate cements). The patient should have an initial 6-month check, followed by yearly recall visits.

Clinicians must familiarize themselves with this new treatment alternative and realize that the radiographic presentation of teeth treated with this treatment modality will appear as if endodontic “filling” or obturation is missing. Therefore, adequate treatment history and current vitality testing must be performed when history of this kind of treatment is suspected to prevent unnecessary retreatment and the violation of a newly formed reparative vital tissue.

The success rate of REPs rivals the success rates of one-step apexification and traditional apexification, when success is defined as resolution of symptoms and apical periodontitis.[33–35] Thus, it is important to point out that the success of REP in resolving apical periodontitis does not seem to depend on the variations of treatment protocols but is determined largely by successful disinfection of the root canal space,[36] recruitment of mesenchymal stem cells (MSCs), sealing ability, and biocompatibility of the coronal restoration.

As stated earlier, both MAP and REPs have shown highly successful outcomes (94.6% and 91.3% for the MAP and REP groups, respectively).[37] However, the criteria for success in the REP group can be stricter by also including root development as a criterion.[38] Root development is seen as a major advantage of REP over apexification.[39] There are three potential advantages associated with this procedure: increases in root length, root thickness, and apical closure, with apical closure being the most common finding.[40] The pooled rate for root development in randomized clinical trials was 79%. The rate of root development varied from 21%[41] to 100%[42,43] in analytic studies. This wide range shows the unpredictability of root development after REP. Figures 3-4 and 3-5 show the successful treatment

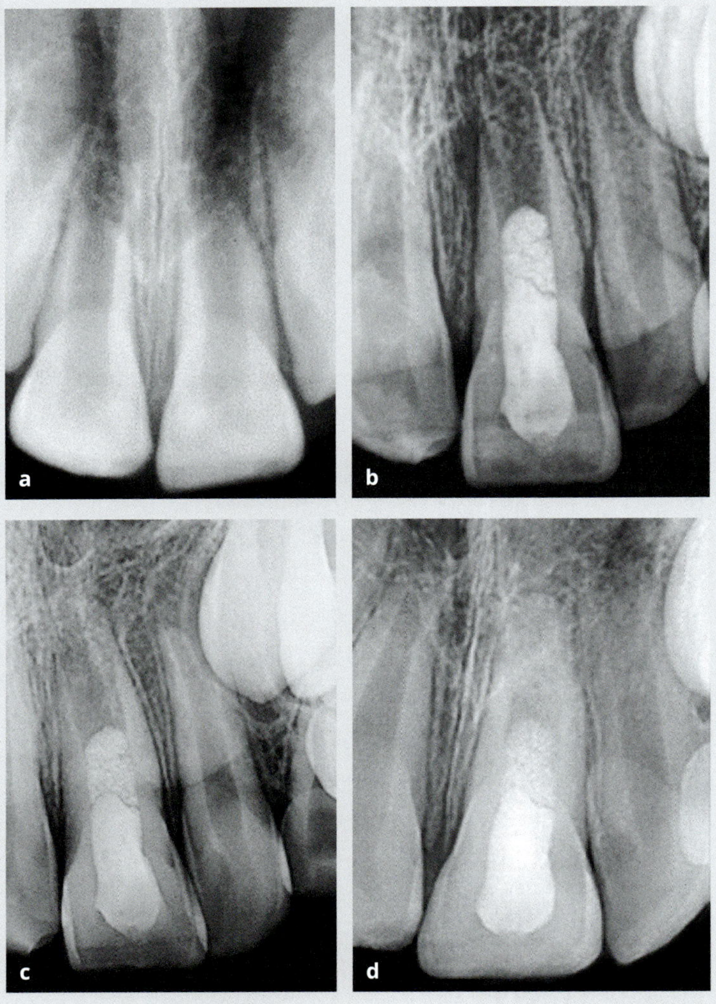

Fig 3-4 *(a)* Preoperative image showing lesion on the mesial aspect of tooth no. 9. *(b)* Regenerative treatment completed. *(c)* The 9-month recall showing increase in root development and root length. *(d)* The 2-year recall showing resolution of the lesion and apical closure.

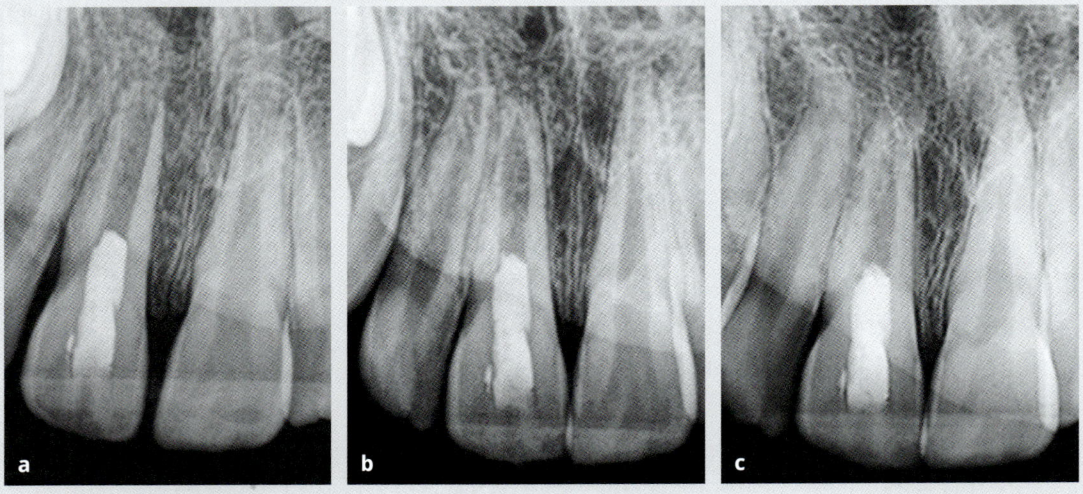

Fig 3-5 *(a)* Postoperative image of regenerative endodontic treatment. *(b)* The 2-year recall displaying changes in root length, width, and apical closure. *(c)* The 5-year recall after regenerative treatment.

of an immature tooth with a necrotic pulp and apical periodontitis, both showing radiographic evidence of root development.

A recent study has revealed that performing regenerative endodontic procedures in a single visit yielded similar clinical and radiographic outcomes compared to completing these regenerative endodontic procedures in two visits with an interappointment dressing with $Ca(OH)_2$.[44] This represents an exciting development if more studies can confirm similar success of one-visit regenerative endodontic procedures.

What is in the canal after an REP?

Once the regenerative endodontic procedure has been completed and evidence of root development has been seen via imaging, the question is raised as to the composition of the tissue(s) in the root. Both animal and human studies have found that the tissue present in the root canals of teeth treated via REPs can be cementum, connective tissue, and bone (Fig 3-6) versus pulpal tissue.[45,46] Shimizu et al and Torabinejad and Faras both published case reports showing that the tissue following regenerative procedures is pulplike.[47–49] A recent study by Torabinejad et al found that true pulpal regeneration is possible if 1 to 4 mm of pulp is present in the apical portion of the tooth.[50] Figure 3-7 shows the ingrowth of pulpal tissue in a ferret cuspid when 1 to 2 mm of pulp is left in the apex.

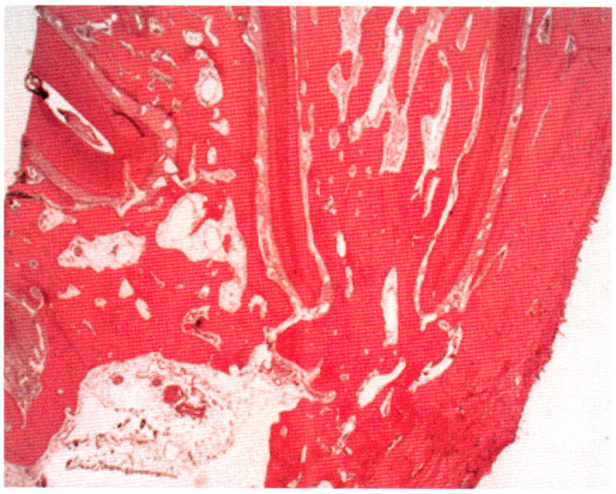

Fig 3-6 Photomicrograph of a ferret root end displaying ingrowth of bone into the canal following regenerative endodontic procedure.

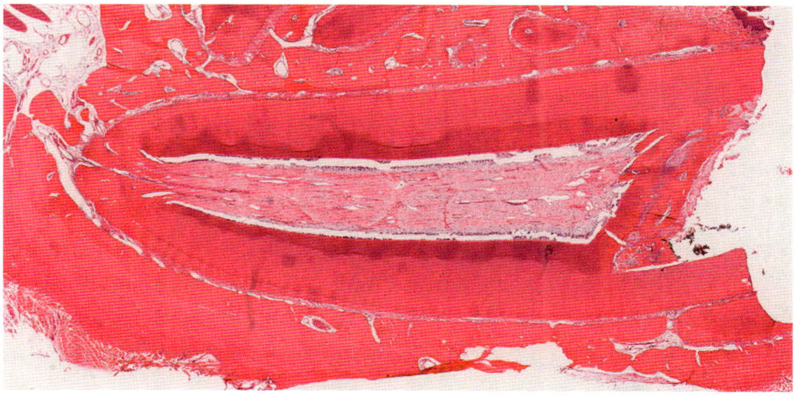

Fig 3-7 Pulp-dentin regeneration in ferret cuspid after leaving 1 to 2 mm of apical pulp and performing REPs using blood clot.

Challenges and Mishaps

Now that we have briefly touched on the management of teeth with necrotic pulps and open apices as well as possible outcomes, it is important to discuss the difficulties associated with the management of these teeth. There are challenges, mistakes, and mishaps that can be classified as occurring during pretreatment, midtreatment, or posttreatment.

Pretreatment

Diagnosis

The defining feature of a regenerative endodontic procedure is that it is performed on a tooth with a necrotic pulp. Any procedure performed in an immature tooth where the pulp has vitality should be considered apexogenesis. Furthermore, if vitality is confirmed when treating a tooth, all efforts should be made to preserve vitality in hopes that the pulp tissue will continue with its development. Obtaining an accurate diagnosis can be difficult with pediatric patients, as the clinician is interpreting cold testing results from a child who may exhibit varying levels of anxiety or may not understand the tests. In these cases, the use of the electronic pulp test (EPT) may help remove any confusion regarding response to testing.

Patient selection

It is important to remember that a vast majority of regenerative endodontic procedures are performed on children, often times children who have sustained trauma to the face and teeth. There are many challenges with treating children, and it is imperative that the clinician identify children who have the temperament for dental treatment. Additionally, it is crucial that the clinician assess parental compliance, as these cases usually take at least two treatment visits and require rigorous follow-up. If the patient is noncompliant in the chair, has difficulty getting to the office, or requires help with varying levels of sedation, it would probably be best to perform MTA apexification rather than regenerative treatment, as the former can be completed in a single visit.

Tooth selection

Next on the list of potential mishaps that can occur prior to treatment is the selection of the tooth. Our best available evidence suggests that regenerative procedures work best when the apical opening is greater than 1 mm, the root itself is short, and there is no need for a post to be included in the restoration.[30] Baseline root development might be a decision-making factor in the treatment of extremely immature teeth with a very short root and very thin root canal walls. MAP is often not viable in these cases, so REP would be the preferred treatment option.

If a clinician attempts a regenerative endodontic procedure on a tooth that has an apex less than 1 mm, they run the risk of not getting sufficient irrigation or delivery of medicaments to the apex. Furthermore, if the apex is less than 1 mm, it is likely that fewer apical stem cells are present, which reduces the regenerative potential. Additionally, if the apex is too constricted, obtaining sufficient bleeding back into the canal space can be difficult if not impossible. Lastly, if a post is needed in a tooth, this requires that the MTA barrier be placed in a more apical position, which would indicate MAP versus REP. As stated earlier, the benefit of REPs is the potential for further development of the root. If the MTA barrier has to be placed more apically, there is minimal if any chance for further root development. A study by Bose et al revealed no changes in root development in MTA apexification and nonsurgical root canal therapy (NSRCT) groups.[51]

Midtreatment

Once the appropriate patient, tooth, and diagnosis have been confirmed, the challenges associated with these procedures do not end. During treatment, there are several pitfalls the clinician can fall into, the first being the selection of an antibiotic paste to help promote disinfection of the canal or to use $Ca(OH)_2$.

$Ca(OH)_2$ vs triple antibiotic paste vs double antibiotic paste

A triple antibiotic paste comprised of minocycline, ciprofloxacin, and metronidazole was introduced by Hoshino et al.[52] Iwaya et al and Banchs and Trope both had case reports that first utilized this triple antibiotic paste in the treatment of immature teeth with necrotic pulps and open apices.[53,54] Since the publication of those papers, several different antibiotics and combinations have been proposed. The challenge is selecting the right antibiotics. The clinician needs to make sure the patient has no allergies to any potential antibiotics. Furthermore, the clinician may have to find a compounding pharmacy to ensure the precise concentrations of antibiotics are present. This makes it difficult to perform these procedures on an emergent basis, as there needs to be time for compounding the antibiotic paste. It is also important to remember that the addition of minocycline to the antibiotic paste carries an increased risk of staining the crown.[55] Omission of minocycline removes this risk. Figure 3-8 represents staining of a tooth following REP due to the use of minocycline in the triple antibiotic paste.

Fig 3-8 Staining of the crown of the right incisor due to the use of minocycline in triple antibiotic paste. (Courtesy of Dr A. Nosrat.)

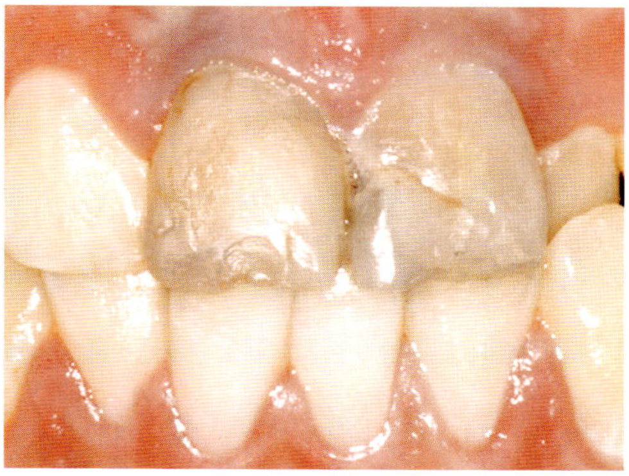

To offset the risks of staining and the time required to compound the antibiotic medicament, $Ca(OH)_2$ can be used. It has been shown that $Ca(OH)_2$ can be removed from the canals more easily than an antibiotic paste.[56] The benefits of $Ca(OH)_2$ are that it is available to every clinician, can be applied easily, and carries no risk associated with staining. However, long-term use (which is rare in regenerative cases), could be associated with an increased risk of root fracture.[2,3] This is critical to remember, as the teeth that are candidates for regenerative endodontic procedures may have an increased susceptibility to fracture due to their thin and weak dentinal walls.[2]

Induction of bleeding

After irrigation and placement of the medicament, the next part of the regenerative procedure is induction of bleeding. The elements present in the blood and blood clot help promote an environment for the further development of the root. Traditionally, this has been performed by over-instrumenting the canal with large files. While it seems like obtaining bleeding would be easy, often it can be difficult. Empirically, bleeding seems to always be easier and more prevalent during the first visit. Bleeding is also easier to obtain when the apex has a larger diameter or when the roots are shorter. To help ensure a favorable environment for bleeding, consider using an anesthetic without epinephrine, as research shows that use of epinephrine results in decreased pulpal blood flow.[57]

If bleeding cannot be successfully induced, the clinician may consider obtaining circulating blood from the patient and placing it into the canal as a scaffold. A study by Alghofaily et al demonstrated that there was no significant radiographic difference in REPs performed with a blood clot or with circulating blood in mandibular sheep incisors.[58] It is possible that bony healing and resolution of symptoms can occur if bleeding is not induced, but it is highly unlikely that further development would occur, as the factors in the blood clot would be absent from the canal. Additionally, without the formation of the blood clot in the canal, placement of the MTA barrier is challenging. Another challenge present at this phase is that the use of mepivacaine may not provide profound anesthesia, which means that the patient could feel pain during instrumentation to induce bleeding.

MTA barrier placement

The placement of the MTA barrier is the most technique-sensitive portion of the regenerative procedure. If the pressure applied to the blood clot is too heavy, the MTA can be forced apically, which gives the appearance of an apical barrier (Fig 3-9). Furthermore, heavy forces could cause disruption of the clot and cause bleeding to start again. If bleeding starts, it may cause a disruption in the setting of the MTA, resulting in an incomplete barrier. To help prevent this, clinicians have advocated for placing a restorable collagen plug over the blood clot to compact the MTA.

To best ensure success, the placement of the barrier should be as coronal as possible. This gives more room for the root to continue to develop. It would seem easier to place the MTA barrier more coronally in a long root; however, induction of bleeding to the coronal third of a long root presents its own challenges.

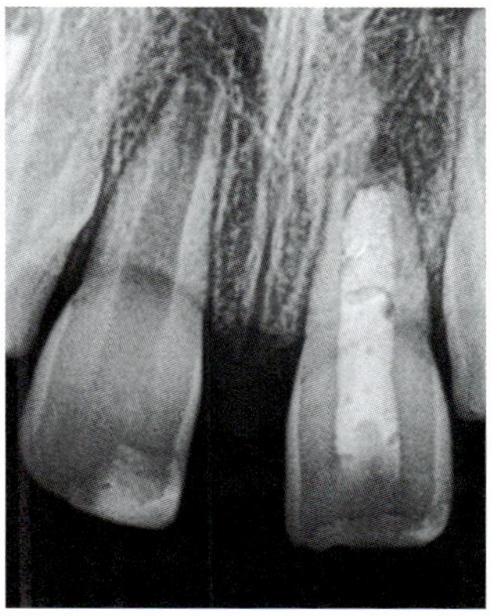

Fig 3-9 Tooth no. 9 was treated with REP. Bleeding was difficult to induce, and the MTA barrier was placed too far apically, giving the appearance of an MAP versus an REP.

Restoration

After the MTA barrier is placed, the next part is the restoration of the tooth. The potential mishaps in this stage include not placing the restoration to the MTA as well as potential washout of the MTA when placing a composite restoration. In general, for most teeth receiving REPs, esthetics becomes a concern, and incorrect color could result in unsatisfied patients or parents. Furthermore, if there is a need to replace the incised edge, the clinician may refer the case back to the restorative dentist, in which case there is a need to at least cover the MTA with an orifice barrier to ensure the MTA sets and has another layer of sealing.

Posttreatment

Once an REP is completed, it is crucial that the patient has regular recall appointments. The clinician is wise to inform all patients and their parents that the prognosis for these teeth is guarded. The biggest mishap at this stage is not informing patients and parents that eventual loss of these teeth or the need for additional treatment may occur. It should be stressed prior to the initiation of treatment that at present REPs do not have a 100% chance of success, so all treatment options and complications should be discussed with patients and/or parents.

Staining

The use of MTA as a barrier against the blood clot has a risk of staining the crown. The main causes of discoloration with MTA are the following: *(1)* the presence of bismuth oxide and its disintegration into oxygen and bismuth, which causes significant color changes once exposed to light in the absence of oxygen[59]; and *(2)* the disintegration of the powder and subsequent release of discoloring molecules such as ferrous oxide.[60] Often this staining causes a grayish discoloration of the crown. This staining can be remedied by internal bleaching (Fig 3-10); however, the staining can recur. To prevent this, the clinician can place a dentin bonding agent prior to placing MTA[60] or use different materials. New materials such as NeoMTA or biodentine can be used, which reduce the risk (if not remove it entirely) of staining the crown.[61,62] However, patients and especially parents should still be informed of the risks of staining when performing these procedures on teeth in the esthetic zone.

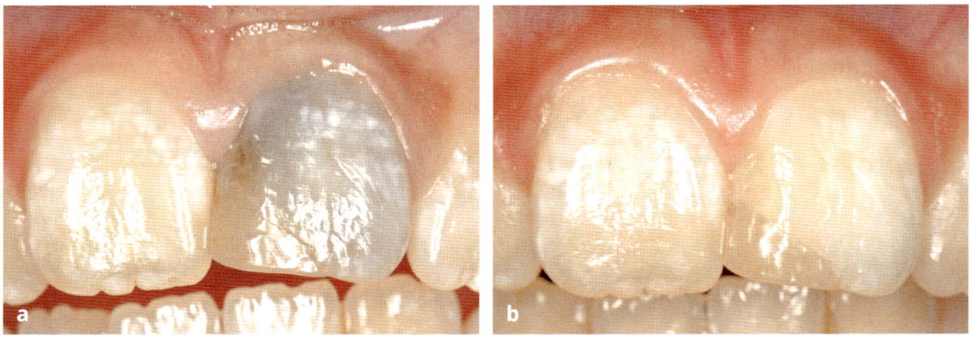

Fig 3-10 *(a)* Clinical view of tooth no. 9 at initial visit after a pulp regeneration procedure showing discoloration. *(b)* Clinical view of this region after bleaching. (Courtesy of Dr Aki Osada.)

Success or failure

The AAE guidelines for regenerative endodontic procedures list three tiers of outcomes. Primary outcomes include resolution of symptoms and sinus tracts (if present) and evidence of bony healing. Secondary outcomes include further development of the root. Tertiary outcomes include a positive response to vitality testing.

One mishap at this stage could be considering the case a failure if it did not meet the secondary or tertiary goals, even if it was successful on the primary goals. It is important to know that not all cases will show increased development of the root. Figure 3-11 shows teeth nos. 8 and 9 with necrotic pulps, immature apices, and apical periodontitis being treated via REPs. The radiographs of these teeth reveal success in the primary outcome of resolution of symptoms and healing but did not show any success in secondary outcomes. It is also crucial to remember that not all cases will show increased root development nor a response to vitality testing; thus, a lack of further root development or of response to cold or EPT should not be viewed as a failure of treatment.

As stated earlier, not all cases will show further root development. It is important at this stage to inform the patient and/or parent that rigorous follow-up is needed to continue to evaluate success or failure. A study by Almutairi et al,[36] which evaluated failure of REPs, found that 63% of cases were deemed a failure after 1 year, and 39% of cases were deemed failures after 2 years. Thus, it seems prudent to inform patients and/or parents that at least 2 years of follow-up will be necessary on teeth treated with REPs.

If a case is deemed a failure, the clinician needs to assess if the tooth has sustained a vertical root fracture or if there was a failure of disinfection or sealing of the canals. The benefit of regenerative treatment is that, should the REP be deemed non-successful, the tooth may still be a candidate for conventional $Ca(OH)_2$ apexification or MTA apical barrier. The reverse, regrettably, is not true. Figure 3-12 represents a case where regenerative endodontics was performed,

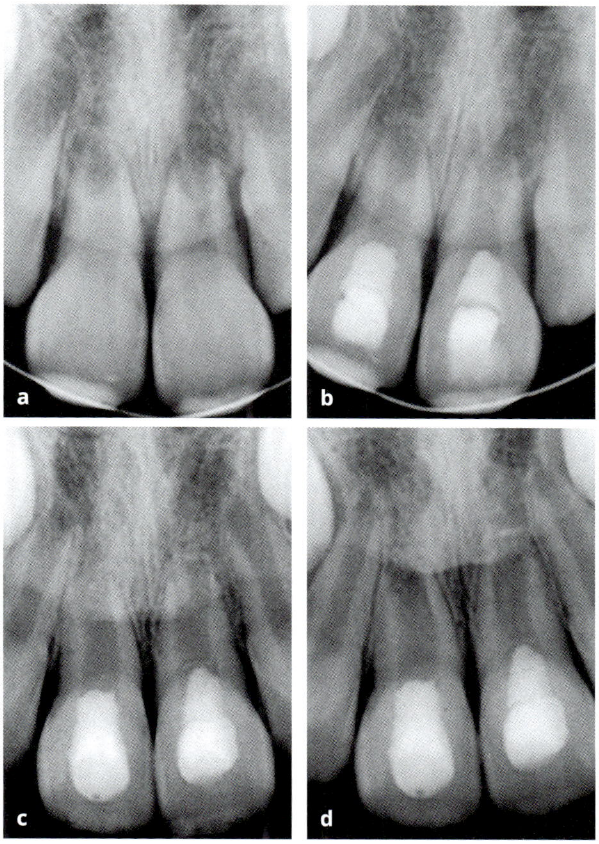

Fig 3-11 *(a)* Preoperative radiograph displaying apical periodontitis and immature apices of teeth nos. 8 and 9. *(b)* Postoperative radiograph following REPs performed on both teeth. *(c)* The 6-month recall displaying resolution of the apical periodontitis on both teeth but no further root development. *(d)* The 1-year recall displaying resolution of lesions but no root development. It is important at this stage to educate patients, parents, and dentists that the treatment is complete despite not having root filings to the apices.

then deemed non-successful because the lesion increased in size. After follow-up examination, the tooth was not deemed to have sustained a fracture, and MTA apexifcation was performed with the use of $Ca(OH)_2$ as an intracanal dressing. As stated earlier, it is important to remember that these cases require strident follow-up, and other teeth may require treatment due to the history of trauma. In Fig 3-12, the recall images show that tooth no. 9 required treatment, and the most recent recall shows tooth no. 10 requires treatment.

However, if there is no option for treatment and the REP has been deemed a failure, the clinician needs to be able to inform the patient and parent of alternative treatments. If the tooth is in the anterior esthetic zone and the patient is closer to completion of growth and development, socket preservation could be performed so a future implant could be placed. If development is far from completion, the clinician could consider replacement via orthodontics if crowding is present or socket preservation in hopes that an implant can later be placed. If the tooth is not in the esthetic zone, other treatments including orthodontics could be considered.

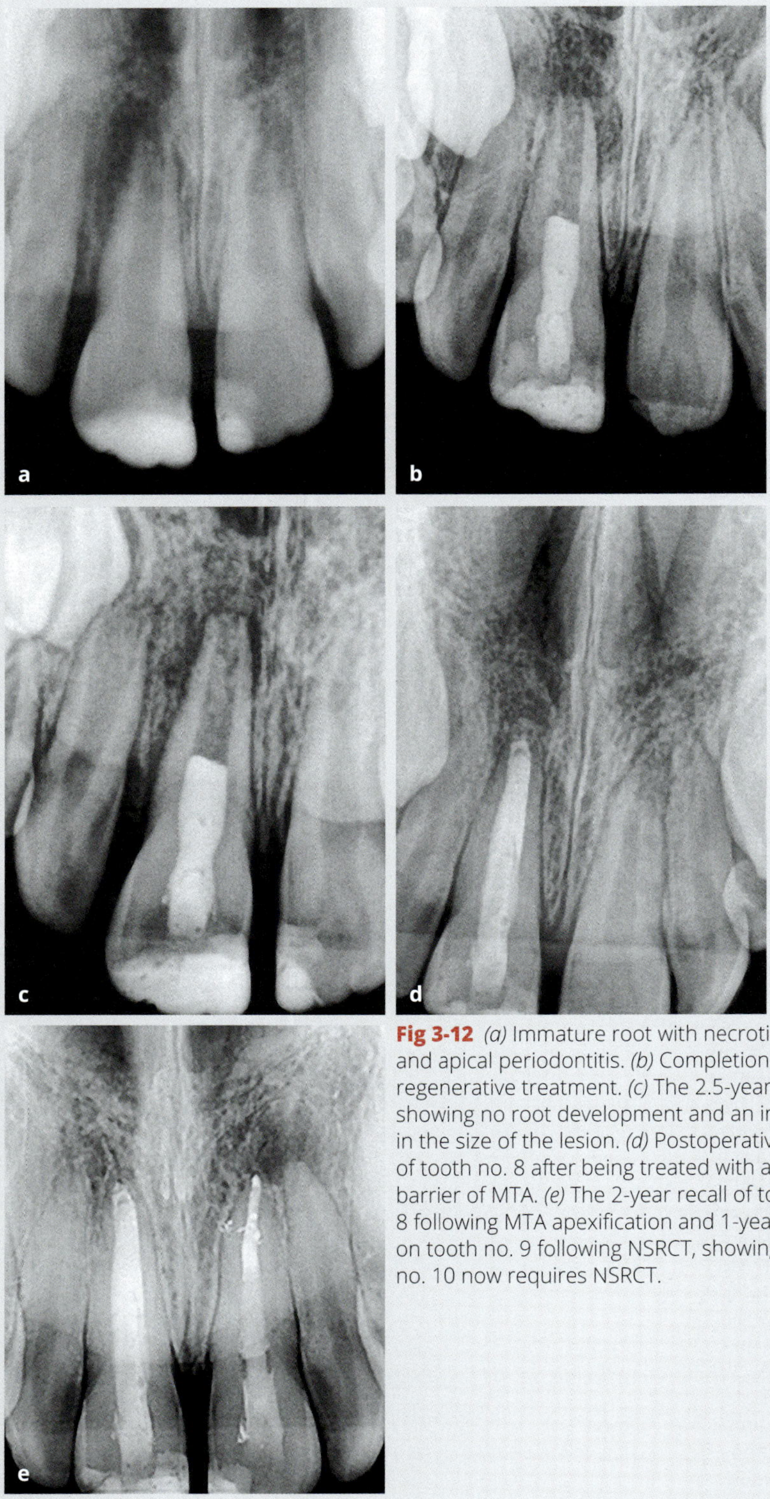

Fig 3-12 *(a)* Immature root with necrotic pulp and apical periodontitis. *(b)* Completion of regenerative treatment. *(c)* The 2.5-year recall showing no root development and an increase in the size of the lesion. *(d)* Postoperative view of tooth no. 8 after being treated with an apical barrier of MTA. *(e)* The 2-year recall of tooth no. 8 following MTA apexification and 1-year recall on tooth no. 9 following NSRCT, showing tooth no. 10 now requires NSRCT.

References

1. Torabinejad M, Anderson P, Bader J, et al. Outcomes of root canal treatment and restoration, implant-supported single crowns, fixed partial dentures, and extraction without replacement: A systematic review. J Prosthet Dent 2007;98:285–311.
2. Andreasen JO, Faric B, Munksgaard EC. Long-term calcium hydroxide as a root canal dressing may increase risk of root fracture. Dent Traumatol 2002;18:134–137.
3. Rosenberg B, Murray PE, Namerow K. The effect of calcium hydroxide root filling on dentin fracture strength. Dent Traumatol 2007;23:26–29.
4. Kerekes K, Heide S, Jacobsen I. Follow-up examination of endodontic treatment in traumatized juvenile incisors. J Endod 1980;6:744–748.
5. Cvek M. Prognosis of luxated non-vital maxillary incisors treated with calcium hydroxide and filled with gutta-percha. A retrospective clinical study. Endod Dent Traumatol 1992;8:45–55.
6. Kakehashi S, Stanley HR, Fitzgerald RJ. The effects of surgical exposures of dental pulps in germ-free and conventional laboratory rats. Oral Surg Oral Med Oral Pathol 1965;20:340–349.
7. Tsukamoto-Tanaka H, Ikegame M, Takagi R, Harada H, Ohshima H. Histochemical and immunocytochemical study of hard tissue formation in dental pulp during the healing process in rat molars after tooth replantation. Cell Tissue Res 2006;325:219–229.
8. Petersson EE, Andersson L, Sörenson S. Traumatic oral vs non-oral injuries. Swed Dent J 1997;21:55–68.
9. Altun C, Ozen B, Esenlik E, et al. Traumatic Injuries to permanent teeth in Turkish children, Ankara. Dent Traumatol 2009;25:309–313.
10. Navabazam A, Farahani SS. Prevalence of traumatic injuries to maxillary permanent teeth in 9- to-14-year-old Ontario schoolchildren. Dent Traumatol 2010;26:154–157.
11. Granville-Garcia AF, de Menezes VA, de Lira PIC. Dental Trauma and associated factors in Brazilian preschoolers. Dent Traumatol 2006;22:318–322.
12. Marcenes W, al Beiruti N, Tayfour D, Issa S. Epidemiology of traumatic injuries to the permanent incisors of 9-12-year-old schoolchildren in Damascus, Syria. Endod Dent Traumatol 1999;15:117–123.
13. Fakhruddin KS, Lawrence HP, Kenny DJ, Locker D. Etiology and environment of dental injuries in 12-to-14-year old Ontario schoolchildren. Dent Traumatol 2008;24:305–308.
14. Kumar A, Bansal V, Veeresha KL, Sogi GM. Pervalanece of traumatic dental injuries among 12- to-15-year-old schoolchildren in Ambala district, Haryana, India. Oral Health Prev Dent 2011;9:301–305.
15. Soriano EP, de França Caldas A Jr, Diniz De Carvalho MV, Amorim Filho HDA. Prevelance and factors related to traumatic dental injuries in Brazilian schoolchildren. Dent Traumatol 2007;23:232–240.
16. Lauridsen E, Hermann NV, Gerds TA, Ahrensburg SS, Kreiborg S, Andreasen JO. Combination injuries 3. The risk of pulp necrosis in permanent teeth with extrusion or lateral luxation and concomitant crown fractures without pulp exposure. Dent Traumatol 2012;28:379–385.
17. Lauridsen E, Hermann NV, Gerds TA, Ahrensburg SS, Kreiborg S, Andreasen JO. Combination injuries 1. The risk of pulp necrosis in permanent teeth with concussion injuries and concomitant crown fractures. Dent Traumatol 2012;28:364–370.
18. Lauridsen E, Hermann NV, Gerds TA, Ahrensburg SS, Kreiborg S, Andreasen JO. Combination injuries 2. The risk of pulp necrosis in permanent teeth with subluxation injuries and concomitant crown fractures. Dent Traumatol 2012;28:371–378.
19. Hecova H, Tzigkounakis V, Merglova V, Netolicky J. A retrospective study of 889 injured permanent teeth. Dent Traumatol 2010;26:466–475.
20. Merrill RG. Occlusal anomalous tubercles on premolars of Alaskan Eskimos and Indians. Oral Surg Oral Med Oral Pathol 1964;17:484–496.
21. Levitan ME, Himel VT. Dens evaginatus: Literature review, pathophysiology, and comprehensive treatment regimen. J Endod 2006;32:1–9.
22. Rao YG, Guo LY, Tao HT. Multiple dens evaginatus of premolars and molars in Chinese dentitition: A case report and literature review. Int J Oral Sci 2010;2:177–180.
23. Alani A, Bishop K. Dens invaginatus. Part 1: Classification, prevalence and aetiology. Int Endod J 2008;41;1123–1136.
24. Hülsman M. Dens invaginatus: Aetiology, classification, prevalence, diagnosis, and treatment considerations. Int Endod J 1997;30:79–90.
25. Oehlers FA. Dens invaginatus (dilated composite odontome). I. Variations of the invagination process and associated crown forms. Oral Surg Oral Med Oral Pathol 1957;10:1204–1218.
26. Frank AL. Therapy for the divergent pulpless tooth by continued apical formation. J Am Dent Assoc 1966;72:87–93.
27. Mente J, Hage N, Pfefferle T, et al. Mineral trioxide aggregate apical plugs in teeth with open apical foramina: A retrospective analysis of treatment outcomes. J Endod 2009;35:1354–1358.
28. Parirokh M, Torabinejad M. Mineral trioxide aggregate: A comprehensive literature review—Part III: Clinical applications, drawbacks, and mechanism of action. J Endod 2010;36:400–413.

29. Torabinejad M, Chivian N. Clinical applications of mineral trioxide aggregate. J Endod 1999;25:197–205.
30. Witherspoon DE, Small JC, Regan JD, Nunn M. Retrospective analysis of open apex teeth obturated with mineral trioxide aggregate. J Endod 2008;34:1171–1176.
31. AAE Clinical Considerations for a Regenerative Procedure. https://f3f142zs0k2w1kg84k5p9i1o-wpengine.netdna-ssl.com/specialty/wpcontent/uploads/sites/2/2021/08/ClinicalConsiderations ApprovedByREC062921.pdf. Accessed 15 December 2022.
32. Galler KM, Krastl G, Simon S, et al. European Society of Endodontology position statement: Revitalization procedures. Int Endod J 2016;49:717–723.
33. Bücher K, Meier F, Diegritz, Kaaden C, Hickel R, Kuhnish J. Long term outcome of MTA apexification in teeth with open apices. Quintessence Int 2016;47:473–482.
34. Chen MYH, Chen KL, Chen CA, Tayebaty F, Rosenberg PA, Lin LM. Responses of immature permanent teeth with infected necrotic pulp tissue and apical periodontitis/abscess to revascularization procedures. Int Endod J 2012;45:294–305.
35. Shah N, Logani A, Bhaskar U, Aggarwal V. Efficacy of revascularization to induce apexification/apexogenesis in infected, nonvital, immature teeth: A pilot clinical study. J Endod 2008:34:919–925.
36. Almutairi W, Yassen GH, Aminoshariae A, Williams KA, Mickel A. Regenerative endodontics: A systematic analysis of the failed cases. J Endod 2019;43:567–577.
37. Torabinejad M, Nosrat A, Verma P, Oyoyo U. Regenerative endodontic treatment or MTA apical plug in teeth with necrotic pulps and open apices: A systematic review and meta-analysis. J Endod 2017;43:1806–1820.
38. Bukhari S, Kohli MR, Setzer F, Karabucak B. Outcome of revascularization procedure: A retrospective case series. J Endod 2016;42:1752–1759.
39. Hargreaves KM, Diogenes A, Teixeira FB. Treatment options: Biological basis of regenerative endodontic procedures. J Endod 2013;39(3 suppl):S30–S43.
40. Saoud TMA, Zaazou A, Nabil A, Moussa S, Lin LM, Gibbs JL. Clinical and radiographic outcomes of traumatized immature permanent necrotic teeth after revascularization/revitalization therapy. J Endod 2014;40:1946–1952.
41. Alobaid AS, Cortes LM, Lo J, et al. Radiographic and clinical outcomes of treatment of immature permanent teeth by revascularization or apexification: A pilot retrospective cohort study. J Endod 2014;40:1063–1070.
42. Jeeruphan T, Jantarat J, Yanpiset K, Suwannapan L, Khewsawai P, Hargreaves KM. Mahidol study 1: Comparison of radiographic and survival outcomes of immature teeth treated with either regenerative endodontic or apexification methods: A retrospective study. J Endod 2012;38:1330–1336.
43. EzEldeen M, Van Gorp G, Van Dessel J, Vandermeulen D, Jacobs R. 3-dimensional analysis of regenerative endodontic treatment outcome. J Endod 2015;41:317–324.
44. Cerqueira-Neto ACCL, Prado MC, Pereira AC, et al. Clinical and radiographic outcomes of regenerative endodontic procedures in traumatized immature permanent teeth: Interappointment dressing or single-visit? J Endod 2021;47:1598–1608.
45. Torabinejad M, Milan M, Shabahang S, Wright KR, Faras H. Histologic examination of teeth with necrotic pulps and periapical lesions treated with 2 scaffolds: An animal investigation. J Endod 2015;41:846–852.
46. Scarparo RK, Dondoni L, Böttcher DE, Grecca FS, Rockenbach MIB, Batista EL Jr. Response to intracanal medication in immature teeth with pulp necrosis: An experimental model in rat molars. J Endod 2011;37:1069–1073.
47. Wang X, Thibodeau B, Trope M, Lin LM, Huang GTJ. Histologic characterization of regenerated tissues in canal space after the revitalization/revascularization procedure of immature dog teeth with apical periodontitis. J Endod 2010;36:56–63.
48. Shimizu E, Jong G, Partridge N, Rosenberg PA, Lin LM. Histologic observation of a human immature permanent tooth with irreversible pulpitis after revascularization/regeneration procedure. J Endod 2012;38:1293–1297.
49. Torabinejad M, Faras H. A clinical and histological report of a tooth with an open apex treated with regenerative endodontics using platelet-rich plasma. J Endod 2012;38:864–868.
50. Torabinejad M, Alexander A, Aliakbar Vahdati S, Grandhi A, Baylink D, Shabahang S. Effect of residual dental pulp tissue on regeneration of dentin-pulp complex: An in vivo investigation. J Endod 2018; 44:1796–1801.
51. Bose R, Nummikoski P, Hargreaves K. A retrospective evaluation of radiographic outcomes in immature teeth with necrotic root canal systems treated with regenerative endodontic procedures. J Endod 2009;35:1343–1349.
52. Hoshino E, Kurihara-Aando N, Sato I, et al. In vitro antibacterial susceptibility of bacteria taken from infected root dentine to a mixture of ciprofloxacin, metronidazole and minocycline. Int Endod J 1996;29:125–130.
53. Iwaya SI, Ikawa M, Kubota M. Revascularization of an immature permanent tooth with apical periodontitis and sinus tract. Dent Traumatol 2001;17:185–187.

54. Banchs F, Trope M. Revascularization of immature permanent teeth with apical periodontitis: New treatment protocol? J Endod 2004;30:196–200.
55. Kim JH, Kim Y, Shin SJ, Park JW, Jung IY. Tooth discoloration of immature permanent incisor associated with triple antibiotic therapy: A case report. J Endod 2010;36:1086–1091.
56. Berkhoff JA, Chen PB, Teixeira FB, Diogenes A. Evalution of triple antibiotic paste removal by different irrigation procedures. J Endod 2014;40:1172–1177.
57. Kim S, Edwall L, Trowbridge H, Chien S. Effects of local anesthetic on pulpal blood flow in dogs. J Dent Res 1984;63:650–652.
58. Alghofaily MM, Torabinejad M, Nosrat A. Regenerative endodontic treatment using periapical blood or circulating blood as scaffold: A volumetric analysis. J Endod 2022;48:625–631.
59. Vallés M, Mercadé M, Duran-Sindreu F, Bourdelande JL, Roig M. Influence of light and oxygen on the color stability of five calcium silicate-based materials. J Endod 2013;39:525–528.
60. Akbari M, Rouhani A, Samiee S, Jafarzadeh H. Effect of dentin bonding agent on the prevention of tooth discoloration produced by mineral trioxide aggregate. Int J Dent 2012;2012:563203.
61. Camilleri J. Staining potential of Neo MTA Plus, MTA Plus, and biodentine used for pulpotomy procedures. J Endod 2015;41:1139–1145.
62. Felman D, Parashos P. Coronal tooth discoloration and white mineral trioxide aggregate. J Endod 2013;39;484–487.

4

Errors During Access Preparation

MOHAMMAD SABETI
MOHSEN RAMAZANI
KIUMARS NAZARI MOGHADAM

Objectives

After reading this chapter, the reader should be able to:

1. Describe the access cavity and the principles of its preparation.
2. Know the importance of access cavity preparation for success of root canal treatment.
3. Anticipate the mishaps encountered in the access cavity preparation.
4. Understand the negative consequences of mishaps of access cavity preparation.
5. Learn how to manage the mishaps of access cavity preparation.
6. Enumerate the techniques and instruments available for prevention or management of mishaps of access cavity preparation in detail.
7. Describe the new approaches to access cavity preparation and their benefits.

The main goal of nonsurgical root canal treatment (NSRCT) is to completely disinfect the root canal system, eliminate microorganisms, and adequately shape the root canals for obturation that allows a hermetic seal. The first step of every root canal treatment is an access cavity preparation, which gives the operator proper visualization and access to the root canal system. Although it is commonly overlooked, a proper access cavity preparation is crucial to achieve a favorable treatment outcome and enhances the stability and longevity of the treated tooth.

A proper access opening allows for straight-line access to the orifices of the root canal(s), which helps facilitate disinfection and complete debridement. While many experts recommend straight-line access, some have scrutinized traditional access cavity preparations for the reduction of sound tooth structure. As a result, minimally invasive access cavity concepts have been proposed to compensate for some of the drawbacks associated with traditional access cavity preparations.[1-3] The purpose of this chapter is to obtain a deep understanding of the steps involved in access cavity preparations, which can help facilitate adequate debridement and prevent procedural mishaps.

Definition

An *access cavity* refers to an opening from the occlusal or incisal aspect of a tooth directed toward the roof of the pulp chamber and corresponding canal orifices. The goals of access cavity preparation are to remove all caries, leaky restorations, unsupported tooth structure, and necrotic tissue and to deroof the pulp chamber in the process, while conserving as much sound tooth structure as possible. Many factors are involved, such as the location of the canal orifices; root curvature; existing restorations; degree of calcification; size and shape of the canals; position of the tooth in the jaw; and the age, sex, and ethnicity of the patient. Anatomical variations in pulp chamber space are also found and therefore need to be taken into consideration.[2,4]

Anatomical landmarks such as the central groove or central fossa, the roof and floor of the pulp chamber, the cementoenamel junction, and the furcation are predictable guides to precisely determine the dimensions of the pulp chamber. Despite the aforementioned factors that affect the design of access cavity preparation, root canal orifices can be located by following a set of basic rules and principles. These aid in guiding the operator on the location of the canal orifices and include, but are not limited to, the law of centrality, law of concentricity, law of cementoenamel junction (CEJ), and laws of symmetry.[5]

- **Law of centrality**: The pulp chamber is always located in the center of the tooth at the level of the CEJ.
- **Law of concentricity**: The walls of the pulp chamber are always concentric to the external surface of the tooth at the level of the CEJ.

- **Law of CEJ**: The CEJ is the most consistent, repeatable landmark for locating the position of the pulp chamber.
- **Laws of orifice location**:
  - The orifices of the root canals are always located at the junction of the walls and the floor of the pulp chamber (Fig 4-1).
  - The orifices of the root canals are always located at the angles in the floor-wall junction.
  - The orifices of the root canals are always located at the terminus of the root developmental fusion lines.
- **Laws of symmetry**:
  - Except for maxillary molars, canal orifices are equidistant from a line drawn in a mesiodistal direction through the pulp chamber floor (Fig 4-2).
  - Except for maxillary molars, canal orifices lie on a line perpendicular to a line drawn in a mesiodistal direction across the center of the pulp chamber floor.
- **Law of color change**: The pulp chamber floor is always darker in color than the walls.

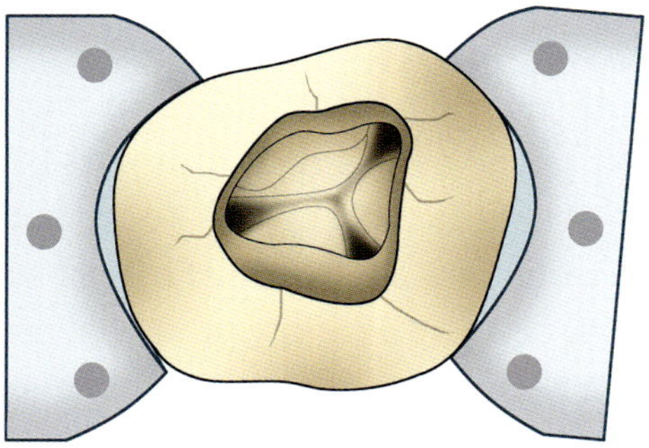

Fig 4-1 Laws of orifice location.

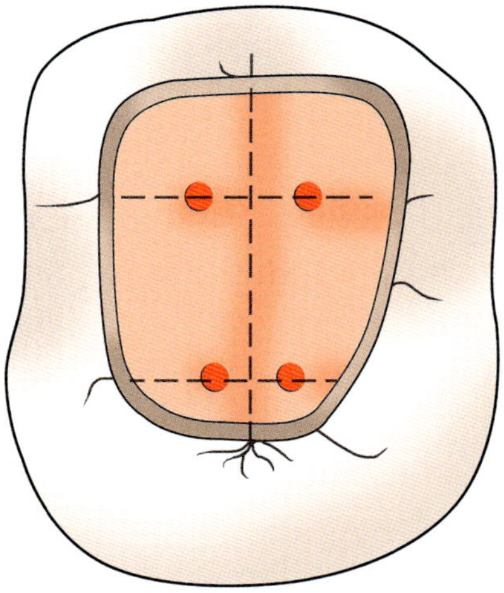

Fig 4-2 A diagrammatic representation of centrality, concentricity, and symmetry of canal orifice location.

Principles for Endodontic Access Cavity Preparation

The clinician should always keep in mind that the primary objective of proper access cavity preparation is to permit a complete, direct visualization to the floor of the pulp chamber and canal orifices. This is especially true in posterior teeth because the floor of the pulp chamber contains natural grooves at the end of which the canal orifices are located. To accomplish the goals of access cavity preparation, it is best that the preparation be completed in a stepwise manner, following the protocol below.[6]

Outline form

Prior to beginning the access cavity, the normal anatomy of the tooth in question should be evaluated by taking a clinically acceptable and undistorted radiograph. There are three important factors to take into account during access cavity preparation:

1. Shape of the pulp chamber
2. Size of the pulp chamber
3. Number of individual root canals, their curvature, and position

The size and shape of the pulp chamber dictate the internal anatomy of the tooth, and it is important for the external outline form of the preparation to follow the internal anatomy. By mechanically projecting the pulpal internal anatomy onto the external surface, the external outline form is created.

Convenience form

The convenience form expands the access cavity to establish straight-line access to the apical third of the canal. This facilitates instrumentation of the apical third of the canal and also ensures that the root canal irrigants reach the apical third of the root canal(s). An access cavity that lacks a proper convenience form leads to limited visual access for the operator and creates friction of the shaft of the instrument with the access cavity walls. This friction can result in an increased compensatory force applied by the operator, which may contribute to weakening of instruments and, ultimately, to their fracture (Fig 4-3). Additionally, the presence of an adequate convenience form allows for the placement of retentive interappointment temporary restorations.

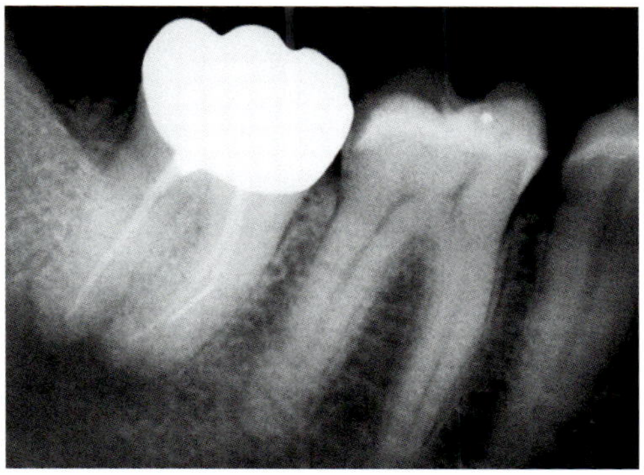

Fig 4-3 Underextended access cavity led to broken file and insufficient debridement and obturation. (Courtesy of Dr Mahmoud Torabinejad.)

Removal of any carious tooth structure and defective restorations

The reasons for removing defective restorations and carious dentin are as follows:

1. To clean and mechanically eliminate as much bacteria as possible from the internal area of the tooth
2. To remove discolored tooth structure, which can contribute to staining
3. To reduce the probability of saliva and bacterial contaminants from leaking into the preparation

Given the porous nature of dentin, incomplete deroofing of the pulp chamber as well as incomplete removal of carious dentin, can result in reinfection of the root canal(s) after root canal therapy, due to microleakage.

Cleaning of the cavity

After removal of residual caries, necrotic tissue, and calcified debris, the access cavity should have a clean appearance. It is important that the access cavity be disinfected with antimicrobial agents, such as sodium hypochlorite, during radicular instrumentation. By using the previously mentioned laws and principles, the canal orifices can be found and instrumentation may be completed.

Common Errors and Misconceptions during Access Cavity Preparation

Access cavity preparation is the first and one of the most important phases of NSRCT. However, it can also be the most challenging and frustrating part of endodontic treatment. Therefore, proper access cavity designs and preparation are imperative for high-quality endodontic treatment and prevention of iatrogenic problems.[7,8]

The following common errors may be encountered during access preparation[9]:

- **Incomplete removal of restorations and caries.** The incomplete removal of restorations and caries can decrease visualization of the pulp chamber and its contents and lead to the next error of incomplete deroofing of the pulp chamber.
- **Incomplete deroofing of the pulp chamber.** This hinders the operator's ability to find the respective canals. Additionally, unexcavated pulpal tissue and decay can significantly increase the amount of microorganisms present in the tooth, which can contribute to reinfection after root canal treatment.
- **Access cavity perforations.** One of the most feared risks during access cavity preparation is perforation, and there are many factors that may contribute to its occurrence. It is recommended to use a non-end-cutting bur to widen the access cavity and search for canals to prevent damage to the pulpal floor.
- **Damage to pulpal floor.** Iatrogenic damage to the pulpal floor may weaken the tooth and increase the chance of a perforation.

Needless to say, root canal therapy, as compared to other dental procedures, is carried out with limited visual guidance. When this is coupled with complex anatomy and the various pathologic conditions that may exist in a tooth, the access cavity becomes the most crucial step of treatment. Most common access preparation mistakes happen due to misconceptions of practitioners, which are highlighted below.

- **Misconception:** The goal of access cavity preparation is to find the canals.
  Fact: The purpose of access cavity preparation is to find the pulp chamber, not the canals.
- **Misconception:** High-speed burs should be used to find the canals.
  Fact: A DG16 slow-speed handpiece and ultrasonic tips should be used for this purpose.
- **Misconception:** Each tooth has a specific access cavity shape that is unique for the tooth.
  Fact: The shape of the access cavity is determined by the pulp chamber morphology rather than that of the individual tooth type. For example, a maxillary second molar may have an ovoid access cavity shape, rather than the common triangular shape, when it has only two canals.
- **Misconception:** The path of accessing the pulp chamber and its contents (lingual for anterior and occlusal for posterior) is applicable to all cases.
  Fact: The path to the pulp chamber varies in cases such as attrition, abrasion, a palatally inclined tooth, and crowding. In such cases, the pulp chamber may be accessed from the labial, rather than the conventional lingual approach, and also from the cusp tip in the case of a peg lateral incisor.[10]

Management of Procedural Mishaps

While the access cavity is the most important step of root canal therapy, errors can also occur during the procedure itself. These errors may be related to the factors listed below.

Treating the wrong tooth

This can occur due to an incorrect diagnosis of the diseased tooth. A common sign of the wrong tooth being treated is that the patient may report new pain symptoms or state that they are experiencing the same symptoms that existed prior to endodontic treatment. To avoid this mishap, one should make sure that thorough clinical and radiographic examinations are performed and that the correct offending tooth is identified. The management of this procedural mishap involves treating both teeth.

Missed canals

The presence of untreated or missed canals has a direct effect on the treatment prognosis. Missed canals are commonly associated with poor access or inadequate unroofing of the pulp chamber.

During treatment, if an instrument or filling material appears to be off-centered in the root, it may indicate the presence of an additional canal. Adequate periapical radiographs with different angulations, use of magnifying loupes or microscopes, and transillumination and use of methylene blue dye for detection of missed canals are beneficial in locating the canals in a tooth.

Dental explorer

Small, sharp endodontic explorers and hard endodontic files can be used to examine the floor of the pulp chamber and to explore any developmental grooves or lines. This should be done with caution, however, as debris or chipped away dentinal shavings may accumulate on the pulp chamber floor, clogging canal orifices.

Dyes

Methylene blue and erythrosine dyes are commonly used to search for canal orifices. It is important that the dye be cleaned out after application, and the operator should look for any dye traces remaining, which can indicate the location of a canal orifice.

Sodium hypochlorite (champagne bubble test)

A drop of sodium hypochlorite may be applied to the floor of the access cavity and observed under magnification and illumination. Sodium hypochlorite induces disintegration of pulpal tissue, and any bubbles that appear to be evading may indicate the presence of a hidden canal.

Crown fractures

When removing an existing crown for endodontic treatment, it may fracture. Therefore, care must be taken when separating or removing a crown.

Underextension

Underextension of the access cavity may result in missing canals, as canals are often hidden under calcified dentin. Even if the canal is found, underextension can lead to a strip perforation, as the instrumenting file will tend to cut away furcal dentin. Another consequence of underextension is that the curvature of the coronal portion of the canal may not be sufficiently removed, which increases the chances of instrument separation, as the operator attempts to go around more than one curve (see Fig 4-3). Furthermore, underextension of the access preparation limits the size to which the apical portion can be prepared.

Overextension

Generally, overextension results in weakening of the tooth and decreases the overall prognosis of treatment. Steps should be taken to conserve as much tooth structure as possible.

Access cavity perforation(s)

While perforations may occur during the preparation of the access cavity, they can also occur during endodontic treatment. In fact, one of the irreversible complications of endodontics is perforation into the furcation area or through the chamber walls. Additionally, perforations may also occur while searching for canals on the floor of the pulp chamber, particularly in molars (Fig 4-4).

The most common cause of perforations is misdirection of the bur during access cavity preparation. This may be due to irregular anatomical configuration or severe inclination of the tooth. Calcifications may also result in narrowing of the pulp chamber, which can lead to missing the pulp chamber entirely and drilling through the chamber floor. The signs of perforation include the following:

- Presence of blood in the access cavity
- Reports of an NaOCl taste by the patient
- Placement of a file in the opening and exposing a radiograph (Fig 4-5)

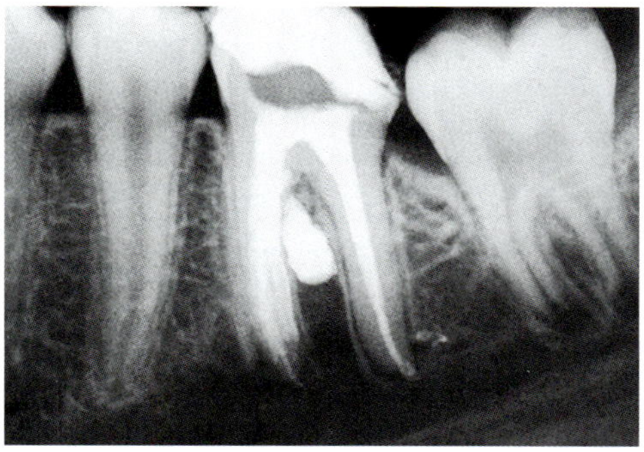

Fig 4-4 Furcation perforation in a mandibular molar, depicted by periapical radiograph. (Courtesy of Dr Mahmoud Torabinejad.)

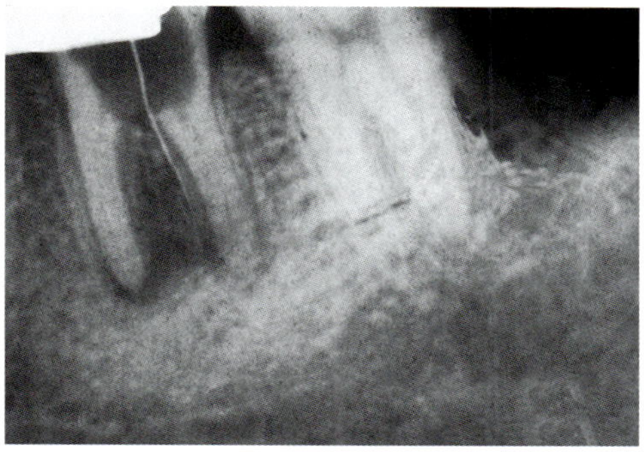

Fig 4-5 Perforation occurred during access cavity preparation. (Courtesy of Dr Mahmoud Torabinejad.)

Prevention

Prevention of access cavity perforation is achieved through the following:

- Making a thorough preoperative assessment, both clinically and radiographically, at different angles.
- Performing access cavity preparation without the use of a rubber dam to adequately visualize the long axis of the tooth.
  - In all teeth, the direction of the bur should be parallel to the long axis of the tooth (Figs 4-6 and 4-7).
  - In posterior teeth, the direction of the bur should be towards the area of the larger canal orifice.

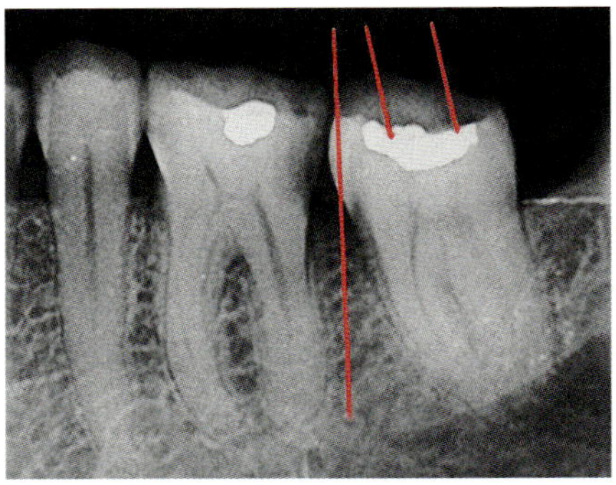

Fig 4-6 Perforation due to misdirection of the instrument.

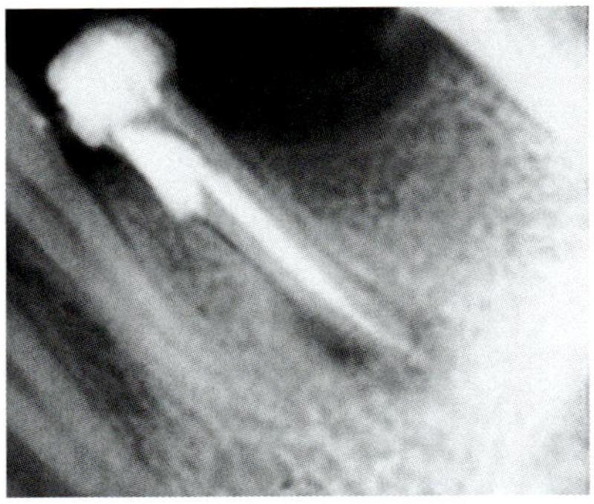

Fig 4-7 Incorrect alignment of the access preparation resulted in coronal perforation in a mandibular premolar tooth.

- Use of a bur should be limited to the roof of the pulp chamber.
- When in doubt about the direction of the preparation, a radiograph should be taken to ensure bur angulation is toward the pulp chamber.

Management

The management of a perforation is to isolate the tooth entirely by using a rubber dam. Among the different materials for perforation repair, mineral trioxide aggregate (MTA) has superior characteristics, including good sealing ability, high alkalinity, and great biocompatibility.[11] Repairing perforations involves locating the site of the perforation (Fig 4-8a), cleaning the floor of the preparation, achieving hemostasis with the application of a hemostatic agent, and applying MTA to obtain a seal at the perforation site (Fig 4-8b). In the unfavorable conditions of the oral cavity, where isolation or contamination may be an issue, glass-ionomer cement (GIC) may be used because GIC, especially light-cured GIC, is less sensitive to moisture (Fig 4-9).[9]

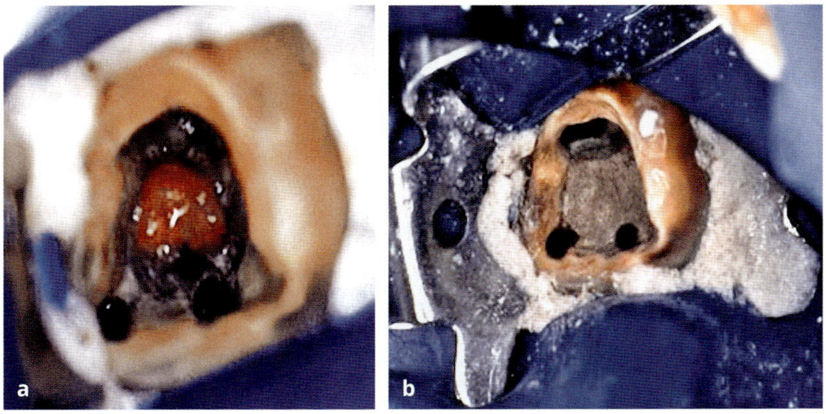

Fig 4-8 *(a)* Furcation perforation in a mandibular molar. *(b)* Repair with MTA. (Courtesy of Dr Mahmoud Torabinejad.)

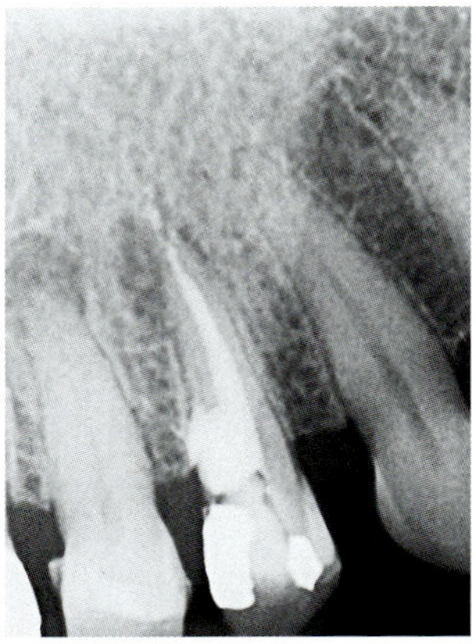

Fig 4-9 Repair of the coronal perforation with glass-ionomer cement.

Preventing Procedural Mishaps

As discussed in the previous section, procedural mishaps are unwanted occurrences during root canal treatment. Familiarity with the complexity of a given root canal can help prevent procedural errors. All clinicians should pay attention to the AAE Endodontic Case Difficulty Assessment Form and Guidelines, which assists in predicting the potential of dental mishaps. The Case Difficulty Assessment Form and Guidelines identifies several factors that contribute to the difficulty of endodontic cases, such as the anticipated number of visits needed, the degree of difficulty for patient selection, treatment completion, and access cavity preparation. Other factors include difficulty in tooth accessibility, especially in the posterior region, limitations in patient opening, patient intolerance, and tooth malposition. Many of these factors can result in non-ideal treatment, which may lead to endodontic mishaps.

Most issues and endodontic mishaps emanate from unfamiliarity with the AAE Endodontic Case Difficulty Assessment Form and Guidelines. Levels of difficulty are categorized into three groups: minimal, moderate, and high difficulty. By placing the endodontic case into one of these groups prior to treatment, the clinician may better anticipate the difficulties that may be encountered during treatment. Levels 2 and 3 address teeth that act as bridge abutments, malpositioned teeth, receded or calcified pulp chamber(s), pulp stones, and high degree of tooth crown inclination. Sufficient knowledge, skill, intuition, and experience are necessary for the successful treatment of level 2 and 3 patients. Otherwise, procedural errors may occur.[9]

Practical guidelines to avoid mishaps during access cavity preparation are as follows:

- Begin by taking a diagnostic two-angled radiograph and inspect the radiograph for the internal anatomy of the tooth, which dictates the size and shape of access preparation (Fig 4-10).

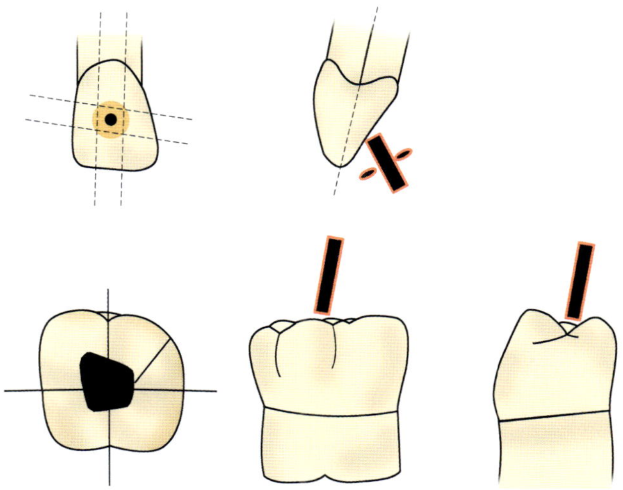

Fig 4-10 The basic direction of bur angulation for entry toward the pulp chamber.

- Remove all caries, unsupported enamel and dentin, and any defective restorations. If the prepared cavity is closer to the chamber, it is better to enter the chamber from the same side. A palatal entry for maxillary anterior teeth, a lingual entry for mandibular anterior teeth, and an occlusal entry for posteriors are advised.
- Begin preparation by orienting the bur parallel to the long axis of the tooth. If the bur is angulated poorly, it can lead to weakening of the tooth structure and contribute to the likelihood of perforations (Figs 4-11 and 4-12).
- Continue drilling until a "bur drop" is felt into the roof of the pulp chamber. The access cavity should be examined to verify that the dark floor of the pulp chamber is visible.

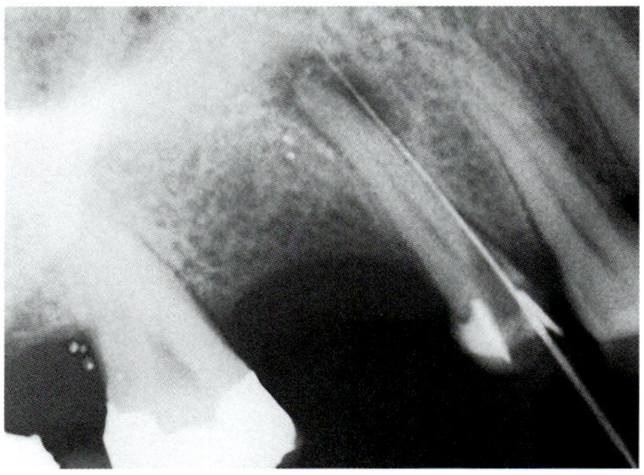

Fig 4-11 An improperly angulated bur during access preparation can lead to weakening of the tooth structure and contribute to crown fracture or even perforations.

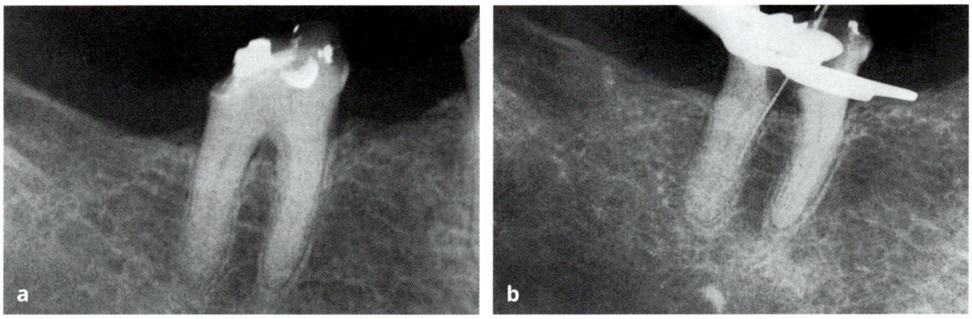

Fig 4-12 *(a)* Initial radiograph of tooth no. 30. *(b)* Postoperative radiograph showing a furcation perforation as a result of miscalculation of depth of access preparation. (Courtesy of Dr Mahmoud Torabinejad.)

- The access cavity may be extended by using a non-end-cutting bur to remove remaining dentin and the roof of the pulp chamber. Complete deroofing of the pulp and removal of the pulp horns is vital to allow for adequate access to the canals. The walls of the access cavity should be probed to ensure that the roof of the pulp chamber has been completely removed, ie, no dentin ledges or lips are present.[10]
- Once the pulp chamber is deroofed, antimicrobial solutions such as sodium hypochlorite and/or chlorhexidine should be used as irrigants to flush the pulp chamber. The coronal or radicular pulp may be extirpated by using a sharp spoon excavator.

- Canal orifices should be located by using a DG16 explorer; do not use round burs. Color changes in the dentin are important to watch for, as they can lead to locating canal orifices. Dark developmental lines may be present, and tracking along these lines can reveal canal orifices. The orifices of canals feel sticky when probed with an endodontic explorer.[10] Once located, a glide path should be established with a #10 K-file or a #6 or #8 K-file in cases of calcification with lubricants, such as RC-Prep.
- After the canal orifices are located and a glide path is established, coronal flaring of the access cavity walls should be completed to ensure straight-line access. The lack of straight-line access can increase the probability of ledges, zips, elbows, and perforation to occur. These issues can be further exacerbated when stiff stainless-steel files are subsequently introduced. Additionally, straight-line access also allows for easier insertion of subsequent rotary instruments during preparation. Straight line access is essential when using nickel-titanium instruments to prevent torsional fracture. Although these instruments are very flexible, poor straight-line access may result in distortion of the files and eventual separation, due to cyclic fatigue[12] (Fig 4-13).

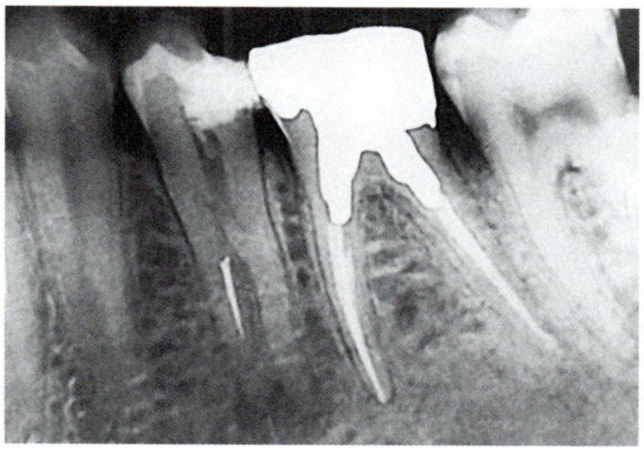

Fig 4-13 Separation of a K-file instrument due to inadequate straight-line access in a mandibular second premolar.

- Evaluate the prepared access cavity. Slight modifications are acceptable based on factors such as case requirements, age, and limited mouth opening. Nonetheless, a modification of the access cavity should allow for the introduction of instruments, as well as any irrigating solutions to the entire working length. A modification can be performed during any stage of the treatment if necessary.

Miscellaneous Factors Affecting Endodontic Treatment

While there are many factors that can influence the success of endodontic treatment, some may not be in the control of the operator. Therefore, recognition and management of such variables is very important. Factors such as limited mouth opening and/or an unfavorably positioned tooth may lead to difficulty in aligning the handpiece along the long axis of the tooth. This can affect the quality of the access cavity and, in turn, decrease the chance of finding canals. Even when the canals have been located in such cases, another challenge could be their negotiation. In cases of limited mouth opening, a pediatric handpiece can be used, and

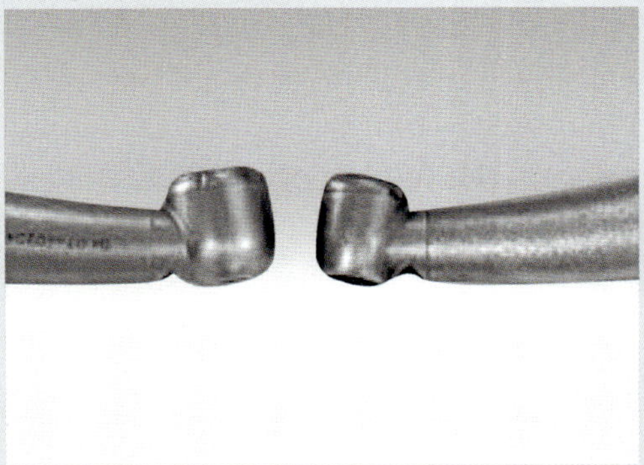

Fig 4-14 The handpiece on the right (KaVo 637 Bellatorque, KaVo Dental) has a smaller head. When used with a shortened bur, it makes accessing molar teeth easier on patients with restricted opening.

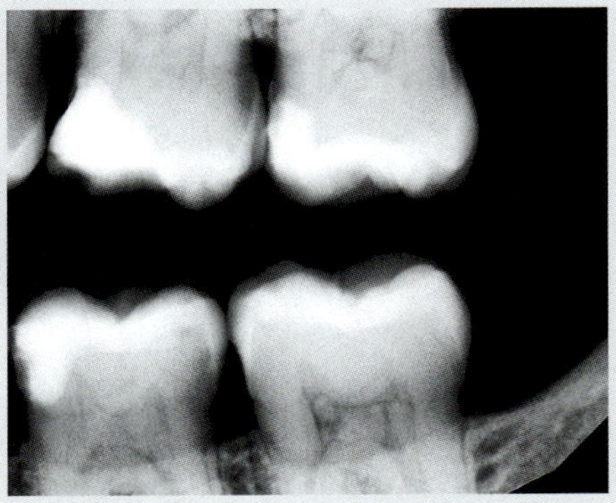

Fig 4-15 Several pulp stones in the maxillary and mandibular molars.

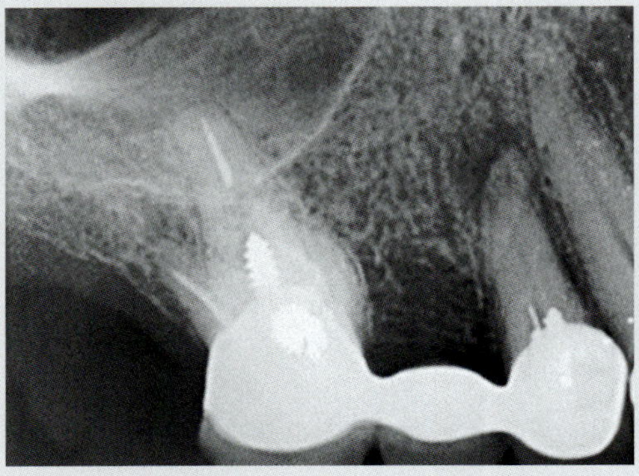

Fig 4-16 Failure to remove the crown makes it impossible to gain access into the canal orifice due to the presence of an intracanal post.

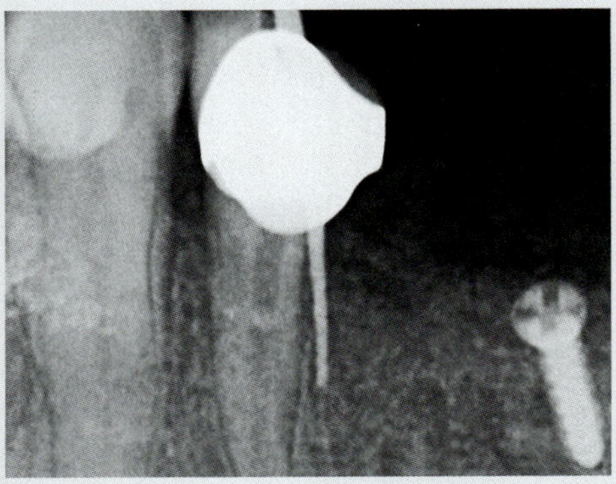

Fig 4-17 Failure to remove the crown has led to a perforation.

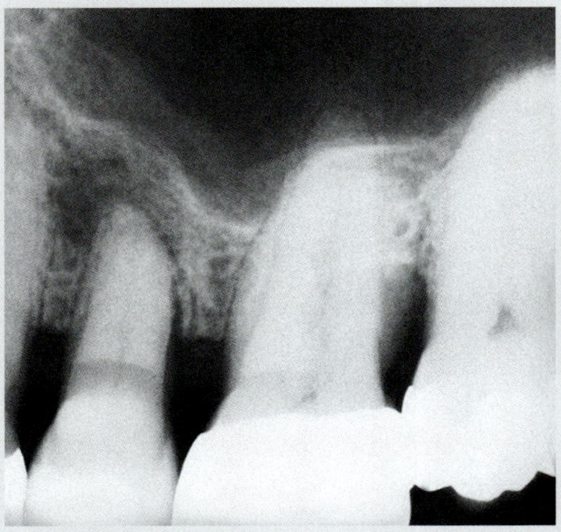

Fig 4-18 The canals in the maxillary left second premolar tooth appear to be calcified.

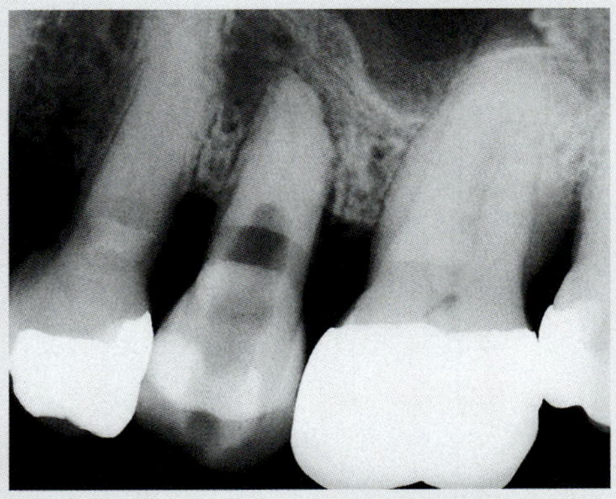

Fig 4-19 As a result of calcification, the operator had difficulty locating the canal.

burs may be shortened by 4 mm to aid in access and treatment. Additionally, the interocclusal distance, and hence visibility, can be increased by shortening the buccal cusps by 3 mm prior to access cavity preparation (Fig 4-14).

Calcifications, including pulp stones, present challenges for locating and instrumenting canals. These can be identified on radiographs (Fig 4-15), and the ease of removal depends on the size and type of pulp stone. Those that are firmly attached to the dentin may require the use of a handpiece to remove, while the lightly attached ones can be removed by using an endodontic explorer. Small instruments, such as pathfinding files, will similarly facilitate the bypassing of pulp stones and aid in locating the orifice in the calcified pulp chamber.

Posterior teeth that are already restored with crowns and need endodontic treatment present a different set of challenges. In such cases, the presence of a crown can make it difficult to visualize the long axis of the tooth. Therefore, it is important to be mindful that the subtle color changes of the pulpal floor may be nonexistent in such cases. If the canals cannot be identified or are impeded by pin restorations, for example, it may be necessary to remove the crown (Fig 4-16). Removing the crown will also contribute to the conservation of sound dentin structure and reduce the likelihood of perforations[12] (Fig 4-17).

Moreover, the volume of the pulp chamber decreases in response to restorative dentistry and with age, as more secondary and tertiary dentin is deposited. With a reduction in volume, the pulp chamber may appear narrower, which can lead to greater difficulty in locating the canal orifices[12] (Figs 4-18 and 4-19). The dentin can be removed by using ultrasonic tips or slow-speed long-shank round burs. Canal entrances can be probed by using an endodontic explorer to feel for stickiness, and any tactile tug back may indicate the presence of a canal orifice. Additionally, the access cavity may be prepared without the use of a rubber dam to help orient the bur toward the long axis of the tooth. During this process, a throat pack may be placed to prevent the accidental swallowing or aspiration of instruments. Radiographs can be taken to ensure the correct direction is being followed, and once canal orifices are located, a rubber dam should be applied.[13]

Newly Introduced Access Cavity Designs

Due to the many innovations in the previous decade, many new access cavity designs have been introduced that limit the amount of tooth structure needing to be removed to gain access to the pulp chamber. This concept originates from the idea that by preserving the roof of the pulp chamber and pericervical dentin, there may be improved fracture resistance of teeth following root canal treatment. Contrary to contemporary beliefs, finding the pulp chamber and canals is not an arbitrary process—one can predictably locate the pulp chamber and canals based on scientific evidence. Previously, access cavities were standardized, mainly dependent on the type of tooth. However, modern endodontic innovations, such as the use of the dental operation microscope and loupes, which allow for better magnification and illumination, as well as the use of CBCT, have allowed the ideal access cavity preparation to evolve from being based on individual tooth type to being based on the shape of the pulp chamber and the overall morphology of the tooth.

It is important to note that a minimal access design may lead to more complications, such as greater difficulty in the visualization and debridement of the pulp chamber as well as in locating, shaping, cleaning, and filling the canals. The risk of iatrogenic complications including missed canals, deviations, instrument fracture,[14] and the absence of a convenience form may pose challenges in ensuring thorough biological debridement.[15] The remaining material including pulpal remnants, dental debris, filling materials, and other residues may cause tooth discoloration, support microbial growth, and have a negative impact on root canal sealers and composites.[16,17]

The different types of access cavity design are outlined below.[18]

- **Traditional access cavity (TradAC).** In posterior teeth, a traditional access cavity is prepared by the complete removal of the pulp chamber roof (Fig 4-20). Then, the cavity is extended so the operator can achieve straight-line access to the canal orifices. The access cavity should have smoothly divergent axial walls so all orifices can be observed within the outline form.
- **Conservative access cavity (ConsAC).** In posterior teeth, preparation begins at the central fossa and extends as far as necessary to find the canal orifices. The walls of this preparation are convergent, and the roof of the pulp chamber is preserved (Fig 4-21). This access type can also be performed with divergent walls (ConsAC.DW). In anterior teeth, this access takes a triangular or oval shape that conserves any pulp horns and pericervical dentin.

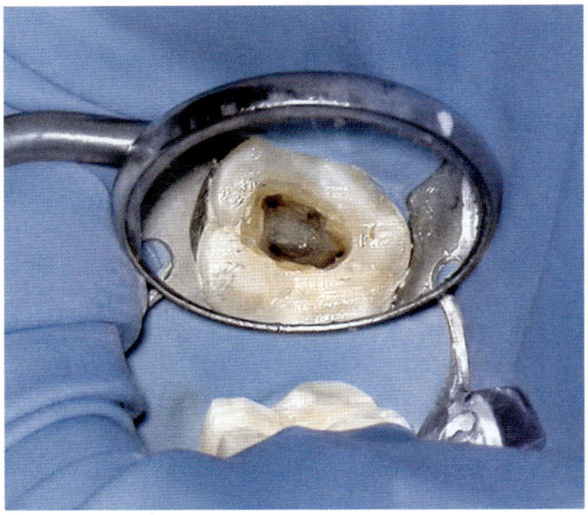

Fig 4-20 Traditional access cavity design.

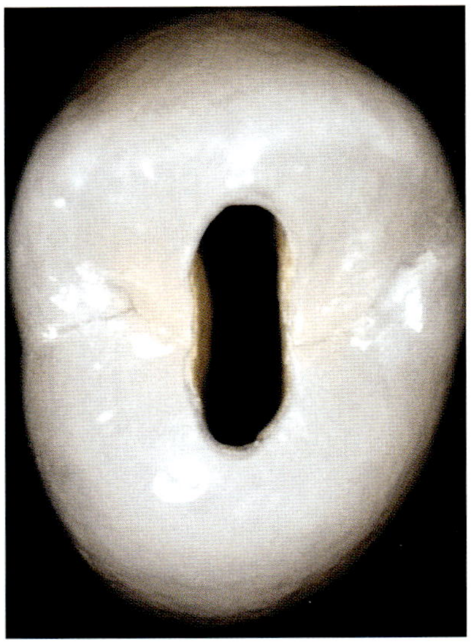

Fig 4-21 Conservative access cavity design. (Courtesy of Dr Mahmoud Torabinejad.)

- **Ultra-conservative access cavity (UltraAC).** This preparation begins the same as ConsAC, but there is no extension, so as much of the roof of the pulp chamber is conserved as possible. These types of access cavities are also termed *ninja preps*.
- **Truss access cavity (TrussAC).** This design involves making small-sized preparations in multi-rooted teeth to find the respective canals while preserving the dentinal bridge between them.
- **Caries-driven access cavity (CariesAC).** This design involves following and removing the caries to reach the pulp chamber while conserving all other tooth structure.
- **Restorative-driven access cavity (RestoAC).** In restored teeth with no caries, access to the pulp chamber is prepared by totally or partially removing existing restorations and preserving all possible remaining tooth structure.

Among the 22 abbreviations reported in the literature, two of them (SLF and SLR) differ from the others because their outlines are derived from pulp space landmarks that are projected onto the occlusal surface of the teeth.[19,20] While the straight-line furcation design (SLF) is based on the location of the center of each canal at the furcation level, the reference for the straight-line radicular (SLR) access is associated with the position of the pulp horns.[19,20]

Impact of Conservative Access Preparation on Treatment/Retreatment

One of the major difficulties when performing conservative access cavities is a limited view of the pulp chamber floor, resulting in greater difficulty in locating the canal orifices. There is a greater chance for detection of second mesiobuccal canals (MB2) in maxillary molars with TradAC compared to ConsAC, with or without magnification.[21] However, no difference was observed when troughing with an ultrasonic tip, along with magnification. Small access cavities (UltraAC) are associated with a greater amount of pulp chamber roof, which may affect the efficiency of irrigation and, consequently, result in greater dentinal debris accumulation within the root canal system.[22,23] Disinfection procedures may also be impaired by the presence of contaminated pulp tissue remnants, which may serve as a source for persistent infection and result in post-treatment disease. It has been demonstrated that ConsAC preparations contain larger amounts of retained pulp tissue in the access chamber of mandibular molars as compared to TradAC after chemomechanical preparation. The remaining pulpal tissue interferes with the mechanical action of the instruments and compromises the flow of irrigants. Consequently, disinfection procedures using conventional syringe irrigation are compromised significantly after root canal preparation of teeth with conservative endodontic cavities.[24]

Current studies suggest that there is no difference between the TradAC and ConsAC in regard to untouched canal walls and accumulated hard tissue debris remaining after preparation.[24] A larger number of canal transportations, however, have been observed in teeth with ConsAC. Additionally, the smallest access cavities, such as TrussAC and UltraAC, were accompanied with negative effects on irrigation efficiency because larger amounts of pulp tissue and hard tissue debris remained after shaping procedures.[25]

Moreover, current studies have suggested that the cross-sectional shape of the canal may have an influence on the outcome of filling procedures and may also lead to the decreased removal of filling material from the pulp chamber in retreatment cases with minimally invasive access cavities.[26] Retreatment procedures in the presence of a ConsAC are more time consuming. However, instruments with asymmetric cutting motions seemed to be more effective than other rotary instruments in the removal of filling materials from oval-shaped canals of single-rooted teeth with TradAC. The minimally invasive concept in endodontics was based on the premise that dentin conservation during access cavity preparation helps to maintain optimal strength and increases fracture resistance and several other characteristics that are needed for the long-term function and survival of endodontically treated teeth. Even though this is yet to be proven, it is likely that the volume of the pulp chamber as well as the thickness, height, and/or volume of the remaining tooth tissue have an effect on the fracture resistance of teeth.[24] Nondestructive 3D imaging tools, such as CBCT or micro-CT technologies, can be utilized to qualify these parameters.

Instruments and Techniques for Detecting and Correcting Access Cavity

Conventional radiography

The complexity of the root canal system can be better understood by having a thorough understanding of root canal anatomy and by taking at least two radiographs from different horizontal angulations. Preoperative radiographs reveal vital information about the size of the pulp chamber, the amount of dentin that occupies the pulp chamber, the distance between existing restorations and the pulp, and the presence and position of pulp stones, as well as additional roots/canals. Bitewing images provide information on the proximity of pulp horns to restorations and the approximate height of the pulp chamber. While very useful, radiographs should be interpreted with caution, because 30% of canal bifurcations are not visible in periapical radiographs.[27]

CBCT scan

When taking a CBCT, a sensor and x-ray source rotate around the patient's head at angles ranging from 180 to 360 degrees. Multiple images (base images) are captured and are highly dependent on the rotation angle, frames per second, resolution, and exposure protocol. In CBCT, the scanned object is reconstructed as a 3D matrix of voxels by the means of special software algorithms. CBCT scans detect lesions of different sizes and their locations more accurately than digital periapical radiographs.[28]

The American Association of Endodontists (AAE) has released a joint statement with the American Academy of Oral and Maxillofacial Radiology (AAOMR) recommending the use of CBCT for diagnosis in patients with nonspecific clinical signs and symptoms, associated with untreated or previously treated teeth, for treating teeth with anomalies or suspected additional or missed root canals, for the localization of calcified canals, and for presurgical evaluation.[29] The CBCT is an invaluable tool in detecting missed canals in molars as well as for identifying complex root canal morphology in premolars (Fig 4-22).

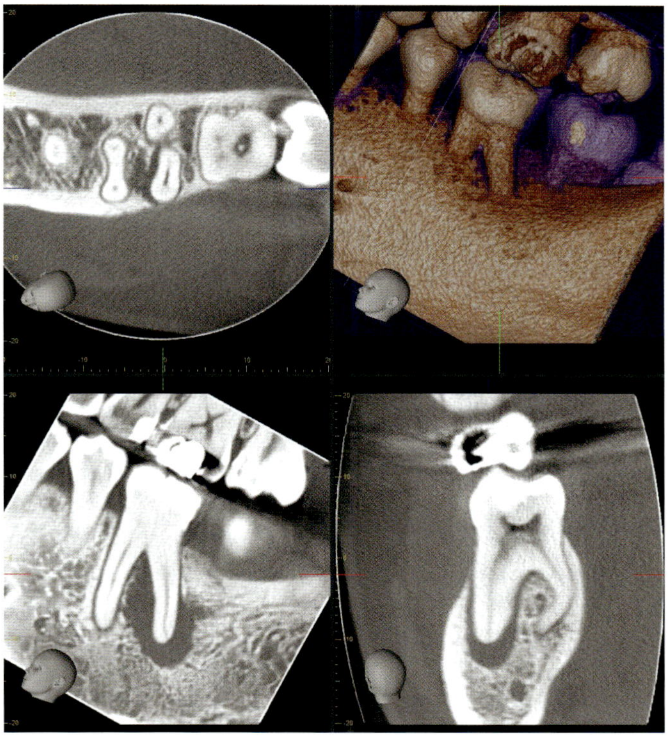

Fig 4-22 The CBCT shows complex root canal morphology in the mandibular first molar.

Burs

Burs are selected depending on tooth type and the presence and type of restorations. Crown removal is generally recommended; however, it is sometimes unfeasible. In such cases, diamond-coated burs with copious water can be implemented to create an access cavity through zirconia restorations, and trans-metal burs can be used for metal or the metallic portions of restorations (eg, porcelain-fused-to-metal [PFM]). For creating the external outline, deroofing the pulp chamber, and removing caries, a round carbide bur (sizes #2, #4, and #6), fissure carbide bur, or diamond bur is suitable (Fig 4-23). If excessive force is applied when creating the access cavity, microfracture or unnecessary loss of tooth structure may occur. Thus, stepwise caries removal is recommended.[17,19]

After penetrating and partially unroofing the pulp chamber, a non-end-cutting bur (eg, Endo-Z, Kerr; LA Axxess, Kerr) or a fissure carbide or diamond bur with a safety tip is best suited to decrease the risk of pulpal floor perforation. Sufficient removal of the tooth structure should be done by the bur to allow instruments to be easily placed into the orifice of each canal without interfering with any impediments (Fig 4-24). By using proper burs for different clinical conditions, the rate of access-related errors will decrease.

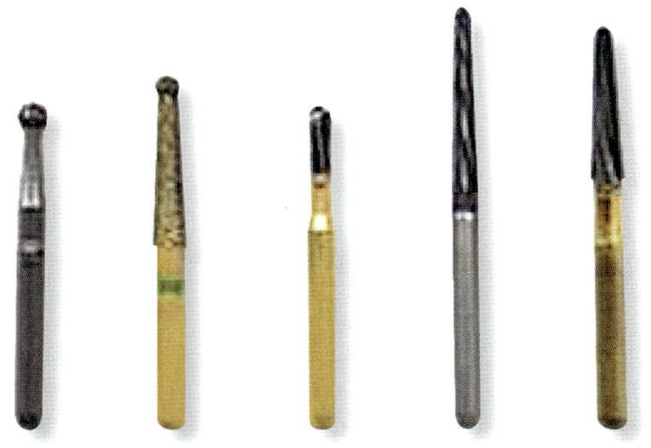

Fig 4-23 *(left to right)* A #2 round diamond bur, a tungsten carbide fissure bur, an Endo-Z bur (Kerr), an LA Axxess bur (Kerr), and a #2 tungsten carbide round bur. The last two burs (SybronEndo) have a longer shank and allow for better vision when used with magnification.

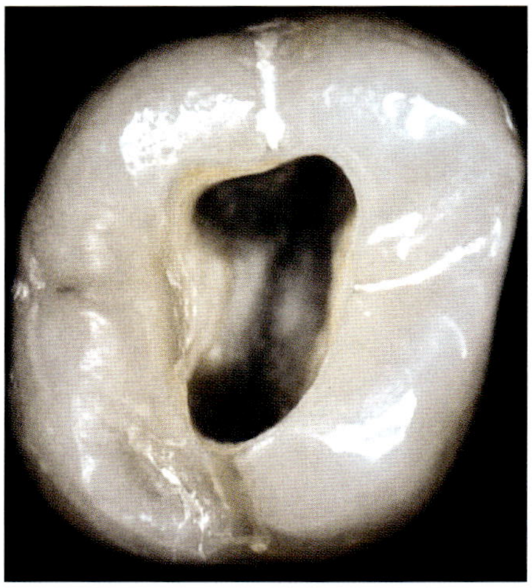

Fig 4-24 Sufficient removal of the tooth structure during access preparation allows instruments to be easily placed into the orifice of each canal. (Courtesy of Dr Mahmoud Torabinejad.)

Ultrasonic units

Different applications for ultrasonic units have been cited in the literature.[30] Access refinement can be completed by using a fine ultrasonic tip to lower the amount of unsupported dentin. Ultrasonic tips can also aid in detecting calcified canals, removing pulp stones or intracanal obstructions, and condensing gutta-percha when obturating. In surgical treatments, ultrasonics can be used to refine the root-end cavity preparation.

References

1. Zehnder MS, Connert T, Weiger R, Krastl G, Kühl S. Guided endodontics: Accuracy of a novel method for guided access cavity preparation and root canal location. Int Endod J 2016;49:966–972.
2. Adams N, Tomson PL. Access cavity preparation. Br Dent J 2014;216:333–339.
3. Gambarini G, Galli M, Morese A, et al. Digital design of minimally invasive endodontic access cavity. Appl Sci 2020;10:3513.
4. Maske A, Weschenfelder VM, Vilella FSG, Burnett LH Jr, Fontoura de Melo TA. Influence of access cavity design on fracture strength of endodontically treated lower molars. Aust Endod J 2021;47:5–10.

5. Krasner P, Rankow HJ. Anatomy of the pulp-chamber floor. J Endod 2004;30:5–16.
6. Castellucci A. Access cavity and endodontic anatomy. Endod 2004;1:245–329.
7. Nikolaidis N, Marras I, Mikrogeorgis G, Lyroudia K, Pitas I. Virtual dental patient: A 3D oral cavity model and its use in haptics-based virtual reality cavity preparation in endodontics. In: Daskalaki A. Dental Computing and Applications: Advanced Techniques for Clinical Dentistry. Hershey, PA: IGI Global, 2009:317–336.
8. Fabricio B, Williamson AE, Shabahang S. Isolation, endodontic access, and length determination. In: Torabinejad M, Fouad A, Shabanhang S (eds). Endodontics: Principles and Practice, ed 6. London: Elsevier, 2020.
9. Jha P. Clinical case 5—Perforation repair with instrument retrieval: Management of multiple endodontic mishaps. In: Chopra V (ed). Clinical Atlas of Retreatment in Endodontics. Hoboken, NJ: Wiley, 2021:32–37.
10. Patel S, Rhodes J. A practical guide to endodontic access cavity preparation in molar teeth. Br Dent J 2007;203:133–140.
11. Torabinejad, M, Parirokh M. Mineral trioxide aggregate: A comprehensive literature review—Part II: Leakage and biocompatibility investigations. J Endod 2010;36:190–202.
12. Connert T, Krug R, Eggmann F. Guided endodontics versus conventional access cavity preparation: A comparative study on substance loss using 3-dimensional–printed teeth. J Endod 2019;45:327–331.
13. Sabeti M, Kazem M, Dianat O, et al. Impact of access cavity design and root canal taper on fracture resistance of endodontically treated teeth: An ex vivo investigation. J Endod 2018;44:1402–1406.
14. Shabbir J, Zehra T, Najmi N, et al. Access cavity preparations: Classification and literature review of traditional and minimally invasive endodontic access cavity designs. J Endod 2021;47:1229–1244.
15. Elkholy MMA, Nawar NN, Ha WN, Saber SM, Kim HC. Impact of canal taper and access cavity design on the life span of an endodontically treated mandibular molar: A finite element analysis. J Endod 2021;47:1472–1480.
16. Perez C, Sayeh A, Etienne O. Microguided endodontics: Accuracy evaluation for access through intraroot fibre-post. Aust Endod J 2021;47:592–598.
17. Silva EJNL, Pinto KP, Ferreira CM, et al. Current status on minimal access cavity preparations: A critical analysis and a proposal for a universal nomenclature. Int Endod J 2020;53:1618–1635.
18. Ballester B, Giraud T, Ahmed HMA, Nabhan MS, Bukiet F, Guivarc'h M. Current strategies for conservative endodontic access cavity preparation techniques—Systematic review, meta-analysis, and decision-making protocol. Clin Oral Investig 2021;25:6027–6044.
19. Aidasani GL, Mulay S. Management of iatrogenic errors: Furcal perforation. J Int Clin Dent Res Organ 2018;10:42–46.
20. Loureiro MAZ, Elias MRA, Capeletti LR, et al. Guided endodontics: Volume of dental tissue removed by guided access cavity preparation—An ex vivo study. J Endod 2020;46:1907–1912.
21. Saygili G, Uysal B, Omar B, Ertas ET, Ertas H. Evaluation of relationship between endodontic access cavity types and secondary mesiobuccal canal detection. BMC Oral Health 2018;18:1–6.
22. Arbiya AS, Swaroop H, Syliva M. Minimally invasive endodontics—A review. J Dent Orofac Res 2019;15:77–88.
23. Connert T, Leontiev W, Dagassan-Berndt D, et al. Real-time guided endodontics with a miniaturized dynamic navigation system versus conventional freehand endodontic access cavity preparation: Substance loss and procedure time. J Endod 2021;47:1651–1656.
24. Silva EJNL, Versiani MA, Souza EM, De-Deues G. Minimally invasive access cavities: Does size really matter? Int Endod J 2021;54:153–155.
25. Saeed M, Al-Obadi M, Salim A, Alsawaf AY, Hadi K. Impact of access cavity design on fracture resistance of endodontically treated molars: A systematic review. Clin Cosmet Investig Dent 2021;13:1–10.
26. Shabbir J, Zehra T, Najmi N, et al. Access cavity preparations: Classification and literature review of traditional and minimally invasive endodontic access cavity designs. J Endod 2021;47:1229–1244.
27. Gröndahl HG, Huumonen S. Radiographic manifestations of periapical inflammatory lesions: How new radiological techniques may improve endodontic diagnosis and treatment planning. Endod Topics 2004;8:55–67.
28. Saidi A, Naaman A, Zogheib C. Accuracy of cone-beam computed tomography and periapical radiography in endodontically treated teeth evaluation: A five-year retrospective study. J Int Oral Health 2015;7:15–19.
29. Bhatt M, Coil J, Chehroudi B, Esteves A, Aleksejuniene J, MacDonald D. Clinical decision-making and importance of the AAE/AAOMR position statement for CBCT examination in endodontic cases. Int Endod J 2021;54:26–37.
30. Liu Z, Zhang D, Li Q, Xu Q. Evaluation of root-end preparation with a new ultrasonic tip. J Endod 2013;39:820–823

5

Cleaning and Shaping

OVE A. PETERS
CHRISTINE I. PETERS

Objectives

After reading this chapter, the reader should be able to:

1. Indicate the correct steps involved in cleaning and shaping procedures.
2. Recognize that procedural mishaps during cleaning and shaping may occur and can alter the outcome of root canal treatments.
3. Register complications during cleaning and shaping and distinguish between reversible and irreversible accidents.
4. Identify methods to prevent such complications.
5. List appropriate approaches for error management.

With improvements in technology, including file design and adjunct devices, root canal preparation has become a quite predictable procedure, even in teeth with complex anatomy. However, procedural mishaps do occur and present challenges to case outcomes, the patient–provider relationship, and the clinician's self-confidence.

This chapter explores accidents and complications specifically related to cleaning and shaping procedures in root canal treatment. Conceivably, the best way to manage potential adverse events is to have strategies in place to prevent them and eliminate risks, but even so, clinicians must be able to diagnose and manage errors when they occur. Therefore, this chapter lists mishaps in the sequence they could occur during a clinical procedure, and it discusses assessment, etiology, prevention, and management of procedural accidents.

Regarding the severity of a problem, mishaps may be described as reversible or irreversible. Irreversible errors or accidents during nonsurgical root canal treatments are rarely life threatening but may cause lasting harm to the patient and can have negative consequences for case outcomes.

Access

In the sequence of root canal treatment, access cavity preparation is the first operative step and is essential in providing an adequate pathway to the root canal system.[1] To avoid treating the wrong tooth, clinicians must first confirm the tooth they are treating is the correct candidate in question. Certain mistakes in charting on referral forms are common, such as transposing numbers or sides of the mouth. Erroneous diagnoses can lead to inappropriate treatments; for example, failure to add supplementary techniques in clinical testing in teeth with mineralized pulps, extensive restorations, or previous trauma may lead to the conclusion that a tooth pulp is necrotic and should receive endodontic therapy. While cold testing is a reliable tool in assessing tooth vitality, each clinician should confirm validity of the treatment request and take any contradictory testing results into consideration.[2] Establishing a solid clinical diagnosis and confirming the need for root canal treatment goes a long way in reducing the chance of unnecessarily accessing a tooth.[3]

Strategies such as time-outs immediately before the procedure to confirm the three C's—correct patient, correct site, and correct procedure—with the dental team and the patient can help the clinician avoid accessing an incorrect tooth.[4]

A well-prepared access cavity must retain sufficient coronal structure yet reveal the anatomy of the pulp. While in many cases access cavity preparation is uneventful, perforation on access is a complication that may reduce the chance for a successful outcome; indeed, perforations have been cited as a main factor affecting the success rate of root canal retreatments.[5]

Perforation during cutting of an access cavity may occur toward the furcation (in multirooted teeth) or toward the outside of the tooth surface, either above or below the periodontal attachment level.[6] Certain clinical conditions, such as a highly mineralized pulp chamber, small mouth-opening, and the presence of full-coverage restorations, are more likely to complicate access preparation. A recent systematic review highlighted practitioner experience, tooth type, and morphology as risk factors associated with perforations during root canal treatment.[7]

It is therefore necessary to plan ahead and conduct an appropriate case assessment prior to accessing a tooth for endodontic treatment. This must include pulpal and apical diagnosis as well as a formal case difficulty assessment. In addition to the American Association of Endodontists (AAE) Case Difficulty Assessment Form,[8] there are now computer and phone apps[9] for this purpose. Diagnostic radiographs and possibly a small field of view (FOV) CBCT image are needed before root canal treatment is commenced.[10]

Assessment

Importantly, a clinician first needs to recognize if a perforation has occurred during access cavity preparation. This may be complicated in cases that present with highly inflamed (pulpitic) conditions that show significant bleeding on access. The best approach in circumventing a perforation is to use non-end-cutting burs and to remove all contents of the pulp chamber.

Bleeding from a perforation site is typically less than from an inflamed pulp, and hemostasis can be achieved with sodium hypochlorite irrigation and pressure.[11,12]

Using magnification, the pulp chamber should be thoroughly inspected, taking into account the typical anatomy of a tooth, including location and number of anticipated root canal orifices. To confirm a suspected perforation, a small file may be connected to an electronic apex locator to determine if an opening detected inside the pulp chamber is a root canal orifice or a de facto perforation.[13] The apex locator would display an apex reading, the location of which can be compared to the expected position of the root tip on a diagnostic radiograph. Lastly, a radiograph with a small file placed in the entrance of a possible perforation site may be obtained to confirm the presence of a perforation (Fig 5-1).

While perforation on access does occur in specific clinical conditions, the erroneous access of an incorrect tooth, one that did not need treatment, may also occur. As stated earlier, this is an avoidable complication; clinicians should be mindful that the correct tooth is isolated, specifically when using a dental dam with the single tooth isolation method. In some cases, such as mandibular anterior teeth or maxillary premolar teeth, adjacent teeth may look very similar, and the dental dam may be placed on the wrong tooth. In addition to using a checklist approach,[4] clinicians can effectively minimize this risk by marking the tooth with a surgical marking pen or by initiating the access cavity without dental dam and continuing to completely unroof the preparation after isolation and disinfection of the tooth to be treated. This approach can also aid in judgment of the long axis of the tooth during access preparation. Another helpful tool is a stent manufactured using

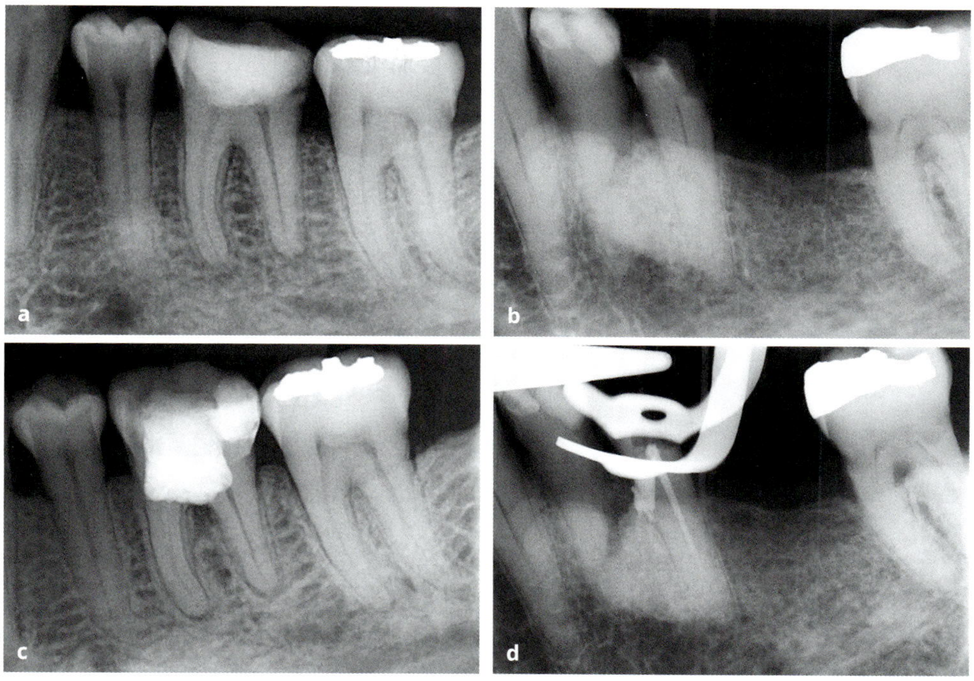

Fig 5-1 Perforation on access is often a result of misorientation in depth *(a)* and direction *(b)*. The opening to the periodontal ligament may be to the furcation in multirooted teeth *(c)*. In single-rooted teeth, perforation on access is often into the PDL, below the osseous margin *(d)*.

CBCT-based planning software. However, operator experience remains the most decisive factor in tooth substance loss during access preparation.[14]

Overpreparation on access may be viewed as a graded occurrence, ranging from minimal deviations from an ideal access, to gross overpreparation/gouging, to perforations that create a communication of the pulp chamber with the oral cavity or the coronal portion of the periodontal ligament.

In this context, it must be mentioned that there is currently a trend toward so-called "minimally invasive access."[15,16] The basis for this strategy is the observation that root canal–treated teeth are more likely to fracture than vital counterparts due to increased substance loss. While the change in fracture resistance is only around 5% for endodontic access only, overpreparation with or without perforation will rapidly decrease resistance to flexure and may consequently facilitate cracking of the remaining walls.[17] However, according to the best available evidence, the most frequently cited reason for the extraction of root canal treated teeth is nonrestorable caries.[18] The ability to restore a tooth after root canal treatment depends on the amount of retained structure, and in this context, the intent to keep access cavities as small as practical is meaningful. Figure 5-2 illustrates variations of access up to the point of a perforation with clinical views and radiographs.

Overall, perforations on access occur with moderate frequency (1% to 5%) but are more frequent with inexperienced clinicians.[7]

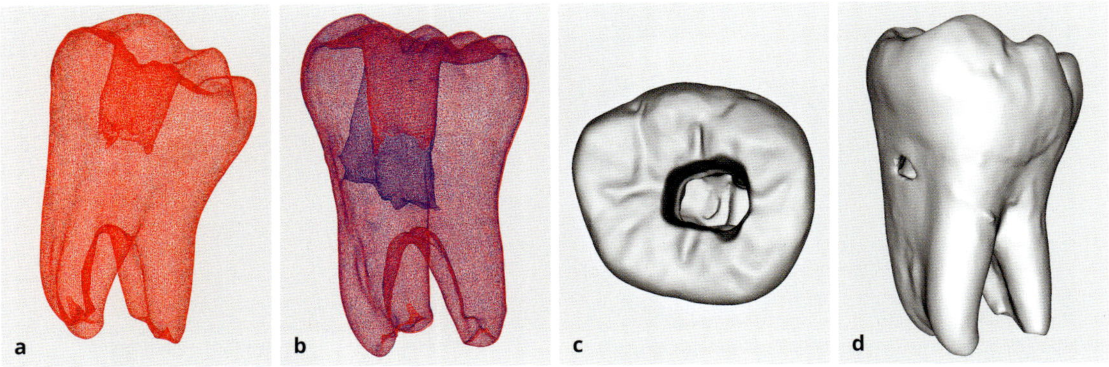

Fig 5-2 Access perforation in a mandibular molar, depicted by integrating surface and volumetric scans using an optical method. In the endodontic literature, it is recommended to probe the CEJ, at which level the pulp is centered for calibration. Starting the access preparation in the mesial groove may be misleading and could result in an access that is located too far mesially. In these images, the access cavity was started correctly *(a)*, but then extended too far mesially *(b and c)*, leading to a perforation *(d)*.

Etiology

Several factors may lead to perforation on access, most significantly incorrect 3D orientation of the bur. The classic paper by Krasner and Rankow[19] established the basic rules of locating the pulp chamber within a crown, based on dentin apposition during development. Because further dentin apposition occurs with aging, caries, and restoration placement, clinicians can appreciate that changes in pulp space, size, and location affect an ideal access cavity. Teeth that are rotated or tilted present an additional challenge for the correct angulation of a bur during endodontic access.

Similarly, the fact that a full-coverage restoration is typically radiopaque and prevents a view of the pulp chamber in a radiograph complicates preparation of an access cavity.

Perhaps the most important factor in the etiology of an access perforation is misguided action of an end-cutting high-speed bur.

Prevention

Proper preoperative assessment and in-depth knowledge of root and root canal anatomy go hand in hand in preventing mishaps on access. An important step in the assessment is to encircle the tooth with a blunt explorer or a periodontal probe, before dental dam placement, in order to appreciate the cross-section at the cementoenamel junction (CEJ). It is this location, not the occlusal table, where the law of symmetry[19] is most relevant, and this determines which direction the access cavity is directed toward. Then it is useful to consider the largest, bulkiest pulp horn and initiate the access towards the space it creates in the pulp chamber (Fig 5-3). This is the most likely area in which a clinician will feel the often cited "drop" of the bur on access, in teeth with nonmineralized pulps.

Another important consideration is the depth in relation to bur length. Most access burs do not have length indicators, but it is useful to relate the location

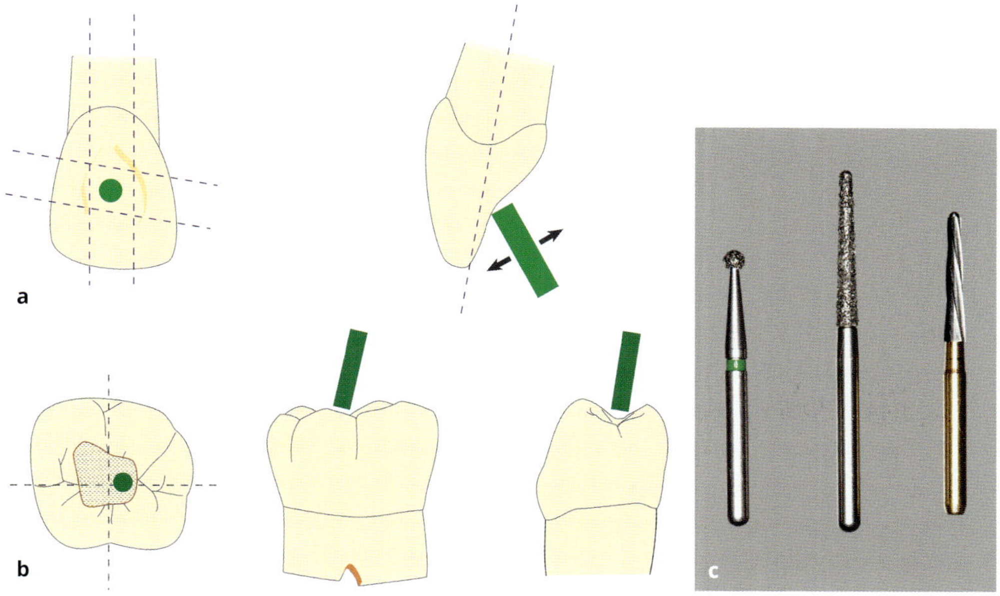

Fig 5-3 *(a and b)* Principles of access cavity preparation ensuring correct alignment in anterior teeth and molars. *(c)* The use of safety-ended burs such as the Endo bur *(right)* prevents furcal perforations.

of certain markings, such as the extent of the cutting surface to the size of the clinical crown. For example, it is well established for intact molars[20] that the distance from an occlusal reference point to the pulpal roof is about 5 to 6 mm, and the vertical extent of the pulp chamber is 1.5 to 2 mm. Again, the CEJ is an important marker as it is located at approximately the level of the pulpal floor. Measurements taken from the preoperative periapical radiograph with calibrated digital calipers help determine the distance of the pulp from occlusal landmarks.

A variety of burs have been recommended for access cavity preparation, and there is one property that is both useful and risky, namely end-cutting ability. Figure 5-3c shows typical burs used for initial access and refinement. Cylindrical long diamonds or fissure burs have been more effective compared to round burs. The Endo-Z bur (Dentsply Maillefer) has proven very useful for refinement, once an initial access into the pulp chamber has been made, due to its domed, non-cutting tip.[10]

Specific situations, such as zirconia restorations or those cast from nonprecious alloy, call for burs with specific cutting efficiency, and care must be taken not to jeopardize remaining tooth structure when using these burs.[21]

Management

Severe gouging with weakening of the remaining tooth structure may require steps to ensure that no crown fracture occurs in the temporary phase until a permanent crown can be placed. This may include reducing occlusal contacts or building the crown up with composite as a pre-endodontic restoration and then reaccessing. The buildup can be completed by closing the endodontic access cavity at the obturation appointment, with or without use of a fiber post.

The main goal when managing a perforation on access is to correctly diagnose and repair the damage as soon as possible. A perforation site may become contaminated via microbial leakage through a temporary restoration within days, and the outcome of any repair will be compromised[12] once a bacterial biofilm is established. Furthermore, it is important to know if the perforation occurs to a site that communicates with the periodontal ligament (PDL), eg, into the furcation or a marginal site; then, two possible avenues to manage a perforation may be considered, if the tooth is restorable:

1. Inclusion of the perforation site into a definitive restoration
2. Restoration of the perforation from the access cavity using appropriate biomaterials

A perforation to the marginal gingiva may be covered by placing a restoration margin more apically; however, the biologic width and any violations of it must be considered in this approach (Fig 5-4). If this is not possible due to the location of the defect, perforation repair involves placement of a calcium silicate material to seal the perforation site. This approach reportedly has a high success rate[23] if accomplished immediately after a perforation is recognized. A delayed repair may require local debridement and calcium hydroxide dressing to reduce microbial contamination.[24]

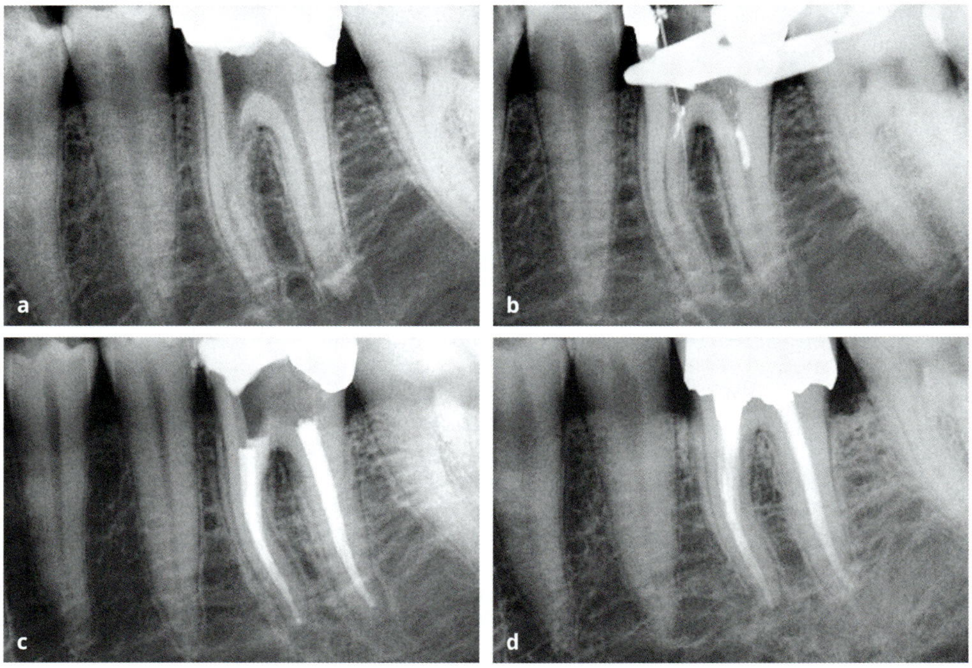

Fig 5-4 In an attempt to find the mesiobuccal canal, a perforation was made in the floor of the pulp chamber. *(a)* Preoperative radiograph. *(b)* A small file has been introduced in the bleeding area and has been connected to an electronic apex locator to confirm the diagnosis of a perforation. *(c)* Postoperative radiograph. The coronal portion of the mesial canal has been filled with mineral trioxide aggregate before obturating the apical part with warm gutta-percha. *(d)* Two-year recall. Case by Dr Arnaldo Castellucci. (Reprinted from Peters[22] with permission.)

For a fresh perforation, there is typically no need for a barrier material, eg, hydroxyapatite, collagen, or others; however, some clinicians may elect to place such a barrier in delayed repairs to ensure the repair material is contained within the perforation site. In aggregate, there is currently no sufficient evidence that the use of a barrier results in superior clinical outcomes.[12]

In summary, perforation on access is a single, irreversible, "catastrophic" event during root canal therapy that is known to reduce clinical outcomes. The best strategy is to use utmost care to prevent this mishap from occurring. If a perforation has been noted and it cannot be included in a restoration margin, repair with a calcium silicate–based material as soon as possible is the best course of action.

Shaping

Root canal preparation, or *shaping*, is the next step in the treatment sequence after access preparation. Procedural errors, collectively known as *canal transportation*,[25] are the basis for many issues that occur during shaping. There are, however, a number of distinct errors that exist in addition to transportation and its sequelae.

Similar to access cavity preparation, canal preparation benefits greatly from adequate diagnosis and treatment planning. A detailed understanding of the prevailing root and root canal anatomy and possible additional root formations, such as *radix entomolaris* or *paramolaris*, is of great importance to ensure that all canals present are treated.

Shaping mishaps can start with not preparing, and therefore not debriding, an overlooked root canal system. In consequence, healing of apical periodontitis is not predictable, as irritants will continue to be present at the periodontal ligament adjacent to the apical foramen. This is evident in the direct correlation of apical periodontitis associated with the mesiobuccal root when a second canal (MB2) is missed.[26]

Additionally, there is a range of issues that can occur during actual canal preparation, such as ledging, apical blockage or perforation, and instrument fracture. Shaping errors of various degrees of severity occur frequently in root canal treatment, specifically in curved canals.[27]

Assessment

Clinicians usually notice the presence of errors during canal preparation by clinical cues (eg, a file cannot reach the working length any more in a blocked or ledged canal). Another cue is a radiograph that reveals a perforation or a retained instrument fragment. The presence of such overt preparation errors may only become obvious in a recall radiograph and may be connected to pathosis such as chronic apical abscess or asymptomatic apical periodontitis.

The fact that a root canal preparation instrument has fractured and a fragment is lodged in the canal becomes evident on a radiograph but may also be noticed visually from the altered appearance of the instrument. Another situation that makes clinicians suspect a fracture is if a previously patent canal length suddenly appears blocked.

More subtle preparation errors such as ledges and dentin blocks may be unnoticed or considered as less relevant, even if they lead to short fill. This is especially true for vital teeth where the apical area is not microbially contaminated. However, ledges at midroot level (Fig 5-5) are often correlated with nonhealing apical periodontitis and overall poor outcomes.

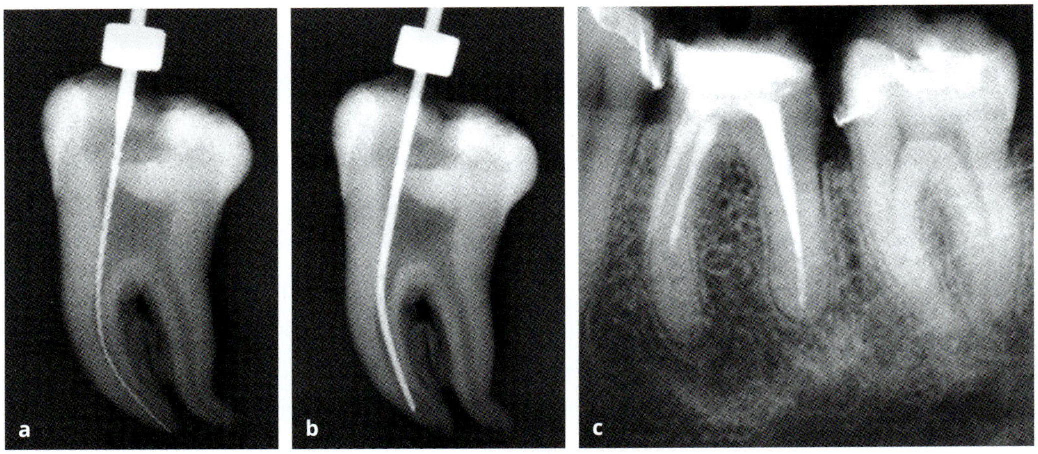

Fig 5-5 *(a and b)* Ledge formation at the beginning of the curvature associated with a marked loss of working length. *(c)* Clinical cases with ledge formation in the mesial root of a mandibular first molar. (Reprinted from Schäfer and Dammaschke[27] with permission.)

Etiology

In essence, typical shaping errors are the consequence of canal transportation—the unequal removal of radicular dentin in a curved canal. The laws of physics dictate that in a curve, an initially straight file will exert more force toward the outer curve apically and to the inner curve at midroot. In consequence, a corono-apical filing action, or translational movement, will tend to remove more dentin on the outside of the curve apically, and this causes canal straightening or transportation of the canal axis.[27] Such straightening also occurs more coronally on the inner curvature; Weine et al[28] described possible endpoints of this typical preparation error as ledge, zip and elbow, and apical perforation.

Perforations during shaping are thus an endpoint of transportation, with the additional complexity that the dentin wall is completely pierced, opening up a new artificial pathway for pathogens to drive changes in the PDL at that location. Root canal perforation can occur laterally with endodontic files or post drills or as long strip perforations in the furcation due to thinning of midroot dentin, as well as apically.

Root canal instruments are delicate and as such may fracture when used inappropriately. Small stainless-steel files typically fracture due to torsional loading at the very tip or through general overuse. Nickel-titanium (NiTi) rotaries are generally believed to fracture at a slightly higher rate than stainless-steel files, with an overall incidence of 2% to 5%.[29] The typical fracture mechanisms for NiTi instruments are described as torsional and flexural (fatigue) failure, which often occur in concert clinically.[30] These two mechanisms translate into overuse (fatigue failure) and excessive apical force (torsional failure).[25]

Prevention

Volumes have been published with approaches to prevent root canal preparation errors, yet no definite system has emerged that can both secure a sufficient preparation size and not in any way compromise radicular integrity. Short of that one ideal system, the following approaches have emerged that minimize canal transportation:

- Use flexible materials, such as heat treated NiTi.
- Design non-cutting tips.
- Select rotary/reciprocation movement over translational filing.
- Limit canal preparation size, depending on canal curvature.
- Follow a specific shaping sequence, ie, include orifice modification and glide path.

In any case and with any system, a specific preoperative analysis of tooth and canal anatomy is important to reduce the incidence of procedural events during shaping. For example, a small FOV CBCT scan gives clinicians the confidence not to miss an entire canal system.

Also, canal curvatures must be determined, particularly their angle, radius, and coronoapical location, prior to canal shaping. Developing and maintaining working length is simplified by using an apex locator. Most current recommendations include the demonstration of apical patency, the ability to extend a small (eg, size #8 or #10) K-file just beyond the apical foramen. While this patency file does not clean the apical foramen, it consistently demonstrates that no ledge or block formation has occurred. Maintaining patency helps reduce the chance of canal transportation.

Clearly, desired apical sizes must be adjusted to canal anatomy; the more curved (large angle, small radius), the more difficult it will be to limit canal transportation. A flexible instrument system and appropriate movement (eg, the balanced force technique for hand files) are important in this regard.

Management

Once canal blockage is suspected, the first important step is to determine the cause of the blockage. In case of a block or ledge, a radiograph can exclude the

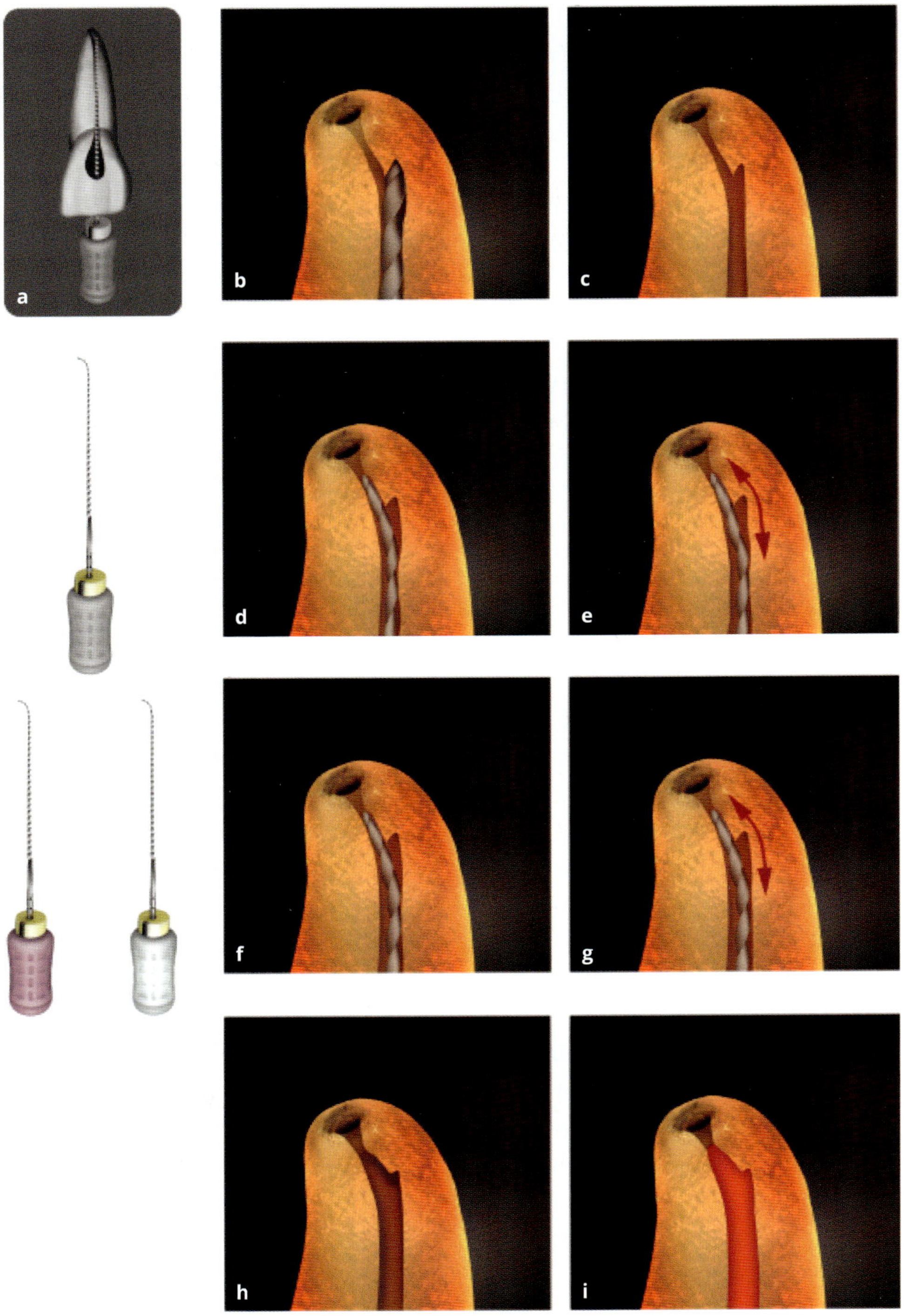

Fig 5-6 Correction of ledge. *(a)* Diagrammatic representation of the radiographic location of the ledge with the help of a small-sized endodontic instrument. Detail of the ledge with *(b)* and without *(c)* the instrument that caused it *(d to g)*. Pre-enlargement of the canal coronal to the ledge and initial bypassing of the ledge with a precurved size #8 K-file, followed by instrumentation up to the established working length with precurved files #10 and #15. Instrumentation with stainless-steel and/or rotary NiTi instruments incorporating the ledge *(h)* into the canal preparation and *(i)* obturation. (Reprinted from Lambrianidis[31] with permission.)

presence of an instrument fragment. For both ledge and block formation, specifically precurved hand files and a diligent manual technique are required (Fig 5-6).

Typically, a ledge gives the manual feedback of a hard stop, while a blockage with collagen and some dentin debris may allow a small penetration by a fine instrument tip, which then generates the impression of what has been termed *rubbery resistance*. To make matters more complicated, both ledge and block often occur concurrently, certainly once the clinician has worked in the area for some time.

Consequently, the approach to management is similar in both cases. A small and stiff file (eg, C-file [Lexicon, Dentsply Sirona]) will be precurved at the tip,[30] without creating a sharp kink (see Fig 5-6). The direction of the curve is marked with the indicator on the silicone stopper, and an effort is made to direct the curve away from the ledge. For example, curved mesial roots in mandibular molars with ledges will require the curve to point toward the distal and the center of the tooth, as the primary curve is toward the distal and the center of the root. It may be necessary to adjust the curve on the file and also to move the file gently into various positions to be able to bypass the ledge. It is imperative to irrigate and bring dentin chips in suspension in order to avoid blocking the canal space apical of the ledge.

Overcoming a confirmed block with collagen or dentin chips requires patience and precision and essentially uses the same approach to overcome the complication to the point that patency can be confirmed. However, the subsequent steps will vary because a ledge must be carefully smoothed out, either using precurved hand instruments or, with care, an engine-driven instrument. Once a blockage is removed, canal preparation may progress as usual.

In regard to instrument fracture, a careful benefit/risk assessment must be made before attempting to remove the fragment. As a general rule, any fragment that is lodged apical of the major curvature and is impossible to be visualized clinically should only be removed by a clinician with experience in this procedure[32] and with specific instruments and techniques.[33] The ultimate endodontic prognosis depends on the initial diagnosis and the extent of chemo-mechanical debridement before the fracture occurred.[29]

If the decision has been made to remove the fragment, the clinician can select from several techniques, all of which include visualization with the operating microscope.[34,35] While the approaches will vary, it is recommended to work with ultrasonic units to generate a graded amount of movement and energy that then dislodges the instrument fragment. Alternatively, a wire loop may be deployed[36] to grab a fragment. Most published cases that document instrument fragment removal show thinned out radicular walls; therefore, the best option in regard to instrument fracture is prevention.[37] Figure 5-7 details a contemporary clinical approach to fragment removal.[33]

In case of an intracanal perforation (as opposed to a perforation on access), elapsed time until repair as well as the size and location of the perforation play

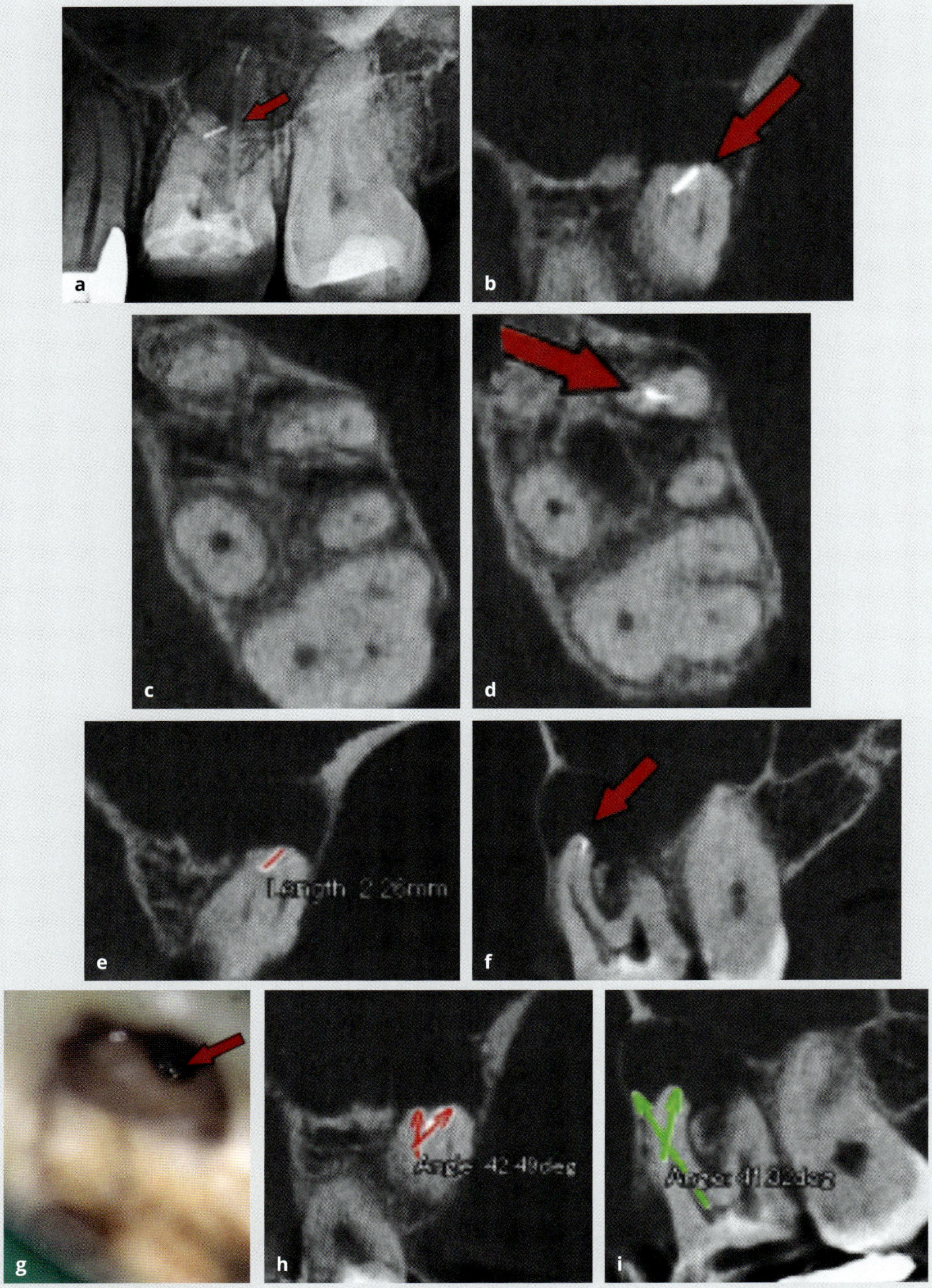

Fig 5-7 *(a)* A preoperative radiograph showing a separated file *(arrow)* in the mesiobuccal root of a maxillary left first molar. *(b)* A coronal CBCT image of the file fragment in the second mesiobuccal (MB2) canal *(arrow)*. *(c and d)* Axial CBCT images showing the location of file fragment in the MB2 canal where it merges with the first mesiobuccal canal in the apical third *(arrow)*. *(e)* A CBCT coronal view allowing the file fragment to be measured (2.26 mm). *(f)* A sagittal CBCT image of the large periapical lesion *(arrow)* associated with the mesiobuccal root elevating the sinus floor. *(g)* A magnified photograph of the separated file partially visible before ultrasonic cavity preparation. *(h)* A coronal CBCT image measuring the MB2 buccopalatal canal curvature at 42.49 degrees. *(i)* A sagittal CBCT image identifying the MB mesiodistal canal curvature at 41.32 degrees.

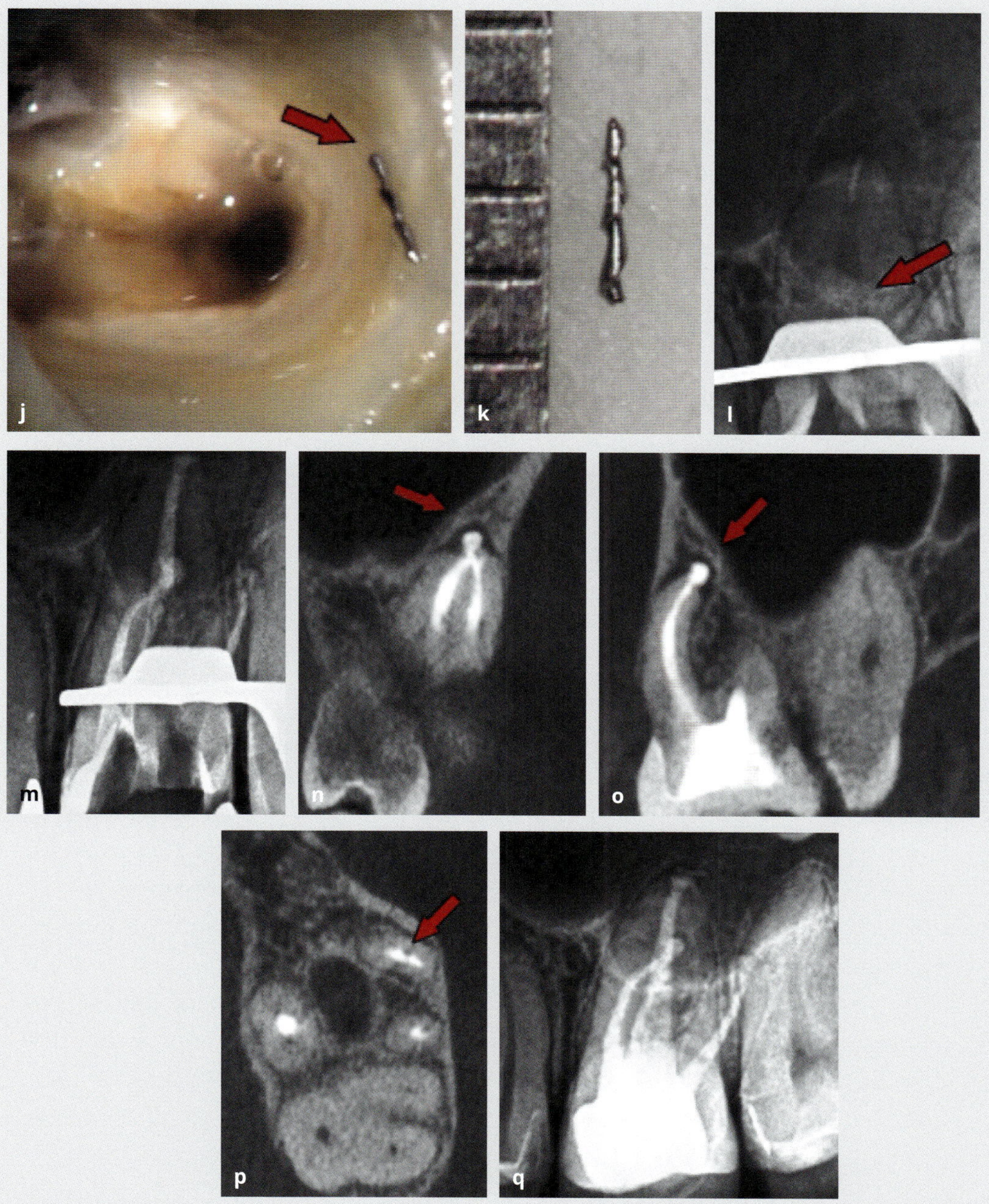

Fig 5-7 *(cont) (j)* A clinical photograph of the ultrasonically ejected file fragment *(arrow)* after removal with an ultrasonic tip at a low-power setting. *(k)* The extracted file fragment measuring 2.26 mm proximal to an endodontic ruler. *(l)* A periapical radiograph confirming the removal of the separated file from the MB2 canal. *(m)* A postoperative radiograph confirming mineral trioxide aggregate obturation of all canals. *(n and o)* Six-month coronal and sagittal CBCT images showing the repair of previous osseous defects *(arrows)*. *(p)* A 6-month axial CBCT image confirming obturation of the first mesiobuccal/MB2 canals *(arrow)*. *(q)* A 6-month postoperative radiograph showing remineralization of supporting bone. (Reprinted from Terauchi et al[33] with permission.)

a crucial role in treatment prognosis. Small lateral perforations in the apical area may be sealed, similar to overprepared apices, by using calcium silicate cement in conjunction with well-fitted gutta-percha points. Depending on the diameter of the artificial communication with periradicular tissues, a cold filling technique, such as lateral condensation, might prevent overfilling through a perforated apex better than warm filling techniques (see chapter 6 for mishaps during obturation). Micro instruments for root perforation repair with calcium silicate cement exist; these allow sealing from inside a root canal under magnification if the defect is visible and accessible. Increased area size of a perforation, eg, strip perforation versus lateral perforation, will heighten the risk of not sealing the site adequately.

If the perforation site is not accessible for repair with micro instruments from an intracoronal approach, endodontic microsurgery may be the method of choice to seal larger fenestrations of the root wall with calcium silicate cement, with or without apicoectomy.

Apical perforations are less likely to become contaminated from a periodontal pocket or the oral cavity than midroot or cervical perforations and therefore have a better outcome after repair.[6]

Irrigation

Assessment

A wide range of irrigation mishaps during root canal treatment has been reported, ranging from damage to patients' clothing to extrusion through a foramen or perforation site. Procedural events in irrigation further include emphysema and allergic reactions to the irrigant or inadvertent injection of an irrigant as an anesthetic solution.[38]

The guiding principle of contemporary root canal therapy is chemo-mechanical canal preparation, with the express goal of debriding the root canal space, that is, reducing microbial burden and removing pulp remnants. To achieve this, sodium hypochlorite is the main irrigant, due to its combination of antimicrobial and tissue-dissolving action.[1] The downside of this irrigant is its reactivity and toxicity in direct contact. Indeed, NaOCl is known for its bleaching effect, owing to the strong oxidation potential of the reactive chlorine ions. At the same time, chlorine is depleted when in contact with organic tissues. This is relevant when it is extruded, as its action is typically self-limiting depending on the concentration of the solution used.

Clinically, irrigation mishaps are often obvious, with sudden pain occurring during an otherwise uneventful root canal treatment, right after deposition of solution. There is typically profuse bleeding for the canal, and a swelling develops (Fig 5-8).[39] Either immediately or with delay, ecchymosis may develop. There have been case reports of nerve damage,[40] which in most cases resolved over time.

Hydrogen peroxide, when injected into periradicular tissues, may lead to accumulation of gas, a phenomenon known as *emphysema*. By itself, an emphysema

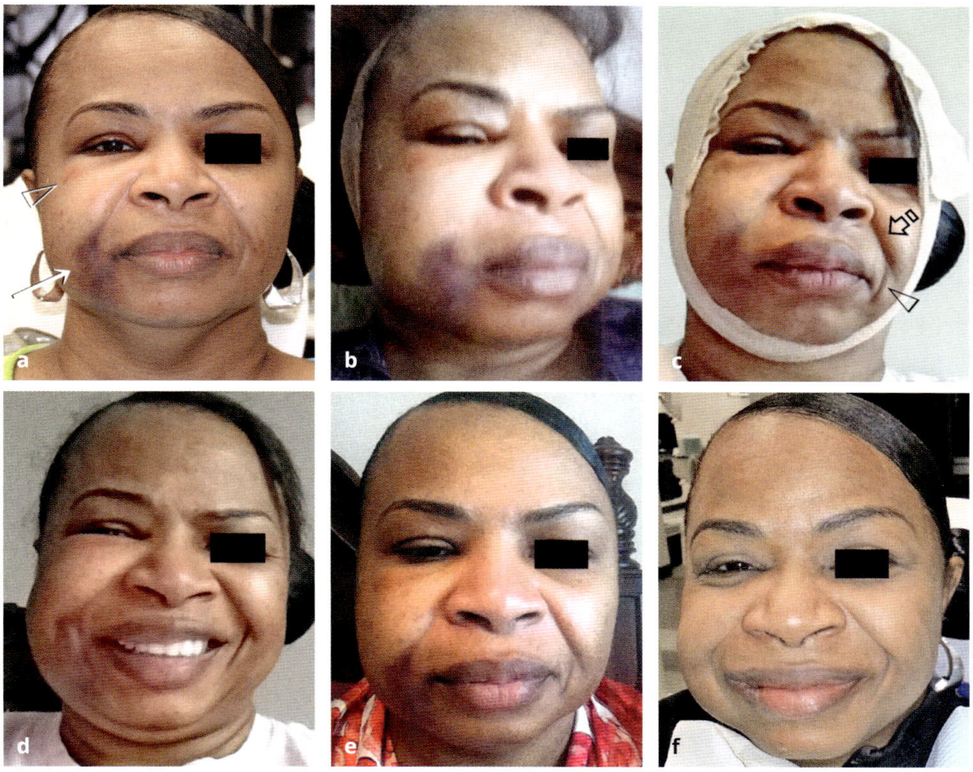

Fig 5-8 A classical sodium hypochlorite accident showing the time course of facial involvement from onset to resolution. *(a)* Immediately after removal of rubber dam. Ecchymosis visible along corner of the mouth *(arrow)* and lower eyelid *(open arrowhead)*. No facial edema. *(b)* Three hours after onset of the accident. *(c)* After 24 hours. Swelling resulted in the disappearance of the nasolabial fold *(open arrow)* as well as marionette lines *(open arrowhead)* on the right side of the face. *(d)* After 48 hours. *(e)* After 4 days. *(f)* After 3 weeks. (Reprinted from Zhu et al[39] with permission.)

will resolve after a few days. The possibility of embolism through an emphysema cannot be completely excluded[41]; however, there are no clinical cases documented for such an occurrence.

Allergy to an irrigation solution is another possible adverse event; published case reports[42] suggest that while an allergic reaction to sodium hypochlorite cannot be completely excluded, it is very rare.

Overall, irrigation incidents that are obvious and present with ecchymosis are an infrequent occurrence in root canal therapy.[39]

Etiology

The conditions inside the root canal system are different from other applications of disinfectants in terms of flow dynamics, in that the root canal space is small and has a natural opening to the surrounding tissues. The size of the irrigation needle is frequently similar to the canal diameter; therefore, there is a risk to wedge the needle into the canal, thus negating or greatly reducing the ability of excess solution to escape coronally.

It has been held that apical pressure counterbalances pressure that develops when irrigant is deposited into the canal space through a pressure-dependent mechanism.[39] Boutsioukis et al[43] argued differently and posited that it is in fact the low conductance provided by the apical canal portion that helps clinicians restrict irrigation to the confines of the root canal system.

Nonetheless, irrigation mishaps occur when there is *(1)* irrigant expressed into the canal space with limited opportunity for backflow and *(2)* an open pathway for the solution to escape the canal system. This pathway could be a foramen or a perforation. Indeed, a number of clinical case reports deal with the latter entity.[44]

Prevention

5

The key to the prevention of irrigation mishaps is to always allow irrigants to escape coronally when deposited.[39] Never must the irrigation needle be placed close to working length and then wedged into the canal. Rather, it is recommended to use a light grip and deposit the irrigant while freely moving the needle inside the canal. Forceful depression of the piston, especially when the needle binds inside the canal, should be avoided to minimize occurrence of overirrigation into the PDL. Using a rubber stopper or a bend of the needle to measure the insertion depth helps avoid expression of irrigants into the PDL.

Also, clinicians should be aware of the potential presence of perforations and wide-open foramina during root canal treatment.

Management

Once an irrigation incident is confirmed, the clinician should reassure the patient and may elect to irrigate with saline to dilute any remaining sodium hypochlorite. Further treatment of irrigation accidents is mainly symptomatic, with interventions such as medication with analgesics and symptomatic therapy such as cold compresses. In cases of expected or proven secondary infection, an antibiotic may be prescribed.[38] In either case, it is important to disclose the nature and extent of the injury and to monitor the posttreatment course appropriately.

Dressing Placement

In the multiple visit approach to root canal therapy, a medication such as calcium hydroxide ($Ca[OH]_2$) is placed into the canal. Because the medication is intended to reduce the microbial burden at the interface to the periodontal ligament, placement close to the apical foramen is desired.

The mode of action for $Ca(OH)_2$ is by pH elevation, clinically up to 12. This pH may be sustained for days and even weeks, and it essentially gives rise to a chemical burn, with potential tissue necrosis. This response is acceptable when $Ca(OH)_2$ is placed on the pulp for vital pulp therapy or in contact with bacteria, but it is potentially harmful in contact with nerve tissue.[45] Recently, there has been discussion in relation to $Ca(OH)_2$ overfills with subsequent permanent nerve damage.[46] According to the literature, the incidence of such mishaps is low when appropriate placement techniques are employed; however, case reports detail the serious consequences that may occur.

Assessment

Most commercial $Ca(OH)_2$ pastes contain a radio-opacifier so that the extent of the fill may be verified by a radiograph. Clinically, some patients, despite local anesthesia, may notice the overfill as a painful incident, but often this occurrence is not noted. If an overfill into a vulnerable structure is suspected, radiographic assessment, potentially including small FOV CBCT, is indicated (Fig 5-9).

In case of an unnoticed overfill into the nerve canal or close to it, the patient may experience altered nerve function within the time frame normally associated with weaning local anesthesia. A prudent clinician would want to review the case as soon as possible and obtain appropriate radiographs.[46]

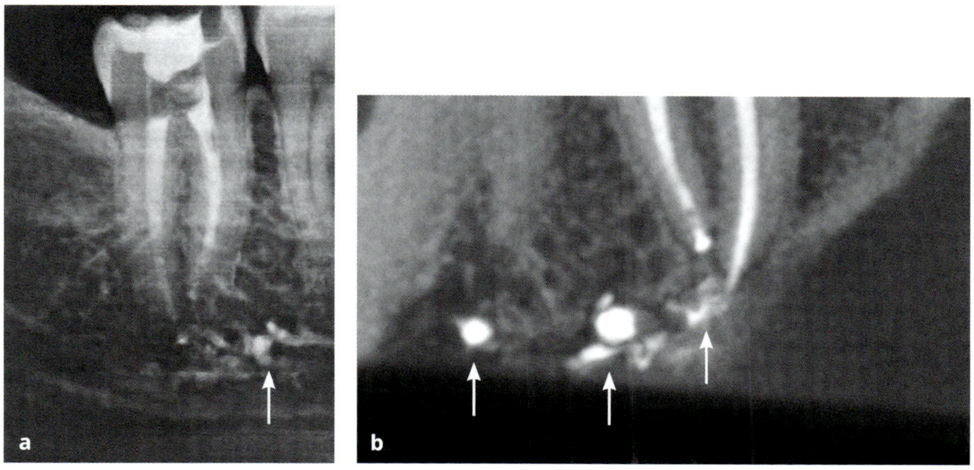

Fig 5-9 Radiographic appearance of overfill with $Ca(OH)_2$ *(arrows)* in *(a)* periapical film and *(b)* small FOV CBCT.

Etiology

Extrusion of $Ca(OH)_2$ into the periapical tissues may occur when there is a patent canal pathway and undue pressure is applied, for example, with products designed for syringe delivery. It is currently not clear which consistency is preferrable; however, cases of extrusion seem to occur more frequently when clinicians try specifically to place medication as apically as possible.

The mechanism of action of $Ca(OH)_2$ on neural tissue is likely not specific but rather a chemical burn,[45,46] resulting in a zone of necrosis and protein denaturation. Neural tissues, within days after contact, develop changes that are similar to signs of so-called "Wallerian degeneration," which describes the interruption of nerve cell bodies leading to cell death.[47]

Prevention

Similar to other mishaps, but perhaps even more importantly for $Ca(OH)_2$ overfills, prevention is important. Clinicians should select a safe placement method to a safe location, that is lentulo spiral and 2 to 3 mm short of working length.[48] Deposition of $Ca(OH)_2$ paste with a syringe or needle system is effective but appears to carry a higher risk of overfills.

Management

Once slow-dissolving $Ca(OH)_2$ is present in tissue, high pH may be present for an extended period of time. As mentioned before, this is damaging to nerve structure, and therefore, a timely (ideally within 48 hours) removal of the paste is indicated.[49] Occasionally, it is possible to remove or dilute the paste via an intracanal approach, but in case of demonstrated nerve damage, early surgical removal is favorable,[46] while delayed surgery does not result in return of nerve function in many cases.[50] There is insufficient evidence to suggest that medication with steroids or vitamin supplements has any benefits after nerve damage associated with $Ca(OH)_2$ extrusion. In case of permanent nerve damage and dysesthesia, further management beyond surgical decompression may include pain specialists and pharmacologic therapy.[51]

Thermal Injury

There are several procedures in root canal treatment that can create potentially damaging temperatures in the periodontal ligament, such as thermoplastic obturation (see chapter 6 for more details) and ultrasonic activation. The threshold temperature beyond which bone damage occurs is believed to be 47°C.[52] Temperatures as high as this and even higher may be reached clinically, for example, during an attempt to remove a metal post with prolonged ultrasonic activation. Consequently, heat injury may result in bone necrosis and significant alterations of the soft tissues.[53,54]

Another procedure that could cause heat-related injuries of the PDL is intracanal heating of irrigation solutions with a System B Heat Source (Kerr Dental).[55] Temperatures close to the critical threshold of 47°C may be reached during this procedure, higher than those described for ultrasonic activation of irrigant solution[56]; however, there are presently no cases reported that suggest permanent injuries.

Overall, heat-related injuries in root canal treatment are rare, but the consequences if they do occur are severe.

Assessment

During treatment, patients and clinicians alike may not immediately notice any effect from ultrasonic-related burns. Some patients have reported significant discomfort during and after heat-related injuries. Alterations in gingiva

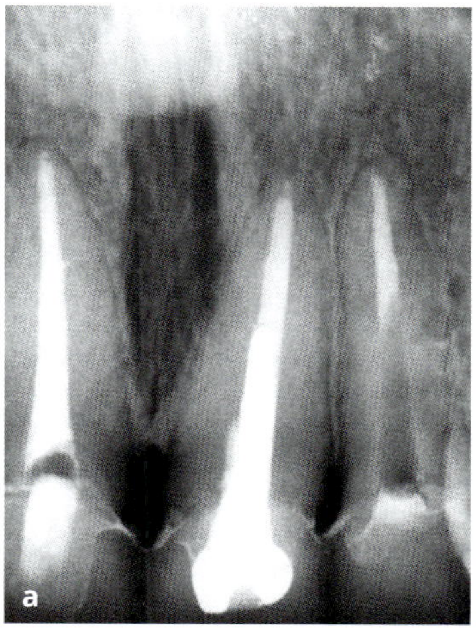

Fig 5-10 *(a)* Preoperative radiograph of a metal post in tooth no. 9. *(b)* Postoperative photograph showing burn injuries to tooth no. 9 and its supporting structures that occurred during heat transfer. *(c)* The tooth was extracted 48 hours after injury took place. *(d)* Extracted tooth shows an absence of viable attachment to the apical one-third of the root. (Reprinted from Gluskin et al[53] with permission.)

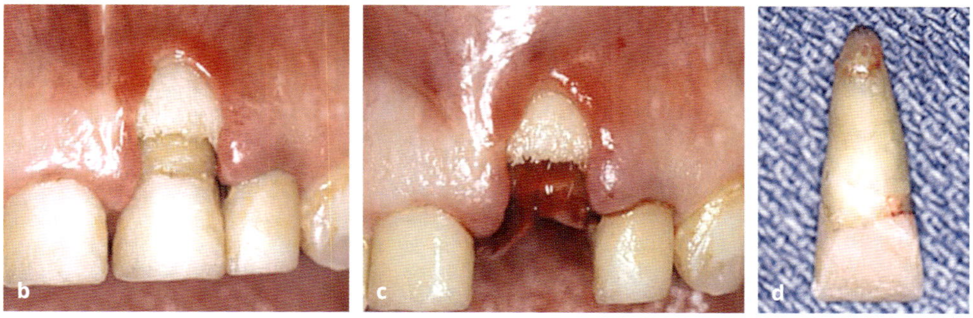

appearance and sloughing of tissue will occur over weeks and ultimately lead to a denuded appearance and mobility (Fig 5-10).

Etiology

The use of ultrasonically powered instruments on metal posts, particularly if continuously activated, introduces significant heat energy into the periodontal ligament and alveolar bone.[57] The energy is dissipated in an area that is close to the source (the ultrasonic tip via the post) and not insulated. Therefore, the facial bone and soft tissue are most affected. According to data reported on rabbits, heating bone to 50°C for 1 minute or 47°C for 5 minutes leads to resorption and replacement with fat cells.[57]

Prevention

The energy transmission during ultrasonically powered post removal may be mitigated by water cooling or by the use of refrigerant spray applied to the post.[58] At a minimum, the time of continuous activation should be monitored, and the temperature of the tip checked. According to in vitro data, there is no relationship between root wall thickness and heat transmission,[59] but heat transfer may be greater in anterior teeth compared to posterior. Regardless, an important step in the prevention of heat-related injuries is adequate planning of the post removal procedure, as most case reports of heat-related injuries detail prolonged attempts at removal.

Management

For suspected initial heat damage, symptomatic therapy (eg, analgesics) may be appropriate. In one case, a gingival graft was considered.[54] Unfortunately, once heat-associated bone necrosis is confirmed, the bone segment and associated teeth will likely have to be removed.[53] Several procedures, including distraction osteogenesis and block grafting, have been proposed to repair a functional and esthetically problematic defect (see Fig 5-10).

5

References

1. Peters OA, Peters CI, Basrani B. Cleaning and shaping of the root canal system. In: Berman LH, Hargreaves KH (eds). Pathways of the Pulp, ed 12. St Louis: Elsevier, 2021:236–303.
2. Mainkar A, Kim SG. Diagnostic accuracy of 5 dental pulp tests: A systematic review and meta-analysis. J Endod 2018;44:694–702.
3. Sirotheau Corrêa Pontes F, Paiva Fonseca F, Souza de Jesus A, et al. Nonendodontic lesions misdiagnosed as apical periodontitis lesions: series of case reports and review of literature. J Endod 2014;40:16–27.
4. Wright S, Ucer TC, Crofts G. The adaption and implementation of the WHO Surgical Safety Checklist for dental procedures. Br Dent J 2018;225:727–729.
5. Farzaneh M, Abitbol S, Friedman S. Treatment outcome in endodontics: The Toronto study. Phases I and II: Orthograde retreatment. J Endod 2004;30:627–633.
6. Fuss Z, Trope M. Root perforations: Classification and treatment choices based on prognostic factors. Endod Dent Traumatol 1996;12:255–264.
7. Sarao SK, Berlin-Broner Y, Levin L. Occurrence and risk factors of dental root perforations: A systematic review. Int Dent J 2020;71:96–105.
8. AAE Endodontic Case Difficulty Assessment Form and Guidelines. https://www.aae.org/specialty/wp-content/uploads/sites/2/2022/01/CaseDifficultyAssessmentFormFINAL2022.pdf. Accessed 31 January 2023.
9. AAE Case Assessment Tools 2020. https://www.aae.org/specialty/clinical-resources/treatment-planning/case-assessment-tools/. Accessed 23 September 2022.
10. Peters OA. Accessing root canal systems: Knowledge base and clinical techniques. Endodontic Practice Today (ENDO) (London) 2008;2:87–104.
11. Saed SM, Ashley MP, Darcey J. Root perforations: Aetiology, management strategies and outcomes. The hole truth. Br Dent J 2016;220:171–180.
12. Clauder T, Shin SJ. Repair of perforations with MTA: Clinical applications and mechanisms of action. Endod Topics 2009;15:32–55.
13. Alhadainy HA. Root perforations. A review of literature. Oral Surg Oral Med Oral Pathol 1994;78:368–374.
14. Christofzik DW, Glandorf P, Conrad J, Fawzy El-Sayed KM, Größner-Schreiber B, Dörfer CE. 2D radiographs, cone-beam computed tomography and 3D CBCT-based planning software in access cavity preparation: A single blinded randomised controlled in vitro study. Aust Endod J 2022;48:283–296.
15. Bóveda C, Kishen A. Contracted endodontic cavities: The foundation for less invasive alternatives in the management of apical periodontitis. Endod Topics 2015;33:169–186.
16. Gluskin AH, Peters CI, Peters OA. Minimally invasive endodontics: Challenging prevailing paradigms. Br Dent J 2014;216:347–353.
17. Reeh ES, Douglas WH, Messer HH. Stiffness of endodontically-treated teeth related to restoration technique. J Dent Res 1989;68:1540–1544.
18. Ng YL, Mann V, Gulabivala K. Tooth survival following non-surgical root canal treatment: A systematic review of the literature. Int Endod J 2010;43:171–189.
19. Krasner P, Rankow HJ. Anatomy of the pulp-chamber floor. J Endod 2004;30:5–16.
20. Deutsch AS, Musikant BL. Morphological measurements of anatomic landmarks in human maxillary and mandibular molar pulp chambers. J Endod 2004;30:388–390.
21. Peters OA, Du D, Ho MY, Chu R, Moule A. Assessing the cutting efficiency of different burs on zirconia substrate. Aust Endod J 2019;45:289–297.
22. Peters OA (ed). The Guidebook to Molar Endodontics. Berlin: Springer, 2017.
23. Bargholz C. Perforation repair with mineral trioxide aggregate: A modified matrix concept. Int Endod J 2005;38:59–69.
24. Ford TR, Torabinejad M, McKendry DJ, Hong CU, Kariyawasam SP. Use of mineral trioxide aggregate for repair of furcal perforations. Oral Surg Oral Med Oral Pathol Oral Radiol Endod 1995;79:756–763.

25. Peters OA. Current challenges and concepts in the preparation of root canal systems: A review. J Endod 2004;30:559–567.
26. Karabucak B, Bunes A, Chehoud C, Kohli MR, Setzer F. Prevalence of apical periodontitis in endodontically treated premolars and molars with untreated canal: A cone-beam computed tomography study. J Endod 2016;42:538–541.
27. Schäfer E, Dammaschke T. Development and sequelae of canal transportation. Endod Topics 2009;15:75–90.
28. Weine FS, Kelly RF, Lio PJ. The effect of preparation procedures on original canal shape and on apical foramen shape. J Endod 1975;1:255–262.
29. Parashos P, Messer HH. Rotary NiTi instrument fracture and its consequences. J Endod 2006;32:1031–1043.
30. Ullmann CJ, Peters OA. Effect of cyclic fatigue on static fracture loads in ProTaper nickel-titanium rotary instruments. J Endod 2005;31:183–186.
31. Lambrianidis T. Ledging and blockage of root canals during canal preparation: Causes, recognition, prevention, management, and outcomes. Endod Topics 2009;15:56–74.
32. Ward JR, Parashos P, Messer HH. Evaluation of an ultrasonic technique to remove fractured rotary nickel-titanium endodontic instruments from root canals: Clinical cases. J Endod 2003;29:764–767.
33. Terauchi Y, Sexton C, Bakland LK, Bogen G. Factors affecting the removal time of separated instruments. J Endod 2021;47:1245–1252.
34. Terauchi Y. Separated file removal. Dent Today 2012;31:108,110–113.
35. Ruddle CJ. Nonsurgical endodontic retreatment. J Calif Dent Assoc 2004;32:474–484.
36. Cheung GSP. Instrument fracture: Mechanisms, removal of fragments, and clinical outcomes. Endod Topics 2009;16:1–26.
37. Di Fiore PM. A dozen ways to prevent nickel-titanium rotary instrument fracture. J Am Dent Assoc 2007;138:196–201.
38. Hülsmann M, Hahn W. Complications during root canal irrigation—Literature review and case reports. Int Endod J 2000;33:186–193.
39. Zhu WC, Gyamfi J, Liu N, et al. Anatomy of sodium hypochlorite accidents involving facial ecchymosis—A review. J Dent 2013;41:935–948.
40. Becking AG. Complications in the use of sodium hypochlorite during endodontic treatment. Report of three cases. Oral Surg Oral Med Oral Pathol 1991;71:346–348.
41. Rickles NH, Joshi BA. A possible case in a human and an investigation in dogs of death from air embolism during root canal therapy. J Am Dent Assoc 1963;67:397–404.
42. Kaufman AY, Keila S. Hypersensitivity to sodium hypochlorite. J Endod 1989;15:224–246.
43. Boutsioukis C, Psimma Z, van der Sluis LWM. Factors affecting irrigant extrusion during root canal irrigation: A systematic review. Int Endod J 2013;46:599–618.
44. Hatton J, Walsh S, Wilson A. Management of the sodium hypochlorite accident: A rare but significant complication of root canal treatment. BMJ Case Rep 2015;2015:bcr2014207480.
45. Brodin P, Orstavik D. Effects of therapeutic and pulp protecting materials on nerve transmission in vitro. Scand J Dent Res 1983;91:46–50.
46. Gluskin AH, Lai G, Peters CI, Peters OA. The double-edged sword of calcium hydroxide in endodontics: Precautions and preventive strategies for extrusion injuries into neurovascular anatomy. J Am Dent Assoc 2020;151:317–326.
47. Nakamura C, Tomida M, Hasegawa H, Kawakami T. Injury and the recovery reaction due to the penetration of material into the mandibular canal. In: Kawakami T (ed). Pathological Basis of Root Canal Restoration: Using Calcium Hydroxide Paste. Tokyo: IDP, 2021:39–51.
48. Lai GS, Davis S, Gluskin AH, Peters CI, Peters OA. Comparison of calcium hydroxide extrusion with syringe vs spiral filler delivery: A pilot study. Aust Endod J 2021;47:408–414.
49. Pogrel MA. Damage to the inferior alveolar nerve as the result of root canal therapy. J Am Dent Assoc 2007;138:65–69.
50. Byun SH, Kim SS, Chung HJ, et al. Surgical management of damaged inferior alveolar nerve caused by endodontic overfilling of calcium hydroxide paste. Int Endod J 2016;49:1020–1029.
51. Rosen E. The diagnosis and management of nerve injury during endodontic treatment. Evid Based Endod 2017;2:7.
52. Eriksson AR, Albrektsson T. Temperature threshold levels for heat-induced bone tissue injury: A vital-microscopic study in the rabbit. J Prosthet Dent 1983;50:101–117.
53. Gluskin AH, Ruddle CJ, Zinman EJ. Thermal injury through intraradicular heat transfer using ultrasonic devices: Precautions and practical preventive strategies. J Am Dent Assoc 2005;136:1286–1293.
54. Walters JD, Rawal SY. Severe periodontal damage by an ultrasonic endodontic device: A case report. Dent Traumatol 2007;23:123–127.
55. Iandolo A, Amato M, Dagna A, et al. Intracanal heating of sodium hypochlorite: Scanning electron microscope evaluation of root canal walls. J Conserv Dent 2018;21:569–573.

56. Zeltner M, Peters OA, Paqué F. Temperature changes during ultrasonic irrigation with different inserts and modes of activation. J Endod 2009;35:573–577.
57. Ettrich CA, Labossière PE, Pitts DL, Johnson JD. An investigation of the heat induced during ultrasonic post removal. J Endod 2007;33:1222–1226.
58. Davis S, Gluskin AH, Livingood PM, Chambers DW. Analysis of temperature rise and the use of coolants in the dissipation of ultrasonic heat buildup during post removal. J Endod 2010;36:1892–1896.
59. Horan BB, Tordik PA, Imamura G, Goodell GG. Effect of dentin thickness on root surface temperature of teeth undergoing ultrasonic removal of posts. J Endod 2008;34:453–455.

6

Errors During Obturation of the Root Canal System

YUJIE HUANG
MOHAMMAD SABETI
MAHMOUD TORABINEJAD

Objectives

After reading this chapter, the reader should be able to:

1. Discuss how obturation contributes to the overall success of root canal treatment.
2. Enumerate common types of obturation techniques and materials.
3. State advantages and disadvantages of each type of technique and material.
4. Enumerate the common mishaps and their possible causes during obturation.
5. Discuss causes and management of mishaps during obturation.
6. Discuss the effects of mishaps during obturation on prognosis of root canal treatment.

Objectives of Obturation in Root Canal Treatment

The aim of nonsurgical root canal treatment (NSRCT) is to prevent and treat apical periodontitis, with the objective of eliminating diseased pulpal tissue and microorganisms with chemomechanical debridement. Subsequently, the instrumented canal space needs to be filled with root filling materials and sealers to prevent reinfection. The purpose of obturation during root canal treatment is to prevent microorganisms from reentering the root canal system and to entomb the remaining microorganisms in the dentinal tubules.

Obturation should be a straightforward step during a successful root canal treatment if the root canal system is appropriately prepared. However, certain errors as a result of improper instrumentation and preparation can happen at this stage. Lack of proper fitting of the obturating material, poor length control, and production of voids are usually associated with poor outcomes. Root canal–treated teeth with periapical pathosis and defects in obturation have 20% more nonhealing outcomes compared to adequately obturated root canals with a similar periapical diagnosis.[1]

Why to Obturate

Causes of endodontic failure

Poor obturation has been reported as one of the major prognostic factors of nonhealing outcomes in NSRCT.[2,3] According to the Washington study, 58.66% of the failures of endodontic treatments were caused by incomplete obturation of the canal, which was far more significant than other factors such as perforation, external root resorption, or coexistence of periodontal-periradicular lesions.[4] This is mainly because the quality of an obturation often reflects a clinician's treatment abilities and attention to the finer details. It may be argued that obturation is the culmination of the root canal treatment and the only part of the treatment that is visible on radiographs. However, the poor quality of obturation or mishaps during obturation were not usually isolated incidents, and they were likely to be consequences of inappropriate access preparation, cleaning, or shaping of root canals. Thus, a poor obturation may lead to a poor endodontic outcome and demonstrates a lack of attention to the art and science of endodontics.

Hollow tube theory

The concept of sealing the root canal system was originally driven by the hollow tube theory proposed by Rickert and Dixon.[5] This theory suggested that an empty space with an open end within a living organism tends to fill with tissue fluids and hence evokes inflammation. This theory was based on observations in experimental animals that when hollow plastic tubes were implanted, inflammatory response was seen at both ends of the tube. Therefore, to prevent inflammation, both ends of the tube must be sealed. The hollow tube theory was refuted by Torneck, who showed no inflammation at the open ends of the implanted tubes when they were sterile,[6] and Klevant and Eggink, who demonstrated that stagnant tissue fluid and necrotic tissue without bacterial contamination did not cause severe inflammation.[7]

Effect of obturation on root canal outcome

Although the hollow tube theory no longer stands, the concept of obturating the root canal system is still believed to be essential for the success of root canal treatment. Prior to obturation, the microorganisms and diseased tissue in the root canal system are removed by instrumentation and irrigation. Peters et al demonstrated that at least 35% of root canals were untouched regardless of the technique used during cleaning and shaping of root canals.[8] The anatomical complexity of the root canal system, such as the presence of isthmus and lateral canals, and the organization of the flora as biofilms impose serious challenges to disinfecting root canals by contemporary armamentaria and techniques. Even with the most rigorous cleaning and shaping protocols, it is impossible to completely clean the entire canal space. The remaining microorganisms may cause reinfection of root canals and periapical tissues later if the root canals are left unfilled. Among six biologic factors—*(1)* intraradicular infection persisting in the complex apical root canal system; *(2)* extraradicular infection, generally in the form of periapical actinomycosis; *(3)* extruded root canal filling or other exogenous materials that cause a foreign body reaction; *(4)* accumulation of endogenous cholesterol crystals that irritate periapical tissues; *(5)* true cystic lesions; and *(6)* scar tissue healing of the periapex—Nair concluded that the residual microbes in the apical portion of the root canal system were the major cause of apical periodontitis persisting posttreatment in both poorly and properly treated cases.[9]

Importance of coronal seal on root canal outcome

Obturation, as a critical step in root canal treatment, is arguably an effective strategy to prevent reinfection of the root canal system. In an animal study, Sabeti et al compared the healing of instrumented and obturated canals versus instrumented and nonobturated root canal systems with apical periodontitis. In their study, it was shown there was no difference in periapical healing in teeth with and without obturation, if the coronal seal of the sterile canal was appropriately maintained.[10] Fabricius et al used monkey teeth to demonstrate that apical healing occurred independently of the quality of the root filling when no bacteria remained in root canals. In contrast, when bacteria remained, there was a greater correlation with nonhealing in poor-quality obturation than in technically well-performed obturation.[11]

The goals of root canal therapy are to completely disinfect root canals, obturate the root canal system in three dimensions, and obtain a hermetic coronal seal following the completion of root canal treatment. Regardless of the quality of obturation, if the coronal portion of the tooth is not appropriately sealed, the microorganisms will invade the root canal system in a short period of time.[12]

The adequate coronal seal prevents saliva, bacteria, and bacterial byproducts in the oral cavity from contaminating the root canal system and invading the periradicular tissues.

In 1961, Marshall and Massler drew attention to the effect of coronal leakage in root-filled teeth. They suggested sealers were essential for effective root canal obturation, and they were also concerned about the overall seal of the root canal if the seal was broken coronally. Using a radioactive tracer, they showed coronal leakage occurred despite the presence of a coronal dressing.[13]

Length of time for contamination of obturated canals

Swanson and Madison were the first to evaluate the length of time the obturation material could be contaminated by artificial saliva with compromised coronal seal. They exposed the coronal portion of the obturated root canals to artificial saliva for various time periods. They found the tracer dye could penetrate from 79% to 85% of the root length in all exposed specimens after 3 days of exposure.[14] Later in 1988, Madison and Wilcox confirmed exposure of root canals to the oral cavity allowed coronal leakage to occur and in some cases along the whole length of the root canals.[15] In 1990, Torabinejad et al used two species of bacteria, *Staphylococcus epidermidis* and *Proteus vulgaris*, to evaluate the coronal leakage of obturated teeth; 80% of root canals were completely contaminated within 30 days of exposure to *S epidermidis* and 85% within 66 days of exposure to *P vulgaris*.[12] Magura et al examined the coronal leakage of human saliva in obturated root canal systems through histologic examination and dye penetrations. They reported that saliva penetration at 3 months was significantly greater than at the four earlier study periods of 2, 7, 14, and 28 days. They recommended to retreat the root canals that have been exposed to the oral cavity for longer than 3 months before placement of a permanent coronal restoration. They also challenged the findings of Madison et al, who had concluded that retreatment should be considered if the obturated canal was exposed to the oral environment for more than 3 days. Their rationale was that aqueous solutions have been shown to penetrate farther than viscous saliva, and dye studies might give inflated values for leakage.[16] Khayat et al studied the length of time for bacteria present in natural human saliva to penetrate through the entire root canal system obturated by lateral and vertical condensation techniques. They reported that root canals were contaminated in less than 30 days and that there was no statistical significance between lateral and vertical condensation techniques.[17]

Quality of coronal seal vs quality of obturation

In 1995, Ray and Trope evaluated the influence of the quality of coronal restoration versus the quality of endodontic treatment for apical periodontal health. Their study showed that patients with adequate restoration and inadequate root canal treatment have higher odds of preserving periapical health compared to patients with inadequate restoration and adequate root canal treatment.[18] This study cast doubt on the importance of canal obturation in creating a barrier against reinfection. However, soon after the Ray and Trope study, Tronstad et al reported an opposite result from their study: that the technical quality of the endodontic treatment as judged radiographically was significantly more important than the technical quality of the coronal restoration when the periapical status of endodontically treated teeth was evaluated.[19] Even with the presence of debates on the importance of obturation versus other factors among endodontic and restorative procedures, the adequate 3D obturation of root canals remains one of the major technical objectives of NSRCT.

When to Obturate

The timing involved with obturation raises the issue of single versus multiple visits for treatment. Selecting between single- and multiple-visit root canal treatment is determined by several biologic, clinical, and technical factors.

Pulp and periapical diagnosis

Pulpal and periapical diagnoses assist the clinician in deciding between single- and multiple-visit root canal treatment. For teeth diagnosed with pulpitis, a single-visit approach may be appropriate. Histologic evidence has shown that teeth diagnosed with pulpitis often only have the coronal portion of pulp tissue infected, and the pulp tissue in the majority of the apical portion of root canals remains uncontaminated.[20,21] Thus, a single-visit approach can allow for greater efficiency in care. For teeth diagnosed with pulp necrosis, even after optimal cleaning and shaping, a small load of microorganisms is likely to remain within the root canal system. In this case, multiple-visit treatment allows interappointment medication like calcium hydroxide ($Ca[OH]_2$) to further disinfect the canals and facilitate apical healing.[22] However, the efficacy of each approach remains controversial at present.

Clinical signs and symptoms

The decision regarding when to obturate is also related to clinical findings, such as the size of periapical lesion, the presence of swelling, the presence of sinus tracts, and the degree of periodontal involvement.[23] Multiple-visit treatment allows providers to assess the effects of treatment on symptom resolution as well as to observe the signs of soft and hard tissue healing. If necessary, more rounds of intracanal medicaments could be applied prior to the obturation of root canals.[24]

Degree of difficulty of the case

Certain preoperative factors such as canal calcifications, broken instruments, or complex anatomy may significantly increase the time of endodontic procedures and thereby preclude single-visit root canal treatment. Obturation should only be carried out after thorough chemomechanical debridement and when the canals are dry. If a dry and clean root canal system that is free from blood or exudate cannot be achieved, then the suggested course of action would be to place an interappointment medicament for a future appointment.[25]

Patient management issues and logistic concerns

Medically comprised patients who are unable to tolerate long procedures or patients with limited mouth opening also may require multiple visits to achieve the objectives of root canal treatment. Patients with symptomatic irreversible pulpitis with a difficulty to achieve pulp anesthesia may also require interappointment medicament and completion of root canal treatment at another appointment.[26,27]

Where to Obturate

To obtain the optimal endodontic outcome and minimize postoperative complications, the obturation material should be placed anywhere between the apical constriction and the anatomical apex. Oftentimes, the radiographic apex and the anatomical apex do not coincide. By using microcomputed tomography, ElAyouti et al showed that the mean distance between apical constriction and apical foramen was 0.2 mm, and the mean distance from apical constriction to apex was 0.9 mm.[28] The consensus is that the ideal obturation material should be confined in the root canal system, 0.5 to 1 mm short of the radiographic apex without any void in three dimensions.[29]

For many decades, the concepts of *overfill* or *underfill* and *overextension* or *underextension* have been subjects of controversy.[30] Schilder contended that the terms *over-* and *underextension* are references to vertical dimensions of obturation, whereas *overfilling* refers to a properly sealed root canal system, and *underfilling* refers to inadequately obturated root canals in any dimension.[31] Clearly, these academic distinctions could not be substantiated solely based on a 2D radiographic image. There is currently no evidence-based information to differentiate these academic terminologies or to justify the preference of one over another. Any obturation beyond or critically short of the apical constriction or any voids throughout the root canal system would deem the treatment inadequate and cast doubt on the clinician's ability to perform quality root canal treatment.[32]

Mishaps: Determining canal length and preparation

As mentioned earlier, it is considered good clinical practice to contain all dental materials within the root canal system. Many authors have attributed poor outcomes to overfilling > 2 mm beyond the apical constriction.[33–36]

Working length determination

Many techniques have been suggested to help identify where this apical constriction actually is. These include 2D radiographs, an electronic apex locator, CBCT image(s), paper points after canal preparation,[37,38] and, at times, a combination of all the above for a more accurate determination.

Electronic apex locators use an electrical circuit through the patient's root canal and oral tissues to determine the location of the apical foramen. Using an apex locator for length determination has been an important advancement in modern endodontics. The technique is highly reliable and accurate and minimizes any unnecessary radiation.[39] Nevertheless, there are several reasons that may cause an electronic apex locator to give inaccurate or nonreproducible readings.[29,40,41] Fluid within the canal can sometimes interfere with the readings, so it is recommended to dry the canal and make sure it is free of sodium hypochlorite, ethylenediaminetetraacetic acid (EDTA), or pus before using the apex locator.[40] If the canal is too large, attaching an apex locator to a small-sized file such as a #10 K-file may render an inaccurate reading as well. A large-sized file should be used until a steady reading is achieved.

The paper point can also be used as a tool to verify the working length upon the completion of cleaning and shaping of canals.[42] After using paper points to completely dry the canal, a new paper point with smaller apical size than master apical size can be inserted slightly beyond the estimated working length. If the canal is patent, the paper point will pick up some body fluid or blood to create a wet/dry interface. Then, the length of paper point from the reference point to the wet/dry interface can be measured to confirm whether the length coincides with the estimated working length.

For years, the routine method has been exposing a periapical radiograph to determine the working length. However, electronic apex locators have been equally advantageous, if not superior to radiographs, because they use no radiation.[43,44] It is always a good idea to confirm the working length using the electronic apex locator or paper point technique with radiographs to avoid mishaps (Fig 6-1). Recently, artificial intelligence (AI) has been used to determine working length in endodontics and more precisely locate the apical constriction/foramen.[45] Saghiri et al used AI in a human cadaver model and reported that AI measurements were the same as the actual measurements and were superior to the periapical radiographs.[46] The future clinical use of this technique remains unknown at this point. However, it has the possibility of being superior to the current approaches.

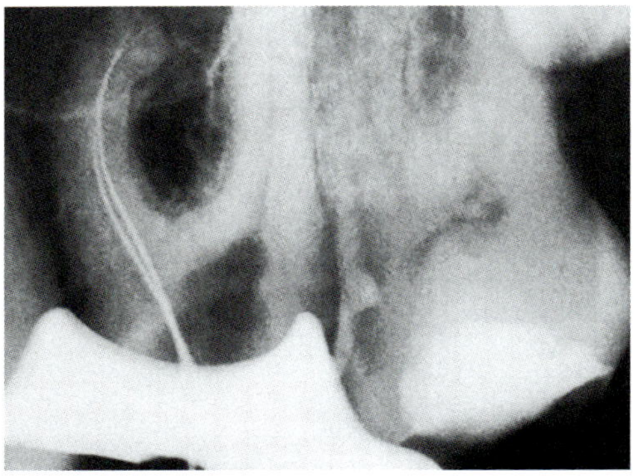

Fig 6-1 A periapical radiograph of tooth no. 14 with a #10 K-file in both MB1 and MB2 canals to confirm the working length after using an apex locator.

Canal preparation

Poor obturation is often a direct result of poor root canal preparation. A root canal system that is well prepared should be easily obturated. Mishaps can occur if, for example, foreign materials, debris, and/or separated instruments obstruct canals during instrumentation, which would affect the subsequent step of obturation. This can easily happen during removal of an amalgam restoration if due diligence is not practiced in protecting the root canal system from amalgam particles.

Mishaps as a result of improper instrumentation of delicate root canals can occur. This can happen if not paying attention to the subtle, complex anatomical pathways and can result in a number of misadventures, including ledging, transportation, perforation, and separation of hand or rotary instruments. A judicious clinician should always start negotiating canals by using the files with small apical sizes (#10 or smaller) to passively negotiate and determine the complexity of the root canal system before attempting to insert larger files.

Mishaps: Violating critical anatomical structures

Many articles have reported accidental injuries to anatomical structures during root canal treatment.[47–49] Having high-quality diagnostic radiographs is paramount to success, and when treating a complex case with close association to anatomical structures, an astute clinician should obtain a CBCT image of the area in question.[50] Care must be taken at all times to avoid damaging the inferior alveolar nerve or the maxillary sinus to prevent unnecessary, and possibly irreversible, negative effects on those structures (Fig 6-2).

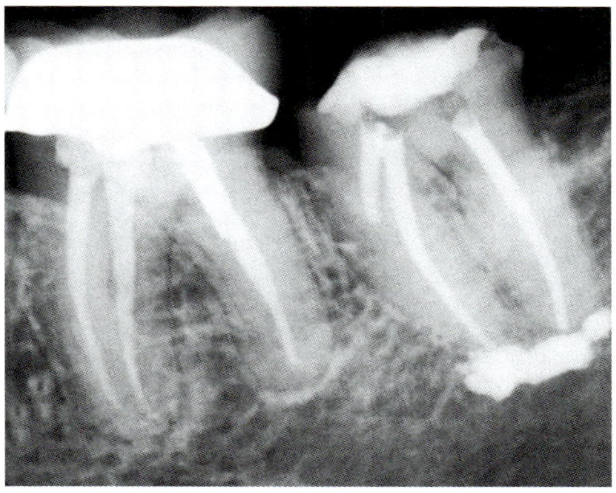

Fig 6-2 A periapical radiograph of tooth no. 18 showing extrusion of excessive root canal sealer above the inferior alveolar canal.

Maxillary sinusitis as a sequela to an endodontic mishap

It is considered poor practice to obturate beyond the apical constriction. Many authors have reported sinusitis resulting from accidental extrusion of obturation materials into the maxillary sinus.[51–53] During obturation, the maxillary sinus may be invaded by sealer or by solid materials such as gutta-percha. Either type of material produces an inflammatory reaction with an area of rarefaction in the periapical tissues. When foreign material invades the maxillary sinus, it may cause chronic inflammation inside the sinus. This inflammation is likely to persist until the foreign object is removed.[54] To prevent such mishaps, the proximity of apices to the maxillary sinus floor should be assessed with CBCT (Fig 6-3). Periapical inflammation sometimes causes perforation of the maxillary sinus floor, which would impose an even higher risk of extruding obturation material into the maxillary

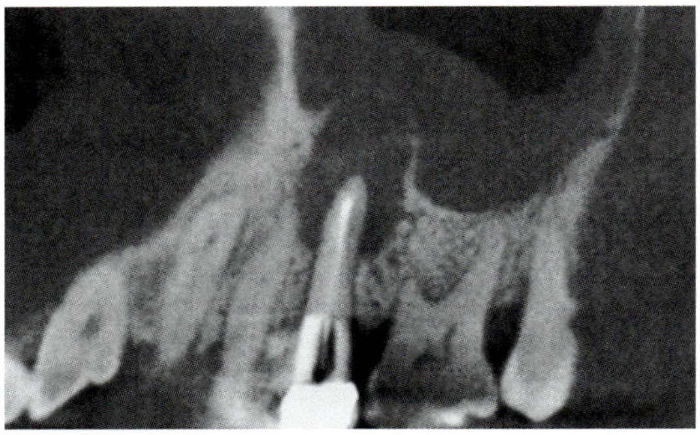

Fig 6-3 Sagittal view of CBCT on tooth no. 13 demonstrating the periapical lesion was associated with the displacement and perforation of the floor of the maxillary left sinus.

sinus. An accurate length determination is also required to avoid any over-instrumentation, which can cause mechanical perforation of the maxillary sinus floor and damage the Schneiderian membrane. Moreover, solid apical stop of master cone needs to be obtained prior to obturation. Avoid using excessive amounts of sealer when the apices are in close proximity to critical anatomical locations (see Fig 6-2).

Inferior alveolar damage as a sequela to an endodontic mishap

Understanding the relationship between the anatomical root apices and the inferior alveolar nerve prior to treatment is of utmost importance in avoiding iatrogenic injury. Obtaining a diagnostic radiograph is critical, and when in doubt, the clinician must expose a CBCT to better appreciate and understand the anatomical complexities.

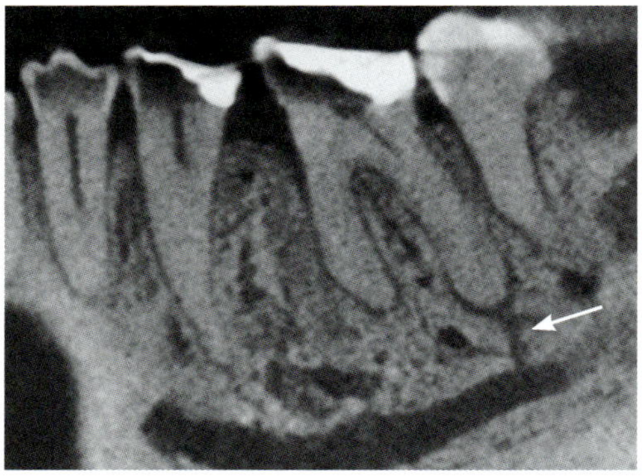

Fig 6-4 Sagittal view of CBCT on tooth no. 19 demonstrating the distance from the apices to the inferior alveolar canal; the *arrow* indicates a possible communication between the periapical lesion on the distal root and the inferior alveolar canal.

Many authors have reported on alveolar nerve damage resulting from endodontic material.[55] These complications can include anesthesia, hypoesthesia, hyperesthesia, or dysesthesia.[56–59] The proximity of the posterior teeth to the inferior alveolar canal demands proper attention and management (Fig 6-4). Examination of the distances from the apices to the mandibular canal can best be accomplished with CBCT.[60]

Although some obturation fillings are more cytotoxic than others, none of the current obturation materials or irrigants are completely biocompatible. Even though the mandibular canal is protected by dense hypermineralized bone, the presence of any foreign material can irritate the nerve function and result in inadvertent complications.

If extrusion of obturation material into the inferior alveolar canal or mental foramen is suspected, CBCT should be taken to obtain more information, including the location and extension of the extruded foreign materials. Treatment of this extrusion remains controversial, varying from a wait-and-see approach, to anti-inflammatory drugs and periodic follow-up, to surgical intervention to remove foreign material from the inferior alveolar canal.[55]

Smear Layer Removal

The goal of obturation is to achieve both good apical and coronal sealing. This sealing prevents residual bacteria and their toxins from reaching the root apex and causing reinfection, which would lead to treatment failure. The smear layer is a substrate of nonhomogenous structure loosely adherent to the root canal walls composed of organic and inorganic particles, coagulated proteins, pulp tissue, blood cells, bacteria, and fungi (Fig 6-5).[61] The smear layer may be a factor supporting the persistence of infection due to the organic and inorganic substrates in its composition. Therefore, it can compromise the intratubular penetration of endodontic sealers and the adhesiveness of luting cements. For these reasons, its removal with chemical substances has been advocated (Fig 6-6).[62]

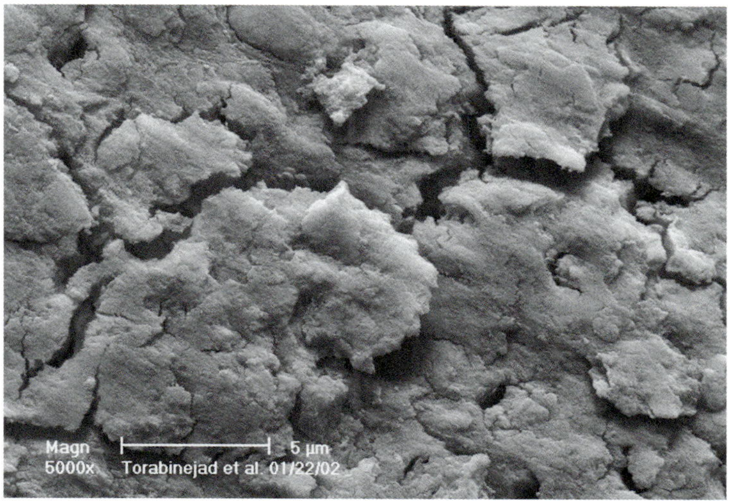

Fig 6-5 A scanning electron microscopic (SEM) picture showing the presence of the smear layer on the root canal walls of a tooth after cleaning and shaping.

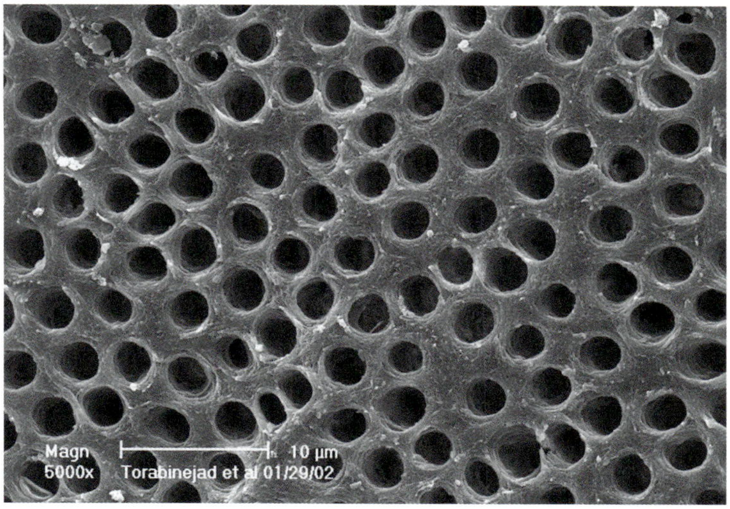

Fig 6-6 An SEM picture showing complete removal of the smear layer from the surface of the root canal walls using a mixture of tetracycline, an acid, and a detergent (MTAD).

The most commonly used irrigation solutions for root canal treatment are sodium hypochlorite (NaOCl) and chlorhexidine (CHX). These are used more specifically because of their antimicrobial properties; however, neither can remove the smear layer effectively. The solution most frequently used to remove the smear layer is EDTA.[61] MTAD was also shown to be very effective in removing the smear layer and disinfecting the root canal system when used as an intracanal irrigant.[63] On top of using irrigants, ultrasonic activation has been proposed to remove the smear layer. This technique is based on the premise that the energy released by the instrument improves the physicochemical properties of the irrigation solutions by cavitation and transmission of acoustic waves.[64]

There is a controversy over the clinical benefit of removing the smear layer. Some clinicians even believe the presence of the smear layer helps increase the success rate of endodontic treatment.[65] However, removing the smear layer is strongly advocated by the majority of clinicians. The smear layer serves as a substrate for microorganisms to multiply and proliferate.[66] In addition, the smear layer can minimize the ability of disinfecting agents and intracanal medicaments to penetrate deeply into the dentinal tubules (Fig 6-7). It also compromises the ability of the sealer or post cements to penetrate the dentinal tubules and adhere properly. The smear layer acts as a sealing barrier between the canal wall and cements. This may compromise the ability of the clinician to achieve a satisfactory seal or to cement a post.[67,68]

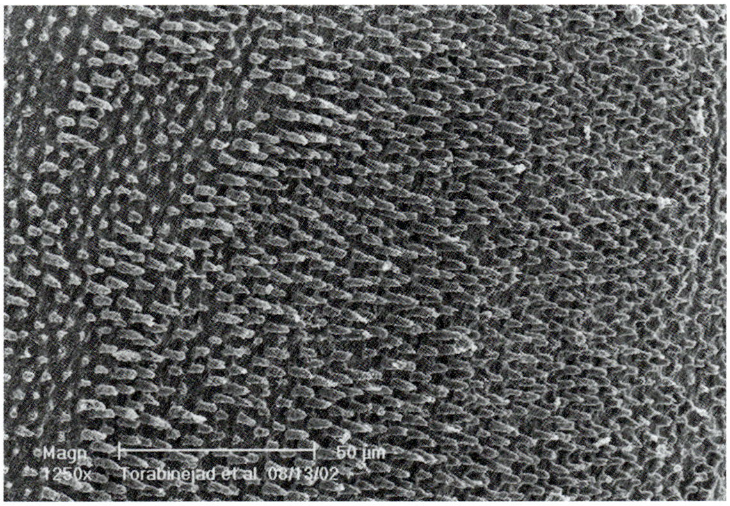

Fig 6-7 An SEM picture showing penetration of AH26 sealer into the dentinal tubules after removal of the smear layer with MTAD and obturation of the root canal with gutta-percha and the AH26 root canal sealer.

Obturation Materials

Obturation was traditionally thought to provide a "hermetic seal" of the root canal system after instrumentation. The goal to obtain a complete and 3D fluid-tight seal of the root canal system continues to drive the development of obturation materials and sealers.

According to Grossman, the ideal root filling should include the following properties[69]: It should not shrink and should be impervious to moisture; should have good adhesion to dentin and root filling materials without staining tooth structure; should be sterile or easily sterilized immediately before insertion and be bacteriostatic or at least not encourage bacterial growth; should stimulate the periapical healing process without irritating the periradicular tissues; should be easily introduced into the root canal(s) as well as easily removed from the root canal(s); and finally, should be radiopaque.

The longest-standing and closest material to fulfill these criteria is gutta-percha. Several materials have been tried and tested as an endodontic filling material, but gutta-percha has been the most extensively used for years and has established itself as the gold standard. Gutta-percha presents the following advantages: It has acceptable biocompatibility and some degree of antibacterial properties (though minimal); it is radiopaque, dimensionally stable, and relatively easy to handle; and it can be easily removed from the root canal system.

However, gutta-percha has a lack of adhesion to dentin, so a sealer is necessary to fill the spaces around the filling material. Gutta-percha shrinks about 1% to 2%, especially after heating. Over the years, different materials have been developed to achieve a true seal of the root canal system. Resilon, a thermoplastic synthetic polyester, is one example. Unfortunately, these other materials all fell out of favor due to worse outcomes. Resilon failures often led to severe flare-ups of endodontic infections, as methacrylate tends to harbor biofilms.[70] Teeth obturated with Resilon were more likely to present with a lesion at follow-up compared to teeth obturated with gutta-percha and sealer.[71]

Although gutta-percha presents important advantages, it exhibits inherent disadvantages that make it less than ideal. The ideal material for root canal obturation has yet to be developed. Mineral trioxide aggregate (MTA) might have a profound advantage when used as a canal obturation material because of its superior physiochemical and bioactive properties. The original MTA material was introduced to seal pathways of communication from the external surface of the tooth in perforation repair and as a root-end filling material in endodontic surgery.[72] When early scientific observations and clinical outcomes demonstrated favorable biologic responses to the material, other uses for MTA were explored and investigated. MTA was found to be effective as a pulp-capping and pulpotomy agent for the repair of internal and external resorptive defects and was also shown to promote root-end induction in teeth with immature apices (apexogenesis).[73] The recently introduced tricalcium silicate cements exhibit many important properties not available in other contemporary materials currently used in endodontics.[74] In conjunction with being sterile, radiopaque, and non-shrinking, these materials are not sensitive to moisture or blood contamination.[74] MTA also provides an effective seal against dentin and cementum and promotes biologic repair and regeneration of the periodontal ligament.[72,75,76] Because perforation repair, root-end induction, and root-end filling are essentially forms of partial canal obturation, the orthograde filling of the apical region or the entire root

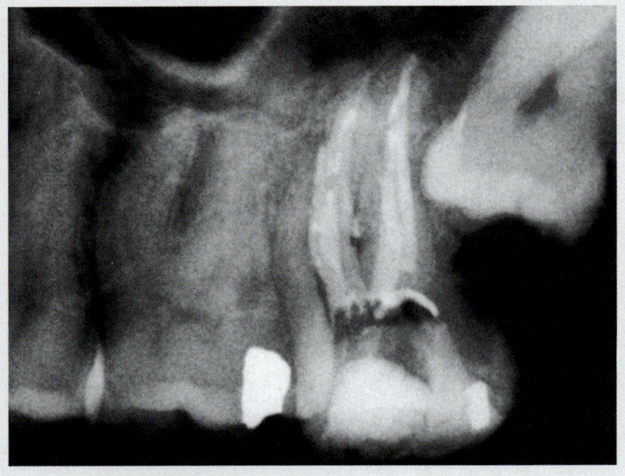

Fig 6-8 A periapical radiograph of tooth no. 15 demonstrating the presence of a void after obturation of the root canals.

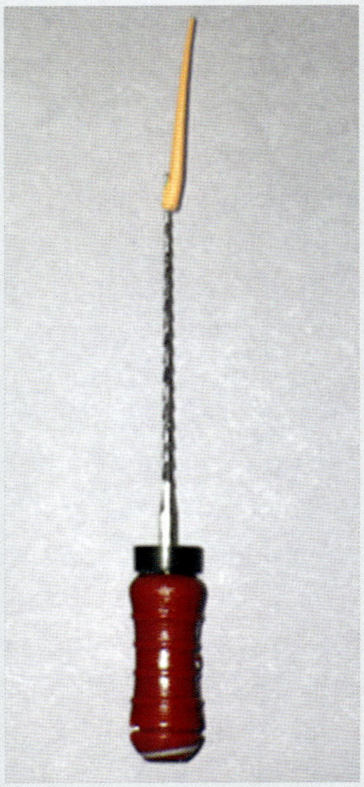

Fig 6-9 A size-25 Hedstrom file was used to engage and remove the gutta-percha cone out of the root canal.

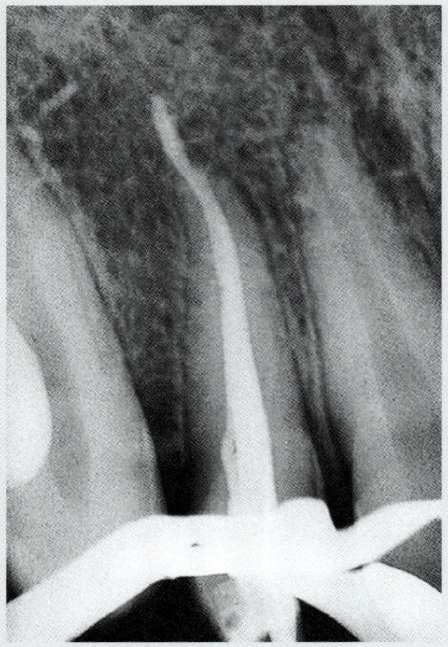

Fig 6-10 The lack of an apical stop resulted in extrusion of the gutta-percha beyond the apical foramen.

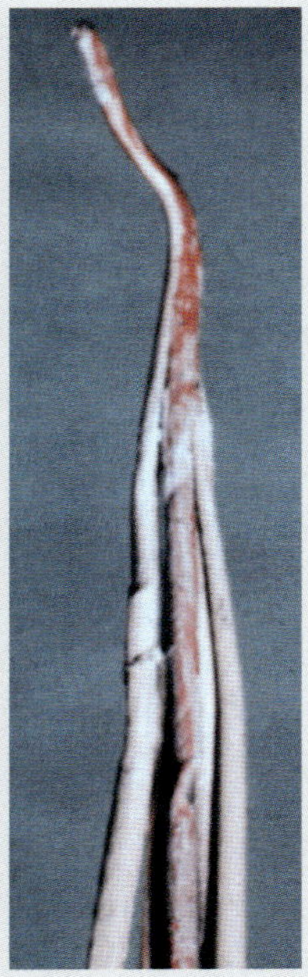

Fig 6-11 Two Hedstrom files were used to retrieve the extruded filling materials from the root canal of this tooth.

canal system with MTA is the next logical progression in the evolutionary application of this material.[77]

As stated in the AAE Position Statement on Use of Silver Points, silver points were historically used as a root canal obturation material in the 1950s and '60s. Silver points have been shown to corrode spontaneously in the presence of serum and blood due to unstable electrochemical behavior.[78] Corrosion byproducts can also cause irreversible staining of the tooth structure and surrounding tissues. Silver points lack plasticity, and the consequent failure to flow and conform to the shape of the root canal system makes them less favorable as filling materials. It is impossible to place post-and-core build-ups with intact silver points. In the case of apical surgery, it becomes more complicated due to the difficulties encountered when attempting a root-end preparation in canals that are filled with a metal. Additionally, corrosion products from silver points have the potential to cause periradicular inflammation and induce inflammatory root resorption.[78]

Despite the shortcomings of silver points relative to newer materials, the AAE does not recommend the prophylactic revision of silver point obturation unless there is clear evidence of endodontic pathosis or if the use of silver points complicate proper restoration of the tooth.

In reality, the obturation material is simply a space filler; in fact, obturation of the root canal system is not a requirement for healing of the periodontium, as discussed previously in this chapter. The obturation material prevents restorative material from blocking the root canal system, which would make retreatment needlessly challenging. To this end, the obturation material should be a material that can be easily removed; while practitioners aim their procedures for success, they also need a plan for failure.

Regardless of the obturation techniques used, a void in sealer mass or core obturation material may occur (Fig 6-8). A void in the middle or coronal third of the root canal can be fixed by removing and downpacking gutta-percha to the level where the void is present and then backfilling with a light layer of sealer to coat the canal walls. If the void occurs in the apical portion due to poor length control of downpack or from cone tips bending, the gutta-percha can be taken out by using the rotary file before the sealer sets or by using a Hedstrom file to engage the coronal portion and remove the cone (Fig 6-9). If the apical size is not gauged appropriately, the gutta-percha cone may extrude beyond the apical foramen (Fig 6-10). The same Hedstrom file technique can be used to retrieve the extruded cone in one piece (Fig 6-11). Alternatively, you can use chloroform at the apex and a slightly long paper point to "wick up" the dissolved gutta-percha.

Sealers

Most root canals are filled with gutta-percha points in combination with an endodontic sealer. An endodontic sealer is an essential component of root canal obturation to establish a fluid-tight seal. The main function of a sealer is to fill the spaces between the core material and the walls of the root canal in an attempt to form a coherent mass of obturating material without voids. Acting as a lubricant, root canal sealer facilitates the placement of the filling core and entombs any remaining bacteria. The sealer is expected to fill irregularities and minor discrepancies between the filling and canal walls, accessory canals, and multiple foramina. Because of the germicidal action of certain types of bioceramic sealers, the sealer is also expected to destroy the remaining bacteria left after cleaning and shaping of the root canal.[79]

Mishaps: Excessive sealer extrusion

Although it is desired that the endodontic sealers remain inside the root canal, excessive use of a sealer may inadvertently push it beyond the apical constriction and into the surrounding tissues (Fig 6-12).

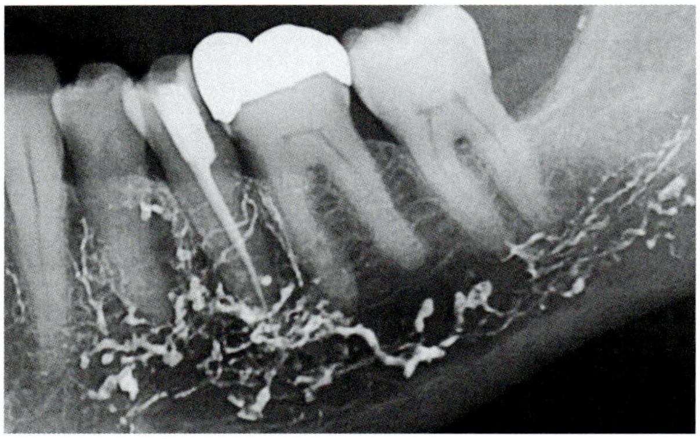

Fig 6-12 An excessive amount of of sealer has been pushed beyond the apical constriction and into the surrounding tissues during root canal treatment for the mandibular second premolar.

When excessive sealer cement comes in contact with soft and hard tissues apically, it can cause persistent inflammation of periradicular tissues and may result in delayed wound healing, manifesting as pain, tenderness, and swelling of the affected area. Therefore, biocompatibility and toxicity of sealers are important considerations for when such mishaps occur.

All currently available sealers exhibit toxicity when freshly mixed; however, their toxicity is greatly reduced on setting.[79] Zinc oxide–eugenol sealers have a history of successful use in root canal obturation for over 100 years. These sealers resorb when extruded into the periapical tissue. However, they have prolonged setting time, shrink on setting, have high solubility, and can stain the tooth structure. The advantages of zinc oxide–eugenol sealer are its antimicrobial activity and popularity among clinicians, especially when used with thermoplasticized obturation technique. However, the eugenol in the zinc oxide–eugenol sealers induces a toxic effect and decreases the transmission in nerve cells. The effect is persistent even after setting of the material. Zinc oxide–eugenol sealer with paraformaldehyde is both cytotoxic and mutagenic.[79] Localized inflammation with zinc oxide–eugenol sealers has been seen in both soft tissues and hard tissues.

$Ca(OH)_2$ sealers exhibit antimicrobial activity and have osteogenic and cementogenic potential.[79] The rationale for the addition of $Ca(OH)_2$ to root canal sealers is from observations of bases and liners containing the material and their antibacterial and tissue-regenerating ability. Solubility is required for release of $Ca(OH)_2$ and for sustained activity, hence it is not consistent with the purpose of an ideal sealer. Soares et al reported that canals overfilled with $Ca(OH)_2$ sealers cause chronic inflammatory reaction in periapical tissues in dog teeth.[80]

Resin sealers also have a long history of use. They provide adhesion and they do not contain eugenol. AH26 is a slow-setting epoxy resin that was found to release formaldehyde when setting.[79] AH Plus is a modified formulation of AH26 in which less formaldehyde is released. The sealing abilities of AH26 and AH Plus are comparable.[81] The extrusion of a methacrylate resin-based sealer through the periapical foramen would create an uncured surface layer for extended time periods. This might alter the toxicity profile of resin-based sealers because the incompletely polymerized monomers present in the exposed sealer are more toxic.[79]

Compared with traditional sealers, the new generation of bioceramic sealers—with benefits such as high pH, hydrophilic properties, no shrinkage, and excellent sealing ability—has gained popularity in the past few years.[82] They have the ability to form hydroxyapatite due to the presence of calcium silicates in the powder, which in a hydration reaction produces a calcium silicate hydrate gel and $Ca(OH)_2$. The $Ca(OH)_2$ reacts with the phosphate ions to precipitate hydroxyapatite and water. Due to their chemical compositions and high pH, bioceramic sealers show a certain degree of toxicity to vital tissue.[83] If the extruded sealer invades critical anatomical structures, immediate attention and appropriate management are needed to avoid significant complications as described earlier (see "Mishaps: Violating critical anatomical structures"). However, there are currently not enough clinical studies or scientific data regarding the long-term use of these sealers and their complications after extrusion.

Obturation Techniques

Depending on the root filling materials, sealers, and the clinician's skills, there are various techniques available to obturate the root canal system, including warm vertical condensation, core techniques, single cone techniques, and cold lateral condensation. Each technique has its pros and cons.

Lateral condensation

Cold lateral condensation is a traditional obturation method. This technique involves placing a single cone of gutta-percha with sealer in the prepared root canal and adding secondary cones that are compacted together with a spreader. The cones stay together due to frictional grip and the presence of the sealer. Although time-consuming, lateral condensation is appreciated for its low cost and its controlled placement of gutta-percha in the canal. This technique relies heavily on sealer to take up the 3D spaces that gutta-percha cannot reach.

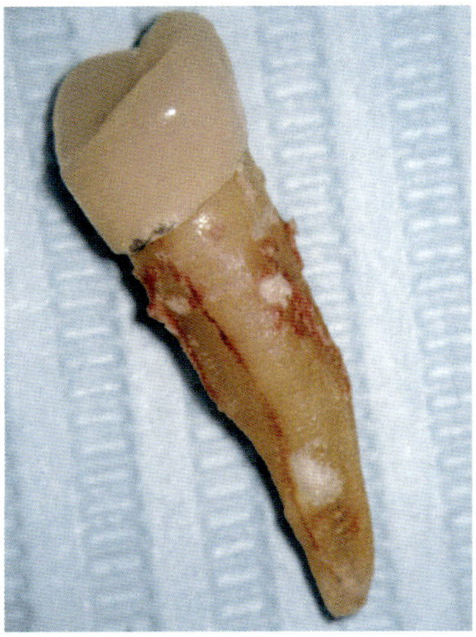

Fig 6-13 The wedging effect of a spreader or plugger can cause vertical root fracture in a tooth during root canal obturation.

Mishaps during lateral condensation

All types of obturation techniques require operator skill. If a technique is not performed well, it can result in under- or overfilling, poor lateral condensation, and voids, which can lead to microleakage and reinfection. If an inappropriate amount of force is used during lateral condensation, it may damage thin root dentin and cause root fracture. The wedging effect of spreader load tends to cause vertical root fractures in the buccolingual dimension (Fig 6-13). Pitts et al showed a spreader load as small as 7.2 kg produced a fracture in a maxillary central incisor.[84] Holcomb et al demonstrated that vertical root fracture can occur in single-canal mandibular incisors at spreader loads as small as 1.5 kg.[85] The biggest advantage of this technique is the ability of the operator to retrieve the extruded filling material during obturation (see Fig 6-11).

Warm vertical condensation

The concept of heating gutta-percha to obtain a uniform tridimensional obturation was introduced by Schilder in the 1960s.[86] He aimed to provide a technique that produced a homogenous, stable, compatible material adapted to the varied and complex anatomy of the root canal system. This technique condenses heated gutta-percha into the canal to adapt it to the prepared root canal walls. This method uses little amounts of sealer to achieve good quality of tridimensional obturation. Variations of this technique have evolved, including the continuous wave obturation and the injectable gutta-percha techniques.[87]

Mishaps during warm vertical condensation

Similar to lateral condensation, warm vertical condensation also requires a certain amount of force to condense the apical portion of gutta-percha. Excessive vertical load of condensation may cause crack and vertical root fractures. Capar et al reported that lateral or warm vertical condensation techniques cause more cracks than canal preparation.[88] The single cone caused fewer cracks compared to the other filling techniques.[88] As mentioned earlier, the extrusion of root filling materials or sealer may occur during warm vertical condensation if an excessive amount of sealer is used or if there is a lack of apical stop on the master cones (Fig 6-14). The biggest disadvantage of this technique is the inability of the operator to retrieve the extruded filling material (Fig 6-15).

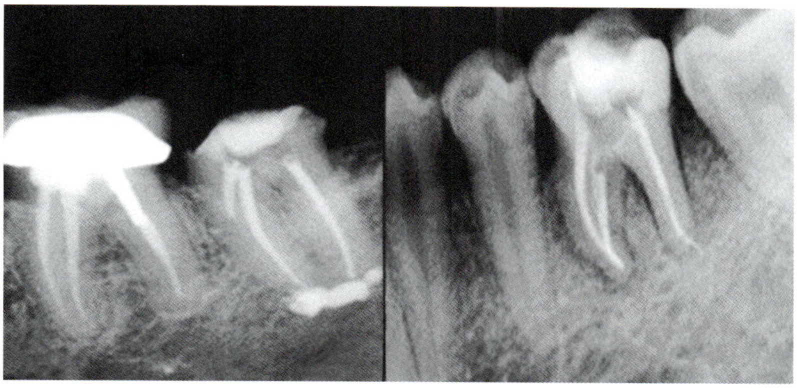

Fig 6-14 An excessive amount of sealer and the lack of an apical stop caused extrusion of root canal sealer beyond the apical foramen during obturation using the vertical condensation technique.

Fig 6-15 The lack of an apical stop caused extrusion of gutta-percha into the maxillary sinus during obturation of the palatal root of a maxillary first molar using the vertical condensation technique.

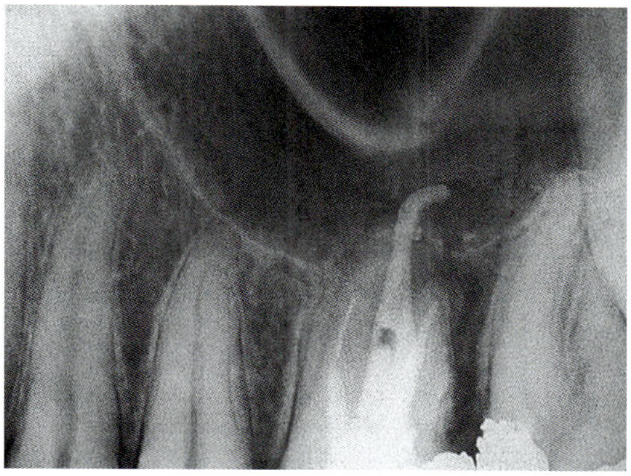

Carrier-based techniques

Carrier-based techniques use a heated plastic carrier coated with gutta-percha to the working length in the canals. Following cleaning and shaping, this technique involves placing a size verifier that will correspond to the correct size obturator to be used. The canal walls are then lightly coated with sealer and a heated obturator is inserted with firm but passive pressure. The plastic carrier is subsequently severed at the canal orifice, leaving the plastic carrier and gutta-percha as the permanent filling. In theory, the carrier is centered in canals and the gutta-percha is circumferentially present around the carrier.

Mishaps during carrier-based techniques

One risk of carrier-based obturation techniques is extruding sealer and gutta-percha from the apical foramen, because after being heated and condensed, gutta-percha may lose its apical stop. Another risk of carrier-based techniques is the possibility of the plastic carrier being stripped of gutta-percha, especially in the apical third, allowing the carrier to be in direct contact with the canal walls. Retreatment of some carriers can be challenging depending on whether the gutta-percha circumferentially surrounds the carrier along its length or if the carrier has become wedged with frictional retention along some length of the canal.

Single cone technique

The single cone technique uses larger master cones that best match the geometry of the nickel-titanium rotary systems. The use of the gutta-percha point does not require either accessory points or lateral condensation when the root canal is enlarged with rotary instruments. The technique speeds the root canal filling while minimizing the pressure applied to the root canal walls. The combination of single cone and endodontic sealer results in a uniform mass that prevents the failures observed with multiple cones.

However, this technique has been considered less effective in sealing root canal systems. Due to the absence of condensation as well as the complexity of the root canal anatomy, even with greater volume sealer, the obturation materials cannot always fill the whole root canal system. Porosities in large volumes, contraction, cement dissolution, and a lower adaptation of the single cone in the middle and coronal thirds of canals with irregular shape are the main disadvantages of this technique.[88]

Budd et al reported that even though high- or low-temperature injectable gutta-percha systems were markedly better than lateral compaction of gutta-percha in replicating the original root canal anatomy, it was very difficult to confine thermoplasticized gutta-percha within the root canal.[89] Once thermoplasticized gutta-percha is injected into the periapical tissues, it is very difficult, if not impossible, to retrieve it. Similarly, if a warm vertical compaction technique is employed, a provider can also inadvertently extrude the heated gutta-percha beyond the apex. A provider must also ensure that the System B plugger is heated to the correct temperature to avoid pulling the cone out or, worse yet, pushing the heated cone beyond the apical foramen.

Although microbial invasion is the primary etiologic reason for periapical pathosis, foreign-body reaction has been considered an evoking consideration leading to a nonhealing outcome.[90] Many different techniques for obturation exist, but they all should reflect the original shape of the root canal system. Errors in obturation are often correctable and might include issues with length control, voids, and gaps. These issues should be immediately corrected before the sealer sets.

Root canal sealers are radiopaque to aid with the core obturation material. Many clinicians have moved to a single-cone technique and calcium silicate sealers because these sealers have shown promising results.[91,92] The advent of calcium silicate sealers and cements that induce bioactivity has been advantageous in challenging cases such as an excessively large apical foramen and/or perforation repair. Although these cements and sealers are biocompatible, extrusion of this material beyond the bounds of the apical foramen is not advisable. For this reason, an astute clinician may decide to place an external matrix against which the calcium silicate cement (internal matrix) would be condensed.[93,94]

Temporization

Teeth undergoing root canal treatment are susceptible to microbial contamination from oral fluids both during and after treatment. After placement of inter-appointment dressing or the completion of obturation, the tooth needs to be immediately restored with either temporary or permanent restorative materials to prevent coronal leakage and contamination of the root canal system.

Upon the completion of obturation, gutta-percha should be cut back to within the canal orifices, and an intermediate restoration (coronal barrier) may be placed to protect it. During temporization, the chamber and cavity walls should be dry. The use of a thin layer of sterile cotton or sponge over canal orifices has both advantages and disadvantages. One advantage is the ease of removal of the temporary restoration without running the risk of unnecessary removal of intact tooth structure or even worse, perforating the floor of the pulp chamber. Placement of a cotton layer can also preclude the accidental blockage of the canal by small fragments of the temporary filling being displaced into the canal.

Mishaps: Failed temporary restoration due to inadequate thickness of temporary materials or delayed placement of final restoration

Using a cotton layer can introduce complications that may seriously compromise the intended seal. First, it may significantly reduce the thickness of the temporary restoration and thereby increase leakage. Second, it may compromise the stability of the restoration by acting as a cushion and allowing displacement during masticatory loading. Third, it may compromise adaptation of the temporary cement during placement. Fourth, fibers of the cotton pellet may inadvertently adhere to the cavity walls and serve as a wick. Finally, there is an increased risk of leakage through exposed lateral canals.[95,96] Another common mistake is when operators do not remove the cotton and put the permanent restoration on top of the cotton pellet.

Cavit is a commercially prepared, premixed, polyvinyl chloride-acetate/calcium-sulfate cement that is catalyzed when it comes in contact with water or oral fluids. It is a hygroscopic material, and its ability to attract and hold water molecules results in a high coefficient of linear expansion with excellent marginal sealing ability. Webber et al found that a thickness of at least 3.5 mm of Cavit is necessary to prevent leakage. Cavit provides a superior seal to other available materials because of its expansion upon setting.[97]

Reinforced zinc oxide–eugenol preparations (IRM) using polymethyl methacrylate provide improved compressive strength and hardness (20% polymethylmethacrylate, zinc oxide powder mixed with eugenol, and 1% acetic acid). IRM has a coefficient of linear expansion only half of Cavit's but a compressive strength nearly double. Thus, while it may leak more due to shrinkage on setting, its increased strength may cause clinicians to favor its use in areas of high occlusal stress.[97]

Glass-ionomer cements can chemically bond to the tooth structures and present with better sealing ability than IRM or Cavit. In endodontics, there are decent temporary restorations that need to be replaced over the long term due to low tensile strength, making them unsuitable in load-bearing areas of the mouth.

The sealing quality of the available endodontic temporary restorative materials deteriorates with time. Imura et al showed that gutta-percha stopping, IRM, and Cavit all permitted bacterial penetration of obturated canals. The average times for contamination in access cavities closed with gutta-percha, IRM, and Cavit were 7.8, 12.9, and 9.8 days, respectively.[98] Safavi et al observed greater endodontic treatment success in teeth restored with permanent restorations within 2 months after the completion of root canal therapy than in teeth with temporary restorations.[99] Due to the possible disintegration of temporary restorations and the potential for canal contamination, it is recommended to restore teeth with an immediate definitive coronal restoration after canal obturation.[98]

References

1. Chugal NM, Clive JM, Spångberg LSW. Endodontic infection: Some biologic and treatment factors associated with outcome. Oral Surg Oral Med Oral Pathol Oral Radiol Endod 2003;96:81–90.
2. Gillen BM, Looney SW, Gu LS, et al. Impact of the quality of coronal restoration versus the quality of root canal fillings on success of root canal treatment: A systematic review and meta-analysis. J Endod 2011;37:895–902.
3. Craveiro MA, Fontana CE, de Martin AS, da Silveira Bueno CE. Influence of coronal restoration and root canal filling quality on periapical status: Clinical and radiographic evaluation. J Endod 2015;41:836–840.
4. Ingle JI, Simon JH, Machtou P, Bogaerts P. Outcome of endodontic treatment and re-treatment. In: Ingle JI, Bakland LK (eds). Endodontics, ed 5. Hamilton, Ontario: Decker, 2002:747–768.
5. Rickert UG, Dixon CM. The controlling of root surgery. In: Transactions of the Eighth International Dental Congress. Paris: Fédération Dentaire Internationale, 1931.
6. Torneck CD. Reaction of rat connective tissue to polyethylene tube implants. I. Oral Surg Oral Med Oral Pathol 1966;21:379–387.
7. Klevant FJ, Eggink CO. The effect of canal preparation on periapical disease. Int Endod J 1983;16:68–75.
8. Peters OA, Laib A, Göhring TN, Barbakow F. Changes in root canal geometry after preparation assessed by high-resolution computed tomography. J Endod 2001;27:1–6.
9. Nair PNR. On the causes of persistent apical periodontitis: A review. Int Endod J 2006;39:249–281.
10. Sabeti MA, Nekofar M, Motahhary P, Ghandi M, Simon JH. Healing of apical periodontitis after endodontic treatment with and without obturation in dogs. J Endod 2006;32:628–633.
11. Fabricius L, Dahlén G, Sundqvist G, Happonen RP, Möller AJR. Influence of residual bacteria on periapical tissue healing after chemomechanical treatment and root filling of experimentally infected monkey teeth. Eur J Oral Sci 2006;114:278–285.
12. Torabinejad M, Ung B, Kettering JD. In vitro bacterial penetration of coronally unsealed endodontically treated teeth. J Endod 1990;16:566–569.
13. Marshall FJ, Massler M. The sealing of pulp less teeth evaluated with radioisotopes. J Dent Med 1961;16:172–184.
14. Swanson K, Madison S. An evaluation of coronal microleakage in endodontically treated teeth. Part I. Time periods. J Endod 1987;13:56–59.
15. Madison S, Wilcox LR. An evaluation of coronal microleakage in endodontically treated teeth. Part III. In vivo study. J Endod 1988;14:455–458.
16. Magura ME, Kafrawy AH, Brown CE Jr, Newton CW. Human saliva coronal microleakage in obturated root canals: An in vitro study. J Endod 1991;17:324–331.
17. Khayat A, Lee SJ, Torabinejad M. Human saliva penetration of coronally unsealed obturated root canals. J Endod 1993;19:458–461.
18. Ray HA, Trope M. Periapical status of endodontically treated teeth in relation to the technical quality of the root filling and the coronal restoration. Int Endod J 1995;28:12–18.

19. Tronstad L, Asbjørnsen K, Døving L, Pedersen I, Eriksen H. Influence of coronal restorations on the periapical health of endodontically treated teeth. Endod Dent Traumatol 2000;16:218–221.
20. Ricucci D, Loghin S, Siqueira JF Jr. Correlation between clinical and histologic pulp diagnoses. J Endod 2014;40:1932–1939.
21. Lin LM, Ricucci D, Saoud TM, Sigurdsson A, Kahler B. Vital pulp therapy of mature permanent teeth with irreversible pulpitis from the perspective of pulp biology. Aust Endod J 2020;46:154–166.
22. Sjögren U, Figdor D, Spångberg L, Sundqvist G. The antimicrobial effect of calcium hydroxide as a short-term intracanal dressing. Int Endod J 1991;24:119–125.
23. Su Y, Wang C, Ye L. Healing rate and post-obturation pain of single-versus multiple-visit endodontic treatment for infected root canals: A systematic review. J Endod 2011;37:125–132.
24. Best S, Ammons CL, Karunanayake GA, Saemundsson SR, Tawil PZ. Outcome assessment of teeth with necrotic pulps and apical periodontitis treated with long-term calcium hydroxide. J Endod 2021;47:11–18.
25. Chong BS, Pitt Ford TP. The role of intracanal medication in root canal treatment. Int Endod J 1992;25:97–106.
26. Figini L, Lodi G, Gorni F, Gagliani M. Single versus multiple visits for endodontic treatment of permanent teeth: A Cochrane systematic review. J Endod 2008;34:1041–1047.
27. Manfredi M, Figini L, Gagliani M, Lodi G. Single versus multiple visits for endodontic treatment of permanent teeth. Cochrane Database Syst Rev 2016;12:CD005296.
28. ElAyouti A, Hülber-J M, Judenhofer MS, et al. Apical constriction: Location and dimensions in molars—A micro-computed tomography study. J Endod 2014;40:1095–1099.
29. Trope M, Rabie G, Tronstad L. Accuracy of an electronic apex locator under controlled clinical conditions. Endod Dent Traumatol 1985;1:142–145.
30. Lin LM, Rosenberg PA, Lin J. Do procedural errors cause endodontic treatment failure? J Am Dent Assoc 2005;136:187–193.
31. Schilder H. Filling root canals in three dimensions. 1967. J Endod 2006;32:281–290.
32. Tabassum S, Khan FR. Failure of endodontic treatment: The usual suspects. Eur J Dent 2016;10:144–147.
33. Ng YL, Mann V, Rahbaran S, Lewsey J, Gulabivala K. Outcome of primary root canal treatment: Systematic review of the literature—Part 2. Influence of clinical factors. Int Endod J 2008;41:6–31.
34. Ng YL, Mann V, Gulabivala K. Outcome of secondary root canal treatment: A systematic review of the literature. Int Endod J 2008;41:1026–1046.
35. Sjögren U, Hägglund B, Sundqvist G, Wing K. Factors affecting the long-term results of endodontic treatment. J Endod 1990;16:498–504.
36. Aminoshariae A, Kulild JC. The impact of sealer extrusion on endodontic outcome: A systematic review with meta-analysis. Aust Endod J 2020;46:123–129.
37. Marcos-Arenal JL, Rivera EM, Caplan DJ, Trope M. Evaluating the paper point technique for locating the apical foramen after canal preparation. Oral Surg Oral Med Oral Pathol Oral Radiol Endod 2009;108:e101–e105.
38. Martins JN, Marques D, Mata A, Caramês J. Clinical efficacy of electronic apex locators: Systematic review. J Endod 2014;40:759–777.
39. Frank AL, Torabinejad M. An in vivo evaluation of Endex electronic apex locator. J Endod 1993;19:177–179.
40. Fan W, Fan B, Gutmann J, Bian Z, Fan MW. Evaluation of the accuracy of three electronic apex locators using glass tubules. Int Endod J 2006;39:127–135.
41. Oishi A, Yoshioka T, Kobayashi C, Suda H. Electronic detection of root canal constrictions. J Endod 2002;28:361–364.
42. Williams CB, Joyce AP, Roberts S. A comparison between in vivo radiographic working length determination and measurement after extraction. J Endod 2006;32:624–627.
43. Khandewal D, Ballal NV, Saraswathi MV. Comparative evaluation of accuracy of 2 electronic apex locators with conventional radiography: An ex vivo study. J Endod 2015;41:201–204.
44. Piasecki L, Carneiro E, da Silva Neto UX, et al. The use of micro-computed tomography to determine the accuracy of 2 electronic apex locators and anatomic variations affecting their precision. J Endod 2016;42:1263–1267.
45. Aminoshariae A, Kulild J, Nagendrababu V. Artificial intelligence in endodontics: Current applications and future directions. J Endod 2021;47:1352–1357.
46. Saghiri MA, Garcia-Godoy F, Gutmann JL, Lotfi M, Asgar K. The reliability of artificial neural network in locating minor apical foramen: A cadaver study. J Endod 2012;38:1130–1134.
47. Gluskin AH, Lai G, Peters CI, Peters OA. The double-edged sword of calcium hydroxide in endodontics: Precautions and preventive strategies for extrusion injuries into neurovascular anatomy. J Am Dent Assoc 2020;151:317–326.
48. Swanljung O, Vehkalahti MM. Root canal irrigants and medicaments in endodontic malpractice cases: A nationwide longitudinal observation. J Endod 2018;44:559–564.

49. Giardino L, Pontieri F, Savoldi E, Tallarigo F. Aspergillus mycetoma of the maxillary sinus secondary to overfilling of a root canal. J Endod 2006;32:692–694.
50. Venskutonis T, Plotino G, Juodzbalys G, Mickevičienė L. The importance of cone-beam computed tomography in the management of endodontic problems: A review of the literature. J Endod 2014;40:1895–1901.
51. Yamaguchi K, Matsunaga T, Hayashi Y. Gross extrusion of endodontic obturation materials into the maxillary sinus: A case report. Oral Surg Oral Med Oral Pathol Oral Radiol Endod 2007;104:131–134.
52. Ishikawa M, Mizuno T, Yamazaki Y, Satoh T, Notani K, Fukuda H. Migration of gutta-percha point from a root canal into the ethmoid sinus. Br J Oral and Maxillofac Surg 2004;42:58–60.
53. Falworth MS, Herold J. Aspergillosis of the paranasal sinuses: A case report and radiographic review. Oral Surg Oral Med Oral Pathol Oral Radiol Endod 1996;81:255–260.
54. Hauman CHJ, Chandler NP, Tong DC. Endodontic implications of the maxillary sinus: A review. Int Endod J 2002;35:127–141.
55. Castro R, Guivarc'h M, Foletti JM, Catherine JH, Chossegros C, Guyot L. Endodontic-related inferior alveolar nerve injuries: A review and a therapeutic flow chart. J Stomatol Oral Maxillofac Surg 2018;119:412–418.
56. Li B, Wang L, Zhao Z, Qian H, Cui H, Li L. Surgical approach to foreign material within the mandibular canal due to iatrogenic factors. J Craniofac Surg 2017;28:1514–1516.
57. Pogrel MA. Damage to the inferior alveolar nerve as the result of root canal therapy. J Am Dent Assoc 2007;138:65–69.
58. López-López J, Estrugo-Devesa A, Jané-Salas E, Segura-Egea JJ. Inferior alveolar nerve injury resulting from overextension of an endodontic sealer: Non-surgical management using the GABA analogue pregabalin. Int Endod J 2012;45:98–104.
59. González-Martín M, Torres-Lagares D, Gutiérrez-Pérez JL, Segura-Egea JJ. Inferior alveolar nerve paresthesia after overfilling of endodontic sealer into the mandibular canal. J Endod 2010;36:1419–1421.
60. Kim TS, Caruso JM, Christensen H, Torabinejad M. A comparison of cone-beam computed tomography and direct measurement in the examination of the mandibular canal and adjacent structures. J Endod 2010;36:1191–1194.
61. Violich D, Chandler NP. The smear layer in endodontics—A review. Int Endod J 2010;43:2–15.
62. Torabinejad M, Handysides R, Khademi AA, Bakland LK. Clinical implications of the smear layer in endodontics: A review. Oral Surg Oral Med Oral Pathol Oral Radiol Endod 2002;94:658–666.
63. Torabinejad M, Cho Y, Khademi AA, Bakland LK, Shabahang S. The effect of various concentrations of sodium hypochlorite on the ability of MTAD to remove the smear layer. J Endod 2003;29:233–239.
64. Poletto D, Poletto AC, Cavalaro A, et al. Smear layer removal by different chemical solutions used with or without ultrasonic activation after post preparation. Restor Dent Endod 2017;42:324–331.
65. Hasheminia SM, Birang R, Feizianfard M, Nasouri M. A comparative study of the removal of smear layer by two endodontic irrigants and Nd: YAG Laser: A scanning electron microscopic study. ISRN Dent 2012;2012:620951.
66. George S, Kishen A, Song KP. The role of environmental changes on monospecies biofilm formation on root canal wall by *Enterococcus faecalis*. J Endod 2005;31:867–872.
67. Kaushal R, Bansal R, Malhan S. A comparative evaluation of smear layer removal by using ethylenediamine tetraacetic acid, citric acid, and maleic acid as root canal irrigants: An in vitro scanning electron microscopic study. J Conserv Dent 2020;23:71–78.
68. Sowjanyaa J, Thomas T, Chandana CS. Comparative evaluation of the efficacy of smear layer removal by ethylenediaminetetraacetic acid, Triphala, and German chamomile as irrigants—A scanning electron microscopy study. J Adv Pharm Educ Res 2017;7:267–271.
69. Grossman LI. Physical properties of root canal cements. J Endod 1976;2:166–175.
70. Whatley JD, Spolnik KJ, Vail MM, et al. Susceptibility of methacrylate-based root canal filling to degradation by bacteria found in endodontic infections. Quintessence Int 2014;45:647–652.
71. Strange KA, Tawil PZ, Phillips C, Walia HD, Fouad AF. Long-term outcomes of endodontic treatment performed with Resilon/Epiphany. J Endod 2019;45:507–512.
72. Torabinejad M, Watson TF, Pitt Ford TR. Sealing ability of a mineral trioxide aggregate when used as a root end filling material. J Endod 1993;19:591–595.
73. Shabahang S. Treatment options: Apexogenesis and apexification. Pediatr Dent 2013;35:125–128.
74. Parirokh M, Torabinejad M, Dummer PMH. Mineral trioxide aggregate and other bioactive endodontic cements: An updated overview—Part I: Vital pulp therapy. Int Endod J 2018;51:177–205.
75. Lee SJ, Monsef M, Torabinejad M. Sealing ability of a mineral trioxide aggregate for repair of lateral root perforations. J Endod 1993;19:541–544.
76. Torabinejad M, Pitt Ford TR, McKendry DJ, Abedi HR, Miller DA, Kariyawasam SP. Histologic assessment of mineral trioxide aggregate as a root-end filling in monkeys. J Endod 1997;23:225–228.
77. Bogen G, Kuttler S. Mineral trioxide aggregate obturation: A review and case series. J Endod 2009;35:777–790.

78. Brady JM, del Rio CE. Corrosion of endodontic silver cones in humans: A scanning electron microscope and X-ray microprobe study. J Endod 1975;1:205–210.
79. Kaur A, Shah N, Logani A, Mishra N. Biotoxicity of commonly used root canal sealers: A meta-analysis. J Conserv Dent 2015;18:83–88.
80. Soares I, Goldberg F, Massone EJ, Soares IM. Periapical tissue response to two calcium hydroxide-containing endodontic sealers. J Endod 1990;16:166–169.
81. De Moor RJG, De Bruyne MAA. The long-term sealing ability of AH 26 and AH plus used with three gutta-percha obturation techniques. Quintessence Int 2004;35:326–331.
82. Al-Haddad A, Che Ab Aziz ZA. Bioceramic-based root canal sealers: A review. Int J Biomater 2016; 2016:9753210.
83. Baraba A, Pezelj-Ribaric S, Roguljić M, Miletic I. Cytotoxicity of two bioactive root canal sealers. Acta Stomatol Croat 2016;50:8–13.
84. Pitts DL, Matheny HE, Nicholls JI. An in vitro study of spreader loads required to cause vertical root fracture during lateral condensation. J Endod 1983;9:544–550.
85. Holcomb JQ, Pitts DL, Nicholls JI. Further investigation of spreader loads required to cause vertical root fracture during lateral condensation. J Endod 1987;13:277–284.
86. Schilder H. Filling root canals in three dimensions. Dent Clin North Am 1967;11:723–744.
87. Bhandi S, Mashyakhy M, Abumelha AS, et al. Complete obturation—Cold lateral condensation vs. thermoplastic techniques: A systematic review of micro-CT studies. Materials (Basel) 2021;14:4013.
88. Capar ID, Saygili G, Ergun H, Gok T, Arslan H, Ertas H. Effects of root canal preparation, various filling techniques and retreatment after filling on vertical root fracture and crack formation. Dent Traumatol 2015;31:302–307.
89. Budd CS, Weller RN, Kulild JC. A comparison of thermoplasticized injectable gutta-percha obturation techniques. J Endod 1991;17:260–264.
90. Nair PR, Sjögren U, Krey G, Sundqvist G. Therapy-resistant foreign body giant cell granuloma at the periapex of a root-filled human tooth. J Endod 1990;16:589–595.
91. Chybowski EA, Glickman GN, Patel Y, Fleury A, Solomon E, He J. Clinical outcome of non-surgical root canal treatment using a single-cone technique with endosequence bioceramic sealer: A retrospective analysis. J Endod 2018;44:941–945.
92. Zavattini A, Knight A, Foschi F, Mannocci F. Outcome of root canal treatments using a new calcium silicate root canal sealer: A non-randomized clinical trial. J Clin Med 2020;9:782.
93. Vanka A, Ravi KS, Shashikiran ND. Apexification with MTA using internal matrix: Report of 2 cases. J Clin Pediatr Dent 2010;34:197–200.
94. Gharechahi M, Ghoddusi J. A nonsurgical endodontic treatment in open-apex and immature teeth affected by dens invaginatus: Using a collagen membrane as an apical barrier. J Am Dent Assoc 2012;143:144–148.
95. Bishop K, Briggs P. Endodontic failure—A problem from top to bottom. Br Dent J 1995;179:35–36.
96. Naoum H, Chandler NP. Temporization for endodontics. Int Endod J 2002;35:964–978.
97. Webber RT, del Rio CE, Brady JM, Segall RO. Sealing quality of a temporary filling material. Oral Surg Oral Med Oral Pathol 1978;46:123–130.
98. Imura N, Otani SM, Campos MJ, Jardim EG Jr, Zuolo ML. Bacterial penetration through temporary restorative materials in root-canal-treated teeth in vitro. Int Endod J 1997;30:381–385.
99. Safavi KE, Dowden WE, Langeland K. Influence of delayed coronal permanent restoration on endodontic prognosis. Endod Dent Traumatol 1987;3:187–191.

7

Complications During Restoration of Endodontically Treated Teeth

SHANE N. WHITE
DANIEL J. BOEHNE

Objectives

After reading this chapter, the reader should be able to:

1. Understand the precepts of endodontic-restorative treatment planning.
2. Prevent bacterial ingress during and after root canal treatment.
3. Conserve tooth structure during root canal treatment and restoration.
4. Apply appropriate restorative techniques to endodontically treated teeth.
5. Avoid endodontic-restorative complications.
6. Recognize and manage endodontic-restorative complications when they occur.

Many factors influence the survival of endodontically treated teeth. Nonetheless, restorative factors are highly influential.[1] Restoration must not be regarded as something separate from root canal treatment but as an integral part of the treatment. Root canal treatment is the beginning of a pathway toward restoration and oral rehabilitation.[2] It is not enough to remove bacteria, their metabolites, toxins, and antigens from the root canal system; a durable restoration must prevent their reentry. Furthermore, a mechanically unsound restoration invites mechanical failure of the restoration, or worse, the tooth itself.

It is noteworthy that endodontically treated teeth tend to be extracted not because of endodontic failure, but due to other reasons, principally periodontal disease, as well as secondary caries, changes in treatment plan or type of prosthesis, tooth fracture, and restorative failure.[3–8]

In most situations, if root canal treatment fails for biologic reasons, bacteria remaining in the root canal system, or reentry, the tooth can be predictably saved through endodontic retreatment and re-restoration or apical surgery.[9] Conversely, mechanical failures of restored endodontically treated teeth can be catastrophic and require extraction of the tooth.

Two key precepts are *(1)* to prevent the ingress of bacteria throughout the process of root canal treatment, restoration, and thereafter, and *(2)* to conserve absolutely as much tooth structure as possible.

Errors in restoration are often irreversible, so prevention is paramount. Errors in restoration leading to bacterial ingress or mechanical failure tend to manifest over time, sometimes many years after the procedure, so follow-up with routine endodontic and restorative evaluation is also very important.[10]

These precepts follow Galen's advice: "In disease, two things must be done: Be useful, or do no harm." Procedures that have no proven benefit to the patient must be avoided; unnecessary removal of tooth structure is intrinsically harmful.[11]

Treatment Planning and Case Selection

Avoiding complications starts with a comprehensive examination that leads to diagnosis, prognosis, and a combined endodontic and restorative treatment plan. Both the restorative dentist and the endodontist must take responsibility for diagnosis and treatment planning. A general dentist must complete at least a preliminary examination, prognosis, and treatment plan before referring a patient to an endodontist. A referral should not be made solely for root canal treatment, but firstly for assessment and advice. Likewise, an endodontist must conduct a comprehensive examination to reach an overall prognosis and plan. Should these plans not concur, it is the responsibility of the endodontist to communicate with the referring dentist, and they should collectively decide on a plan before initiating treatment. An endodontist must not assume that a referral is a mandate for root canal treatment. Concomitantly, the referring dentist must not assume that completion of root canal treatment indicates a good endodontic or restorative

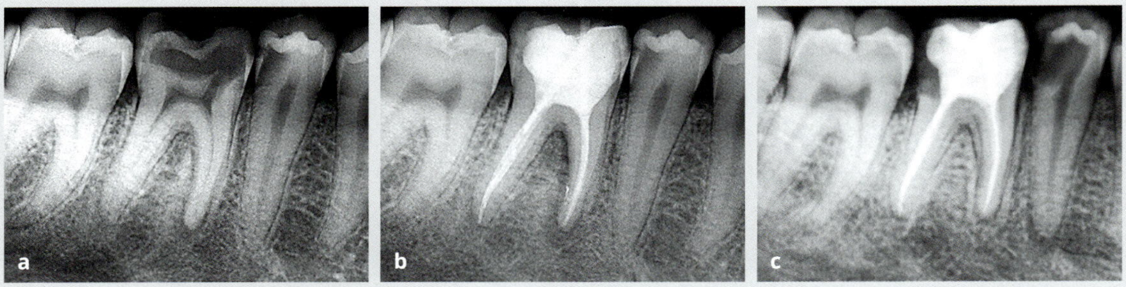

Fig 7-1 Caries susceptibility must be considered a key restorative issue in its own right. *(a)* This patient presented because he had unbearable pain on tooth no. 30. *(b)* He was treated and *(c)* returned 3 years later only when he had unbearable pain on tooth no. 29, as well as new decay elsewhere. Although the apical periodontitis on tooth no. 30 had healed and the build-up was intact, substantial new decay would have ultimately led to its failure. He elected to have tooth no. 29 extracted because he knew that he wouldn't complete the restorative treatment; he expects more decay.

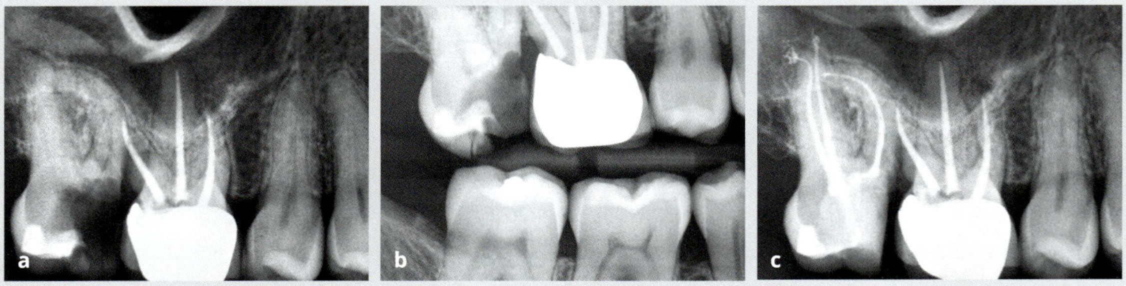

Fig 7-2 Bitewing radiographs are useful for the preoperative assessment of interproximal caries. *(a)* Although the periapical view suggested that tooth no. 2 is nonrestorable, *(b)* the bitewing view showed that several millimeters of tooth structure remained above the bony crest and furcation and that *(c)* sufficient bulk remained.

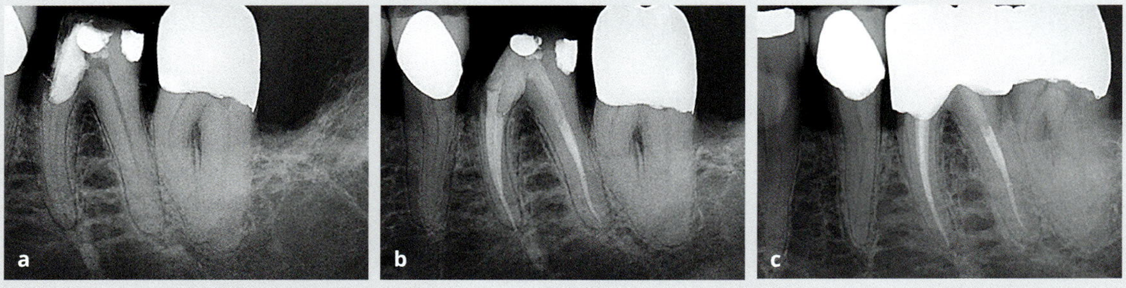

Fig 7-3 Case selection and treatment planning failure. *(a)* The general dentist deferred to the endodontist, and *(b)* the endodontist deferred to the general dentist on prognosis and treatment planning. *(c)* Although sufficient height of tooth structure remained on the distal part of the tooth, little remained on the mesial, and minimal thickness remained in the furcation, so the tooth's prognosis is poor.

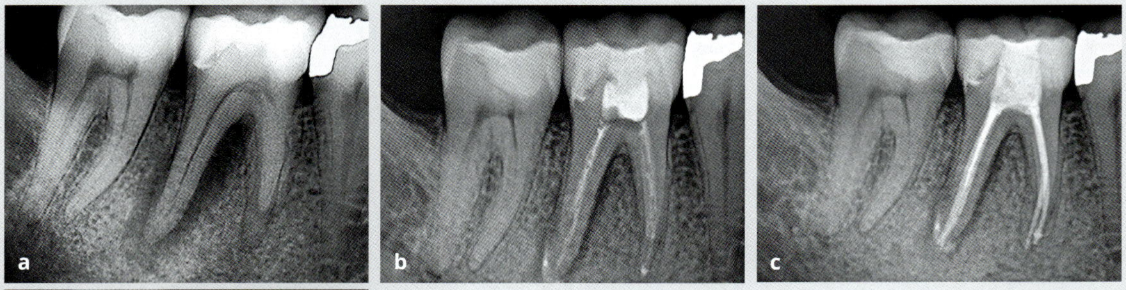

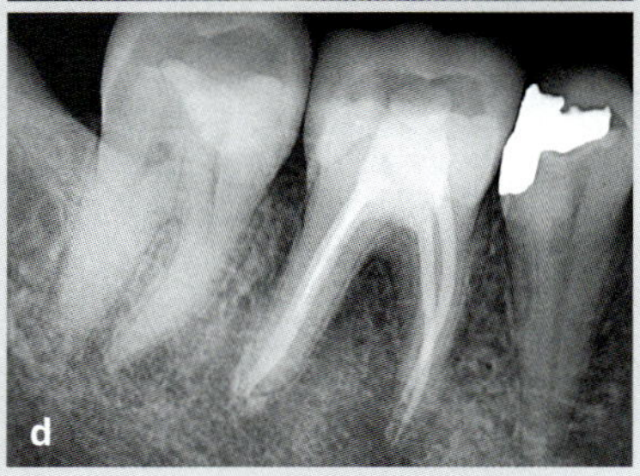

Fig 7-4 *(a)* Extensive bone loss was suggestive of a vertical crack on tooth no. 30, but a crack was not positively identified. *(b)* The tooth was observed for some months after cleaning, shaping, and calcium hydroxide intracanal medicament placement. Tempit (Centrix) was used as a base layer of the provisional restoration, covered with a bonded resin-composite surface layer. *(c)* After some initial healing occurred, the tooth was obturated and an immediate definitive restoration placed; *(d)* healing continued.

prognosis. There is no place for anyone involved to dismiss diagnosis and planning as "not my responsibility." Time must be made for communication and the building of trust among all care partners.

Restorative prognosis and planning must be based upon endodontic, periodontic, caries, and restorative considerations.[1]

A careful radiographic assessment is needed to understand the endodontic prognosis and to identify technical challenges, but it also provides important information relating to the extent of caries and remaining tooth structure (Fig 7-1). Bitewing views best depict the pulp chamber, the cervix of the tooth, and the extent of coronal caries, particularly as it impinges on root structure and nears the bone crest and the furcation (Fig 7-2). As well as showing the height of the tooth structure relative to the bony crest, they also show the width of the remaining root (Fig 7-3). Teeth usually get much narrower below the dentino-enamel junction, so even a loss of ~1 mm horizontally can dramatically decrease the root's thickness.

An evaluation should include periodontal probing and assessment of gingival health. Isolated vertical probing defects may be indicative of a draining chronic abscess or a cracked root in a tooth with a necrotic pulp. Restorability may not be clearly assessed until potential cracks are evaluated through symptomology, staining with methylene blue, transillumination, using a Tooth Slooth, and radiography; additionally, all caries must be removed so that the height and thickness of the remaining natural crown or stump can be assessed for adequacy (Fig 7-4).

Consideration must be given to the role of the tooth in the patient's rehabilitation.[11–17] Does sufficient tooth structure remain for the tooth's future role? An abutment for a long-span bridge or fixed dental prosthesis (FDP) must have a substantial bulk, height, and thickness; likewise, a terminal abutment for a free-end saddle removable partial denture (RPD) bears substantial loads, whereas an overdenture abutment may be successful with a minimal amount of remaining tooth structure, just enough to form or facilitate placement of a dome. Moreover, the consequences of mechanical failure must be considered; the loss of a key bridge abutment may be devastating, but the loss of one of a few overdenture abutments may be trivial.

In many cases, attention to the patient's occlusal scheme can minimize lateral and protrusive contacts and therefore minimize tipping or jiggling forces on an endodontically treated tooth. For example, canine rise may protect adjacent endodontically treated premolars or molars. Alternatively, if an endodontically treated canine is to be restored, spreading the excursive contacts over the adjacent teeth and achieving group function may protect that canine. It appears that endodontically treated teeth that have mesial and distal proximal contacts with other remaining natural teeth enjoy some advantage.[17,18]

Sometimes a tooth with a very poor restorative prognosis should still be retained to avoid an extraction in a vulnerable patient, eg, those who have bleeding disorders or those who have received high doses of bisphosphonates or head and neck radiation, etc. In such cases, masticatory function may be less important, but the restoration must seal the access preparation and prevent tooth fracture.

Complications and corrective actions

There is little that can be done after the fact to address an error in prognosis or treatment planning. Should an error in diagnosis or treatment planning be recognized, a new comprehensive evaluation should be initiated and a new plan created. The sooner any error is identified and addressed, the better. Alertness to potential issues, reflection, and communication among restorative dentists and endodontists is essential.

Prevention of Bacterial Ingress, Coronal Leakage

Prevention of bacterial ingress from the mouth to the root canal system is critically important from the initiation of root canal treatment onward. The oral flora comprises of a complex and dynamic ecosystem that can quickly adapt to opportunities provided by disease processes, carious, endodontic and periodontal, and the availability of new niches. Successful endodontic treatment is dependent on creating and maintaining an effective coronal seal.[19–32] Most current obturation methods are ineffective in forming a biologic barrier between the oral cavity and the periapical tissues.[33–36] Calcium-silicate sealers (EndoSequence BC Sealer HiFLow, Brasseler) may be more effective at reducing leakage than other sealer types, but there is not enough evidence for such an assumption. A durable coronal restoration is necessary to keep pathogens from contaminating or recontaminating the obturated root canal system and ultimately causing apical periodontitis.[37–39] The only substantive controversy regarding coronal leakage is how long it takes for microbial penetration to occur once a protective restorative seal is lost; estimates range from 3 days to 3 months.[37,39]

Rubber dam isolation

Rubber dam isolation must be provided whenever the root canal system is accessible or potentially accessible by the oral flora. Rubber dam isolation should be initiated during caries removal, whenever it is possible that caries might extend to the pulp or root canal system, as well as during build-up placement, post preparation, and post placement. The importance of rubber dam isolation is overwhelming; it prevents bacterial ingress, provides improved mechanical and visual access, prevents leakage of irrigants into the patient's mouth, protects the airway and gastrointestinal system from inhalation or ingestion of instruments and posts, and prevents salivary contamination during adhesive procedures. However, rubber dam isolation is not universally used during root canal or restorative treatments when bacterial ingress may occur. This appears to be more than a knowledge or cognitive problem, but one rooted in dentists' attitudes and behaviors.[40] Minor defects in rubber dam isolation, eg, in deep proximal boxes, can be addressed using a water-based caulking material (OraSeal, Ultradent).

Provisional or temporary restorations

If root canal treatment is not to be completed in a single visit, eg, to receive the benefit of the antimicrobial effects of a calcium-hydroxide intracanal medicament (UltraCal XS, Ultradent), a provisional or temporary restoration will be needed. This must be of sufficient thickness and durability to resist microbial ingress. Soft materials that can be removed using a spoon excavator tend to be inadequate with respect to strength, wear resistance, and leakage (Fig 7-5).[41,42] For up to a

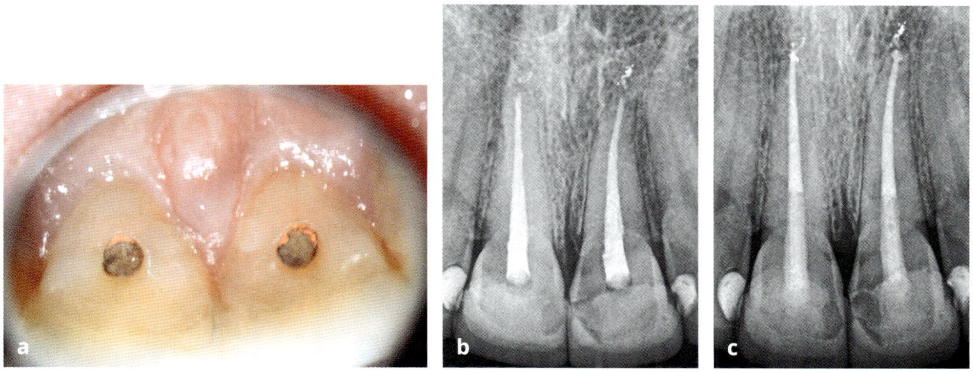

Fig 7-5 This patient's dentist completed root canal treatment on teeth nos. 8 and 9 and placed cotton and Cavit (3M) instead of a permanent restoration. The patient did not understand that this was a temporary restoration and did not return for permanent restorations. *(a and b)* One year later, she presented with symptomatic apical periodontitis. *(c)* Both teeth received nonsurgical retreatment and immediate resin-composite restorations.

couple weeks, a reinforced zinc oxide–eugenol-based material may be adequate. For longer periods, a glass-ionomer, a resin-modified glass-ionomer, or even a resin-composite material is preferred (see Fig 7-4). A soft pledget can be placed in the floor of the access preparation, but this should be thin so as to maximize the thickness of the provisional restoration. Synthetic pledgets, foam (Pele Tim, VOCO Dental), or polytetrafluoroethylene (PTFE) tape are preferred over cotton, because they do not support microbial growth. Whatever type of pledget is used, care must be taken to remember to remove it prior to definitive restoration; a niche for bacterial colonization must not be left, and a mechanically sound foundation is a necessity (Fig 7-6). Likewise, all soft and flexible gutta-percha must be removed from the pulpal floor.

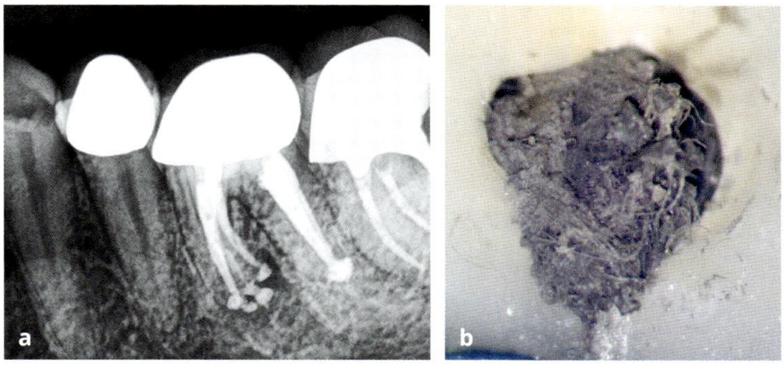

Fig 7-6 *(a)* Although all five canals were treated and obturated, a cotton pledget was not removed from the bottom of the pulp chamber before restoration and healing did not occur. *(b)* A smelly, contaminated cotton pledget was found inside the failing root-canal-treated tooth's access cavity. Correction included retreatment of the entire root canal system and an immediate build-up.

7

Orifice barriers

If there will be a delay before definitive restoration, orifice barriers, divots of an adhesive or bonded restorative material, can be placed over or in the coronal 1 to 2 mm of obturated canals to minimize the potential for microbial ingress if the temporary restoration leaks.[43] Alternatively, a liner, typically glass ionomer, can be used to cover the floor of the pulp chamber. An orifice barrier should not be placed over a canal that is planned to have a post.

Foundational restorations and build-ups

Foundational restorations or build-ups should be placed at the time of obturation, before the rubber dam is removed (Fig 7-7). Bacterial ingress will be prevented, and the remaining tooth structure will be at least somewhat protected.[7,24,44–48] Delaying the definitive restoration only brings disadvantages.

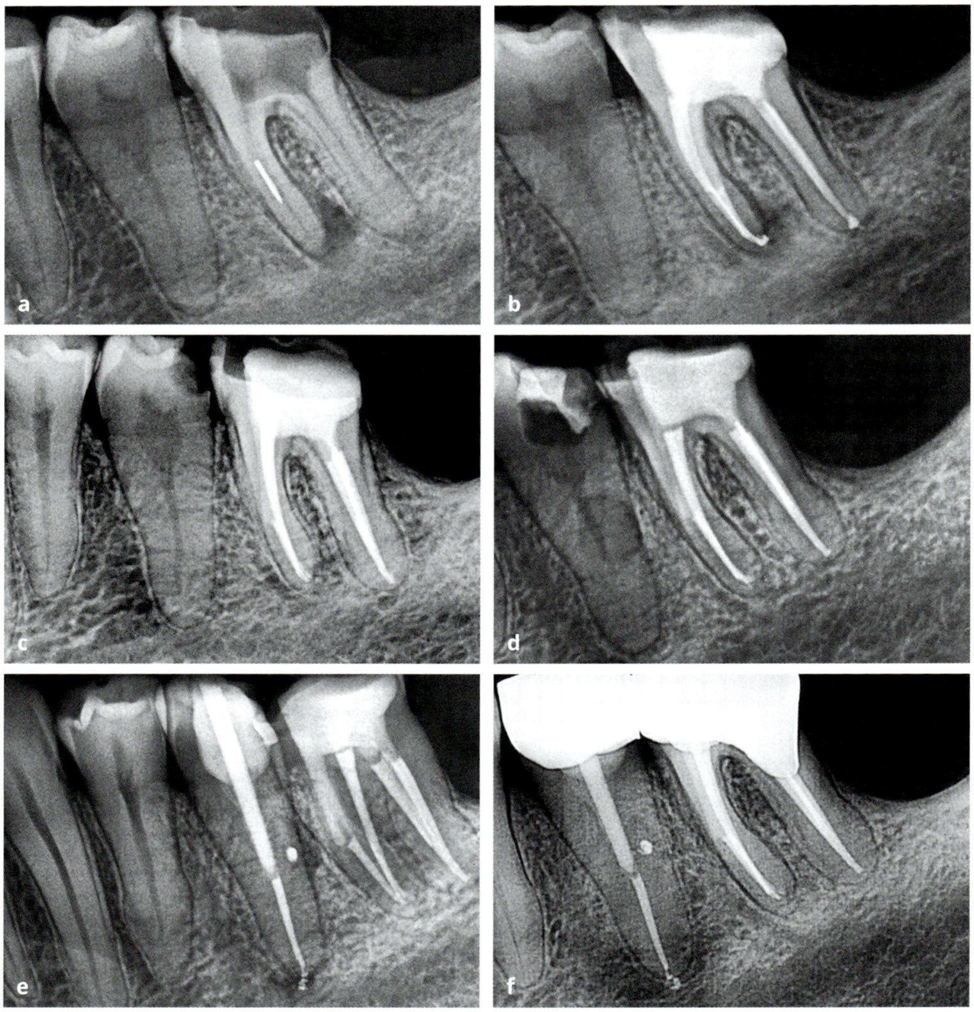

Fig 7-7 A complicated root canal treatment. *(a)* After removal of a separated instrument, *(b)* an immediate build-up was placed on tooth no. 19, and the patient was referred back to their general dentist for a crown. *(c)* Four years later, the patient returned for endodontic recall and was referred to their general dentist again for restoration of teeth nos. 19 and 20. *(d)* Eleven years later, the patient returned due to incomplete root canal treatment and pain in tooth no. 20. *(e)* The immediate permanent build-up had allowed apical healing and saved tooth no. 19. *(f)* Finally, both teeth received definitive restorations; complete periradicular healing had occurred.

A build-up restores damaged or missing parts of the tooth to full contour or creates an ideal form for crown preparation so that the artificial crown can be of uniform thickness. The build-up provides an opportunity to increase axial wall height to provide better resistance and retention form for the artificial crown.

From a practical standpoint, it barely requires more effort to place a build-up than it does to temporize, but this small difference in procedure can have a significant impact on the outcome. Patients will appreciate that they don't need another dental visit just to close an endodontic access preparation. Also, the crown preparation appointments will be straightforward and predictable. It is much easier to prepare the built-up tooth for a crown than it is to isolate the tooth, remove the temporary material, and build the tooth up prior to preparing the crown. Using a build-up material that is not dentin colored, eg, opaque white (Core Paste, DenMat), will make it easier for the restorative dentist to ensure the crown margins will be placed on dentin and to be conservative in their tooth preparation (Fig 7-8). Crown margins, deep and interproximal, can be prepared at the time of build-up placement when the gingiva has been retracted by the rubber dam and the endodontic microscope is available (see Fig 7-8). The endodontist must communicate the value of immediate build-up placement to the patient and to the restorative dentist.

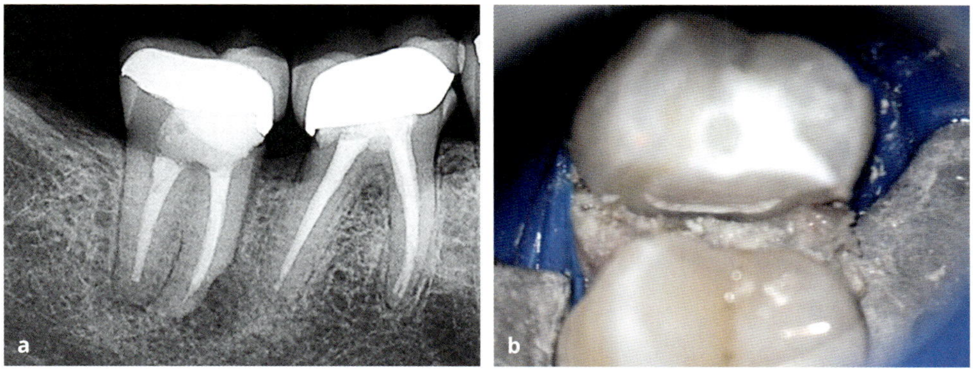

Fig 7-8 Crown margins must be placed on solid tooth structure, but dentin and tooth-colored resin-composite can be difficult to distinguish. *(a)* Sometimes margins are inadvertently placed on the build-up, not on dentin. *(b)* In this case, the endodontist used a bright white build-up material and prepared the deep margin using a microscope while the tooth was isolated by a rubber dam.

Complications and corrective actions

If apical or periradicular healing does not occur after root canal treatment and restoration or if bacteria reenter due to an ineffective restoration or through a new caries lesion, nonsurgical retreatment is generally the first-line treatment choice. Retreatment should generally include thorough reinstrumentation, long duration of irrigation, "the soak," replenishing sodium hypochlorite, and placement of a calcium hydroxide ($Ca[OH]_2$) intracanal medicament for at least 1 week before reobturation (Pulpdent Paste, Pulpdent). This will generally necessitate access through careful and conservative disassembly. This should be performed with

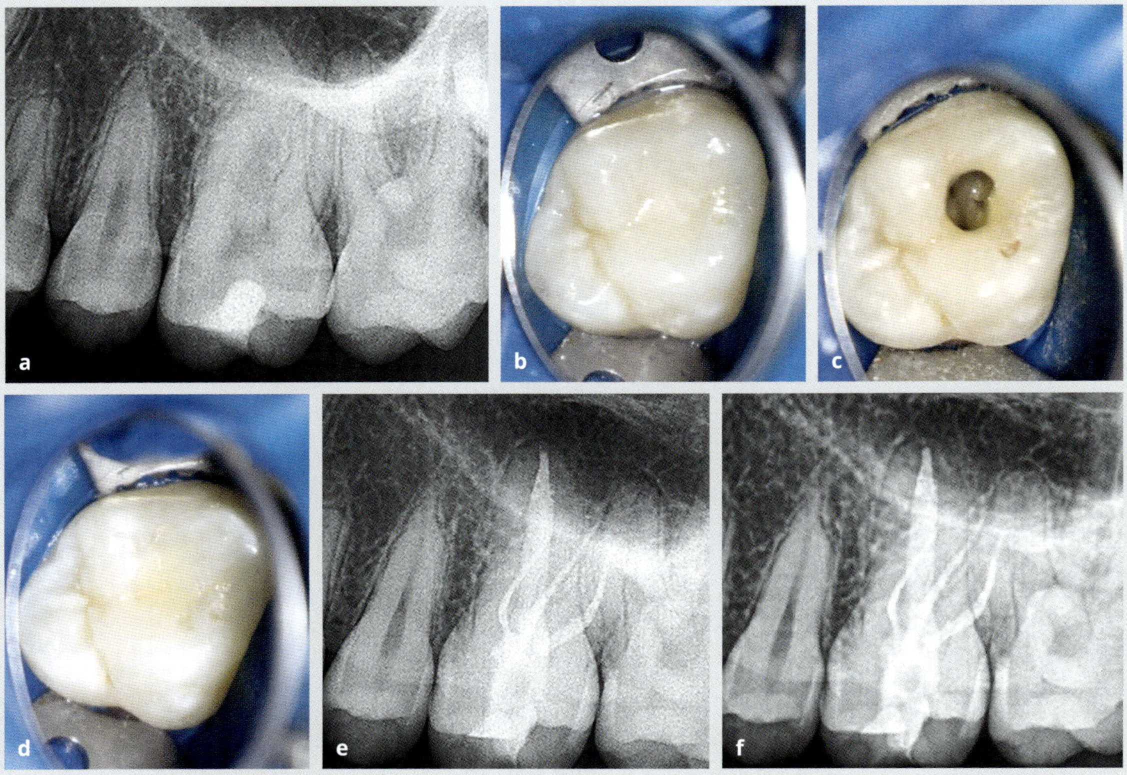

Fig 7-9 Most molars that require RCT have extensive damage from caries and will require coronal coverage after root canal treatment. *(a and b)* However, in this case, the prior restoration was narrow, and *(c)* a conservative endodontic access preparation gave straight-line access to all canals and left all the marginal ridges intact. *(d and e)* Therefore, coronal coverage was not considered to be necessary; *(f)* 4-year recall.

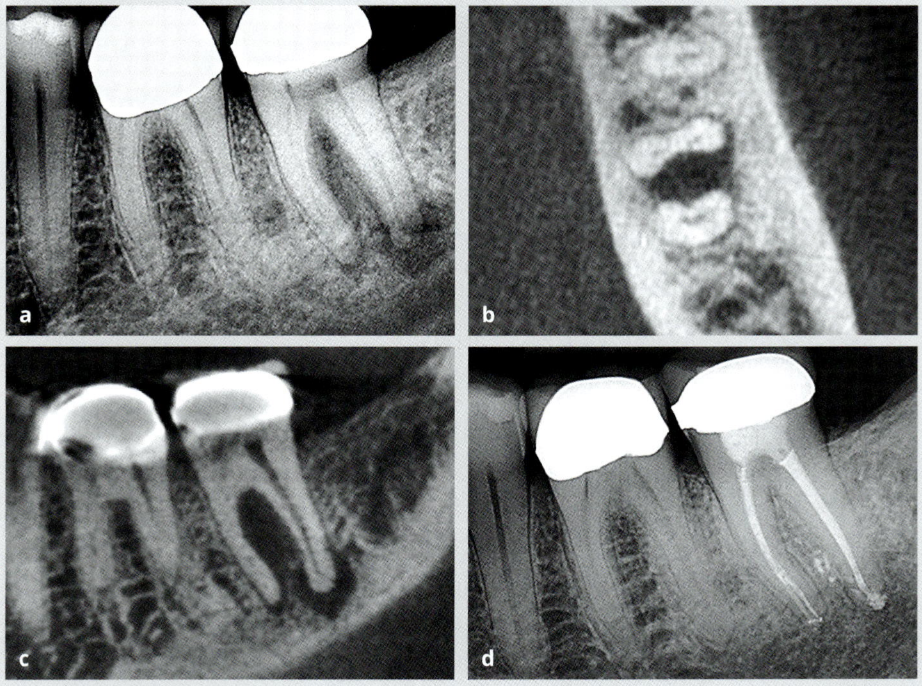

Fig 7-10 *(a)* The periapical view made it appear that the walls of the mesial of tooth no. 18 were bulky, but this root had pronounced biconcavities; *(b and c)* only 0.2 mm of dentinal thickness was present on the furcal side of the mesial canals as viewed by CBCT. *(d)* Undue flaring or post preparation would have produced perforations. With appropriate minimal instrumentation, irrigation, and intracanal medicament, healing of the J-shaped lesion occurred.

rubber dam using ultrasonic instrumentation and magnification. Restorations are replaceable, but natural tooth structure is irreplaceable. Of course, conservative and carefully planned re-restoration will be needed after endodontic retreatment.

If apical or periradicular healing does not occur after nonsurgical retreatment and re-restoration—a rare outcome—apical surgery is generally the second-line response. If healing still does not occur—another rare outcome—tooth replacement using an osseointegrated implant is the preferred third-line response.

Conservation of Tooth Structure

Many in vitro and in vivo studies have found that the amount of remaining tooth structure is strongly related to the mechanical strength and survival of endodontically treated teeth.[47,49,50] Tooth structure must be conserved during caries removal for routine restorative tooth preparations; this will reduce the need for root canal treatment and improve the tooth's long-term prognosis. Tooth structure must also be conserved during endodontic access preparation, canal preparation, and subsequent restoration.

Restorations that undergo mechanical failure typically do so through repeated fatigue loading that stresses the interfaces between natural tooth structure and its artificial substitutes, causing microstrain and micromovement that eventually transitions to long-crack growth and catastrophic fracture.[51] The most effective way to diminish such strain is to minimize the size and volume of the artificial restoration by conserving all possible tooth structure.

Access preparation

Access preparation must be conducted with conservation and restoration in mind (see chapter 4). Only the tooth structure to attain straight-line access to the coronal third of each canal is needed (Fig 7-9). Larger access preparations are not necessary and can greatly weaken the tooth. A conservative access preparation may have only minimal deleterious impact on the mechanical behavior of the tooth; however, teeth that need root canal treatment have usually been ravaged by caries, so retaining all possible tooth structure must be prioritized.[52] Canal preparation must be sufficient to achieve the biologic goals described in the introduction to this section; however, removing tooth structure beyond what is necessary only weakens teeth and predisposes them to fracture. An overenlarged access preparation combined with excessive coronal flaring and unwarranted tooth reduction is a recipe for disaster (Fig 7-10).

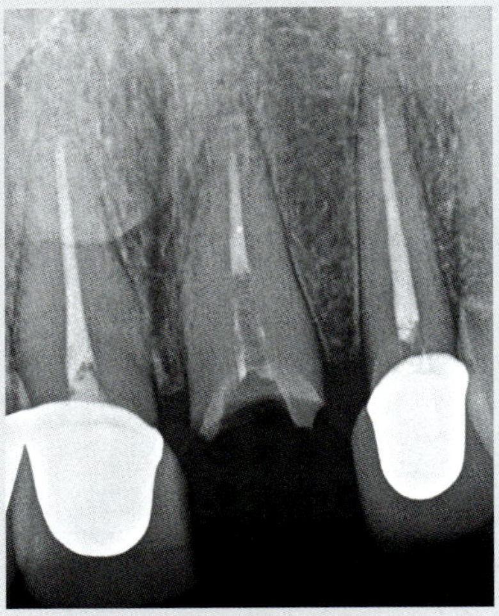

Fig 7-11 Ferrule height and thickness are both important in providing resistance and retention form; both are minimal for tooth no. 9. Also, tooth no. 9 will not have a post that is longer than the clinical crown; however, it is fortunate that the walls of the root are thick. Voids between the obturations and restorative materials provide a niche for bacteria on teeth nos. 8 and 10.

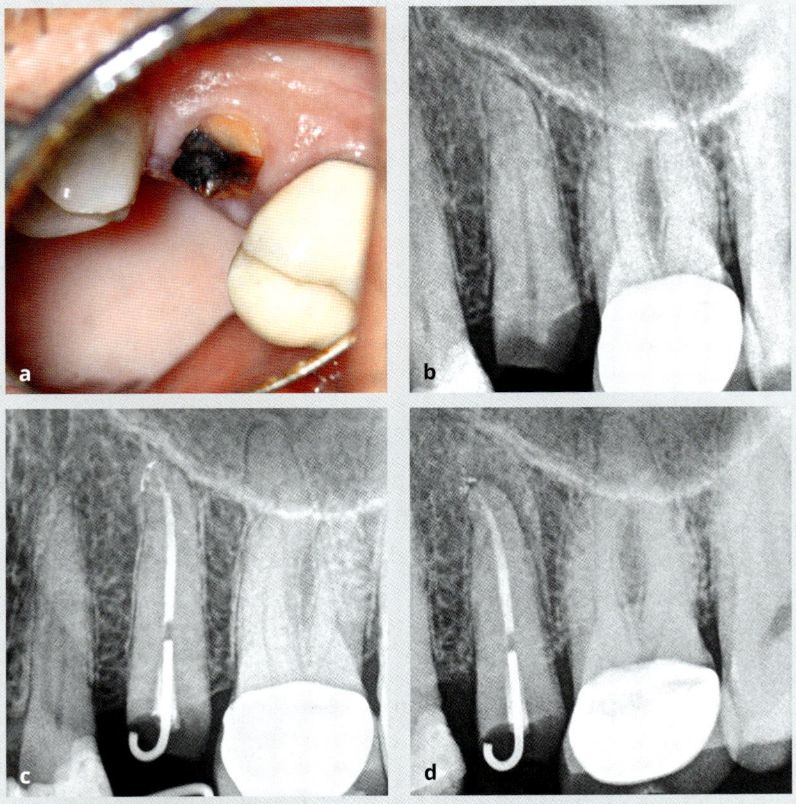

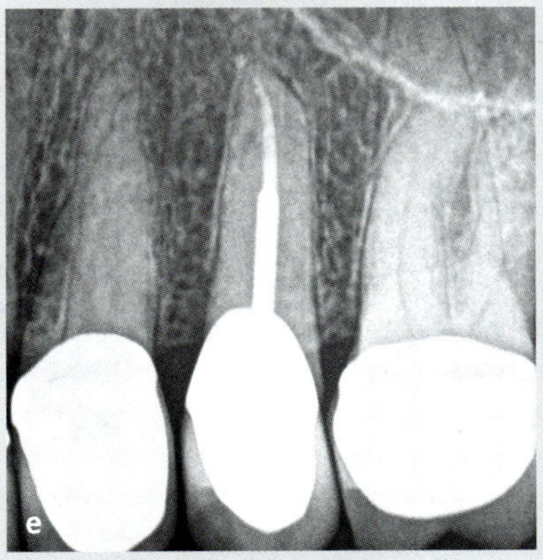

Fig 7-12 *(a and b)* The stump of tooth no. 13 was mostly level with the gingiva, and its distal aspect was level with the bony crest. *(c)* Root canal treatment was completed, and a J-shaped hook was cemented into the post space and connected by an elastic ligature to a thick wire bonded to teeth nos. 12 and 14. *(d)* The tooth was extruded within a couple of months, providing 3 mm of ferrule. *(e)* The tooth then received a parallel-sided, passive, serrated, vented post that was luted with an auto-curing resinous cement, a resin-composite build-up, and a full crown. (Case courtesy of Dr Mary Chien.)

Ferrule

The ferrule concept, when a band or ring is used to encompass the natural root or crown of a tooth, should be considered when an artificial full crown is necessitated for a severely damaged tooth (Fig 7-11).[53] The height of the ferrule, or the remaining tooth stump, is of paramount importance.[51,54–57] The thickness of the walls of the remaining stump is also important, as is their number and distribution.[49,55] The higher the stump, the thicker the remaining walls, and the greater the number of intact walls, the better. Even if the remaining stump is irregular in height form, it should not be shortened to make its form more regular or elegant.

Fokkinga et al reported that the 10-year survival rate for restoration of endodontically treated molars was 92% to 95% when substantial dentin remained, defined as follows: > 75% of the circumferential dentin wall had > 1 mm thickness and a height of > 1 mm above gingival level; < 25% of the circumference had < 1 mm above the gingiva, but a ferrule of 1 to 2 mm could be achieved.[49] If these conditions were not met, the 10-year restoration survival rate fell to between 83% and 87%. Clearly, the amount of solid ferrule is very important, but the long-term survival rates for restorations where minimal ferrule existed are still substantial. It is important to note that adequate ferrule can still be achieved by the remaining buccal and lingual walls of a tooth preparation even when deep proximal boxes are present. Ferrule height may be more important for the restoration of anterior teeth, because they are primarily subjected to horizontal tipping forces. If inadequate ferrule exists, crown lengthening or orthodontic extrusion can provide a longer ferrule, though at the cost of a slightly decreased crown-to-root ratio (Fig 7-12). Orthodontic extrusion is preferred in situations where the gingival architecture is visible when the patient smiles. If coronal cracks are present, including them within the ferrule is likely to be beneficial.

Complications and corrective actions

There is nothing that can be done after the fact to address a failure to conserve tooth structure; the tooth's prognosis is irreversibly lessened. The tooth should be restored with respect to the principles outlined above and below. Overall planning for the patient's long-term rehabilitation should be extended to include contingencies for the possibility of tooth loss. For example, a terminal RPD abutment with a full crown can be converted to a dome underneath a distal extension, which can be predictably retained while it provides key vertical support to the prosthesis and shortens the length of the tissue-supported distal extension. Long-term transition from one type of prosthesis to another may be considered, such as partial denture to complete overdenture, tooth-supported to implant-supported or mixed, etc. Even though a tooth's prognosis has been lessened by failure to maximally conserve tooth structure, it is important to recognize that a restoration with minimal remaining coronal structure can still have a good long-term survival rate.[49]

Access Preparation Through Restorations

Preexisting coronal restorations should generally be removed before or during access preparation due to the possibilities of coronal leakage, microbial ingress, and secondary caries. However, if the restoration is known to be new and sound, it may be retained.

Access through metallic restorations should be accomplished using new carbide burs, copious water spray, and light pressure. Several burs may be needed because metals are tougher than tooth enamel.

Access through porcelain-fused-to-metal (PFM) restorations should start by using fine diamond burs until the metal coping is reached, and then carbide burs should be used.

Access through all-ceramic restorations, either zirconia or lithium disilicate, demands patience, multiple fine diamond burs, copious water spray, and light pressure, because these materials are extremely hard and brittle. The inherent brittleness of ceramics means that sufficient bulk must remain after access preparation if the restoration is to be predictably retained.

Complications and corrective actions

If leakage is recognized after access through an existing restoration, it should be immediately removed so as to prevent further microbial contamination. If the previously existing restoration fractures, it should be removed. In both situations, a provisional restoration is needed to prevent microbial ingress and to prevent drift of adjacent or opposing teeth.

Internal Bleaching

Internal bleaching, also known as *walking bleaching*, is a valuable adjunct to the restoration of stained anterior teeth. Internal bleaching and direct resin-composite restorations are extremely conservative of tooth structure. Full-crown preparations should be avoided whenever possible in anterior teeth, especially those that have received access preparations for root canal treatment. The remaining tooth structure is extremely precious.

Internal bleaching is effective in increasing color value or lightness. Value is considered more important to the viewer than both *hue*, ie, the place of a color on the visual spectrum, and *chroma*, ie, the saturation or intensity of the hue. Value can also be increased by using an opaque white resin-composite build-up material in the deeper part of the access restoration. Internal bleaching is effective against many stains, notably those caused by blood degradation products during pulpal death. Internal bleaching is generally not effective against stains from metallic restorations or severe tetracycline staining.

Sodium perborate can be packed as a slurry into an access cavity and replaced weekly for a few weeks. But first, a liner should be placed to above the level of periodontal attachment to reduce the risk of damaging the periodontal ligament or of external resorption. Even though sodium perborate is bactericidal, a robust provisional restoration is needed to prevent washout and subsequent microbial ingress. It has been suggested that heat and hydrogen peroxide (eg, Superoxol, Sultan) not be used because they elevate the risk of external resorption.[59-61]

Complications and corrective actions

If an unacceptable esthetic result occurs despite internal bleaching and replacement of indirect resin-composite restorations, then a porcelain veneer should be considered. Full-crown restorations should only be placed as a last resort.

If heat and hydrogen peroxide are not used, it is unlikely that external resorption will occur. If external resorption does occur, it can be recognized through periodontal probing, the use of a curved explorer tip, and the presence of a radiolucency that moves laterally when an off-angle radiograph or CBCT is used. Often, external resorption following bleaching is self-limiting, making hygiene the primary problem. External resorption can be addressed through periodontal flap surgery and the placement of a resin-modified glass-ionomer restoration.[62]

The Coronoradicular Build-up and Access Preparation Closure

A coronoradicular build-up without a post is an excellent core foundation restoration for most root-canal-treated molars. Sufficient resistance and retention form can generally be attained from the opposing walls of the pulp chamber, even if undercuts are not present, and even if only 2 to 3 walls remain.[63-65] It is also possible to engage the coronal 1 or 2 mm of the canals,[63] but there is no utility in placing a build-up deeper into the canals because both amalgam and composite are weak in tension. It is important that there be no void between obturation and restoration (Fig 7-13; see also Fig 7-11). As explained above, the coronoradicular build-up is best placed at the time of obturation, before the rubber dam is removed (see Fig 7-7).[24,45,48]

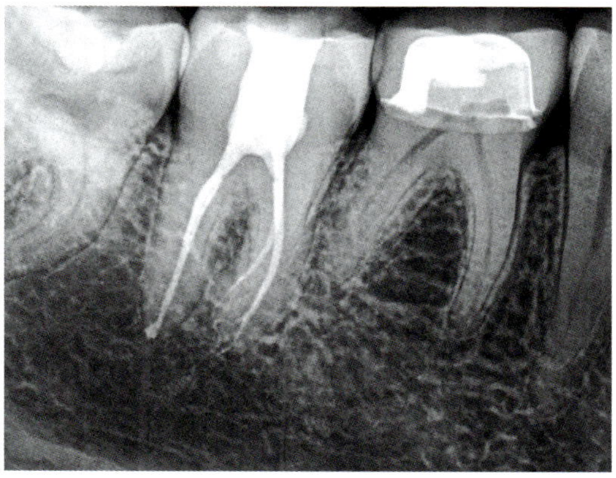

Fig 7-13 Voids between obturation material and build-up should be avoided. Excess radiolucent bonding resin can pool in the canal orifices, but this can be dabbed away using inverted or trimmed paper points.

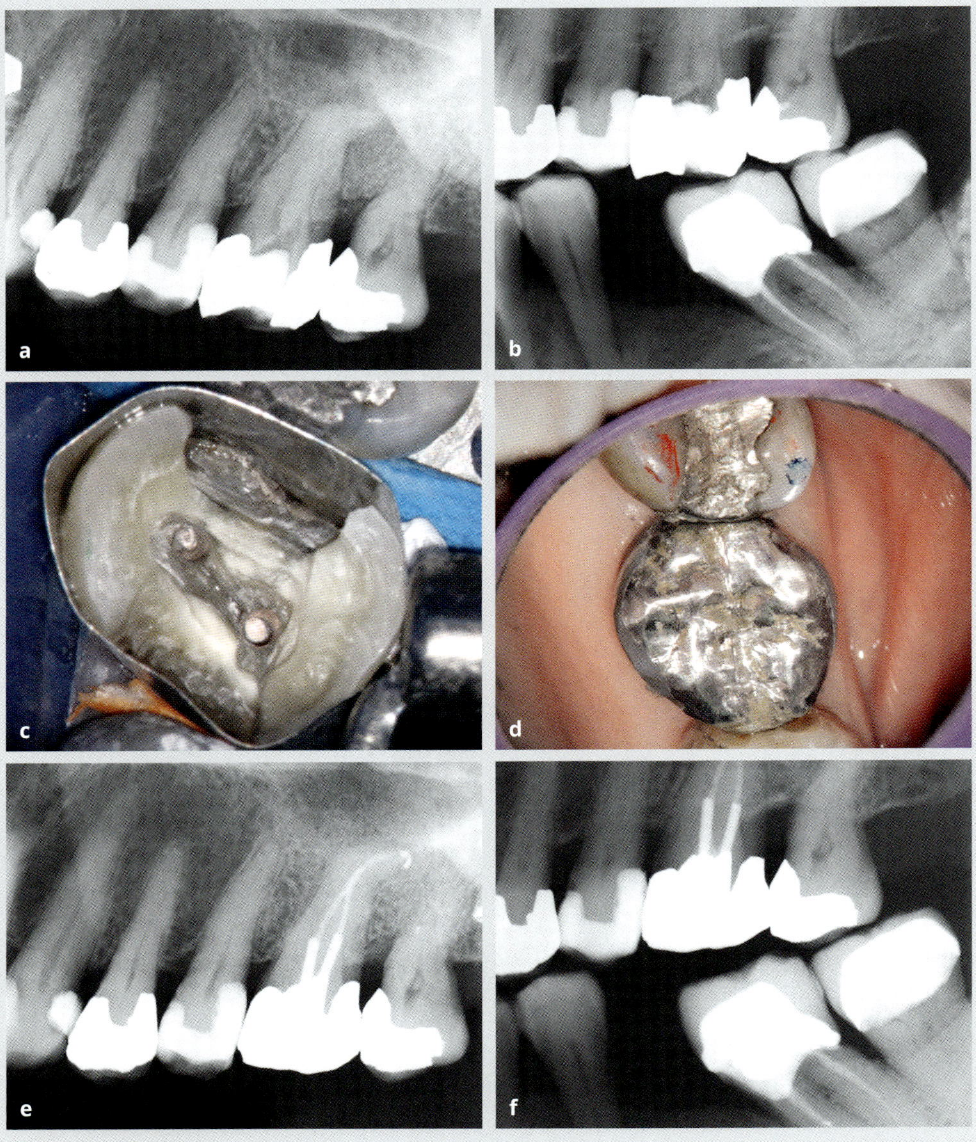

Fig 7-14 *(a)* Tooth no. 14 required root canal treatment and extensive restoration; the patient had additional pressing needs. *(b)* A bitewing view indicated that adequate coronal tooth structure remained. *(c and d)* An amalgam coronoradicular build-up, including two conservative parallel-sided, vented, and serrated posts, was used to provide an immediate restoration, with coronal coverage obtained by shoeing all the cusps. *(e and f)* Recall demonstrated health and provided opportunity for polishing. (Courtesy of Dr Dale Jung.)

Amalgam or resin-composite can be used, but the glass-ionomer family is too weak to be used as a bulk build-up material.[66,67] Glass-ionomer is better suited to be used as a liner or a base; it has good sealing ability and potential for fluoride release, both desirable properties for a liner or base in endodontically treated teeth. Amalgam has many advantages—it is strong, stable, and user friendly.[66] It can also be used to shoe or cover cusps when an indirect restoration is not planned (Fig 7-14).[63] Amalgam is the authors' first choice for posterior teeth. One disadvantage is that even fast-setting amalgams need 45 minutes or longer to set before they should be prepared using a handpiece.

Resin-composite is widely used for build-ups and the restoration of access preparations (Fig 7-15). Its principal advantages are that it is tooth colored and can be prepared with a handpiece shortly after polymerization. Posterior resin-composite restorations are considered highly technique sensitive. Polymerization shrinkage is a problem inherent to all resin-composite restorations, but the issue becomes more acute the deeper the restoration becomes and the less free unbonded surface area is available for stress relaxation through deformation, giving a more unfavorable configuration factor (C-factor). An unfavorable C-factor fights against the efforts of the bonding agent to adhere the restoration to the walls of the preparation.

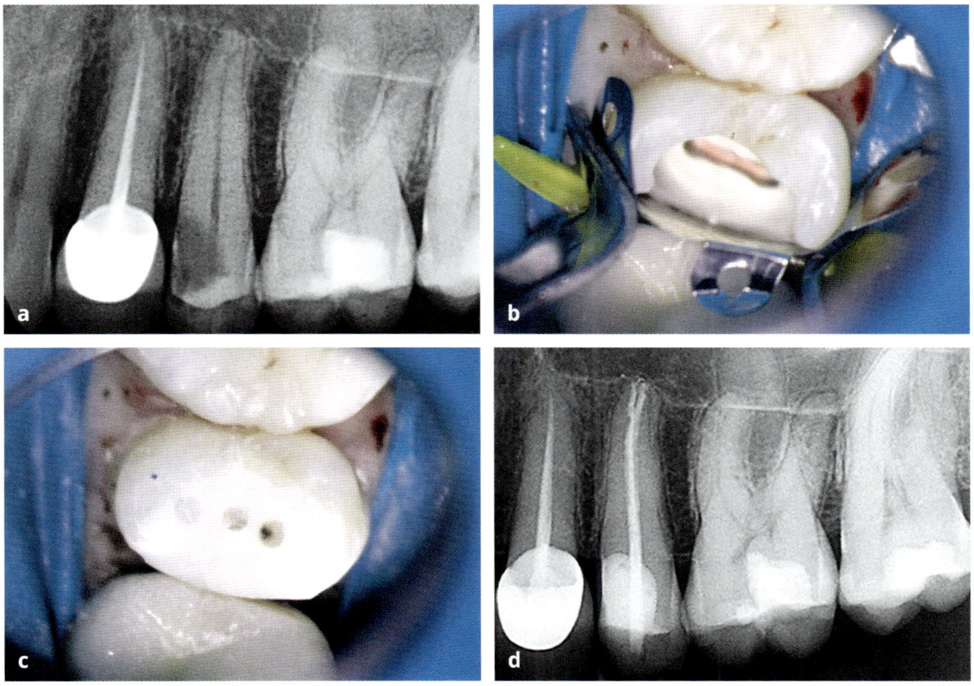

Fig 7-15 *(a and b)* Tooth no. 13 suffered extensive caries, undermining both cusps. *(c)* Small 0.6-mm diameter fiber posts (Size 0, Ultradent) were placed, along with a resin-composite material (LuxaCore Z Dual, DMG America) to form an immediate core build-up. In this case, the form of the coronal defect facilitated curing-light penetration, and the relative abundance of free unbonded surface area reduced the consequences of polymerization shrinkage. *(d)* No additional tooth structure was removed for post placement.

An endodontic access cavity presents the worst possible C-factor of all direct restorations. A glass-ionomer base will help to ameliorate the C-factor somewhat. If a light-cured resin composite is used, many layers are needed to ensure that the full depth of the restoration is fully cured. This is time consuming, but layering may help to reduce net shrinkage. Alternatively, if an auto-curing resin composite is to be used, the dentist can be assured that setting will be achieved through the full depth of the restoration, but the effects of polymerization shrinkage cannot be modulated. Most dual-curing resin composites will not achieve optimal levels of polymerization unless they are layered, so they have little if any advantage. Flowable composites contain less filler than regular composites, so they tend to have lesser mechanical properties and lesser dimensional stability; therefore, their use is not recommended for build-up restorations for endodontically treated teeth. Although resin composites shrink upon polymerization, they also tend to imbibe water over time, leading to some dimensional instability and degradation of mechanical properties. Furthermore, the resin-to-dentin bond is inherently weaker and less predictable than the bond to enamel, and it tends to degrade over time, so fundamental restorative principles not dependent upon the resin-to-dentin bond must be followed.

Dentin bonding procedures for resin composites in endodontic restorations present additional challenges. Dentinal tubule density tends to decrease in deeper dentin and radicular dentin, making dentin bonding less effective. Performing the multiple steps necessary for resin bonding becomes more difficult the deeper the preparation; access preparations are the deepest of all. Any residual sealer may prevent adhesion. Eugenol, a component of all zinc oxide–eugenol sealers, poisons resinous polymerization. Sodium hypochlorite irrigants, preferred for their antimicrobial activity, tend to produce a mushy and oxygen-rich smear layer, preventing micromechanical adhesion and inhibiting polymerization of bonding agents. Carefully cleaning the pulp chamber and the entire preparation using an ethylenediaminetetraacetic acid (EDTA) rinse to remove the oxygen-rich smear layer, using a glass-ionomer base to cover the obturations and decrease restoration depth before commencing bonding procedures, and paying attention to technical detail are all helpful in improving the effectiveness of adhesive resinous procedures.

Adhesion of composite to preexisting coronal restorations, to seal access preparations, primarily uses the ability of multipurpose bonding agents to engage micromechanical roughness. Exposed porcelain can be etched using hydrofluoric acid gel, an intrinsically dangerous material, but stronger all-ceramic substrates such as lithium disilicate and zirconia are resistant to acid etching.[68]

Gingival management is important when build-up or crown margins are adjacent to or below the gingival crest. Again, using a rubber dam is helpful. Hemostatic agents can also be helpful, as can judicious cauterization; gingivectomy may be needed sometimes as well. Prerestoration, eg, using a resin-modified glass ionomer, is sometimes needed to achieve isolation and gingival health before the tooth can be isolated and root canal treatment initiated.

Complications and corrective actions

If insufficient tooth structure remains to provide resistance form after caries removal and access preparation, either for a coronoradicular build-up or for a crown preparation, posting is indicated. Lack of retention form may also sometimes indicate the need for a post, particularly for full-crown restorations. However, care to achieve parallelism in ferrule preparation may improve both resistance form and retention form and thereby may decrease the need for a post.

Pins should generally be avoided in the restoration of endodontically treated teeth because little room remains between the periodontium and the pulp chamber. Also, pins are actively placed into dentin and tend to cause microcracks.[69,70]

If adhesive resinous procedures are planned, using an endodontic sealer that does not contain eugenol should be considered. Resin-based sealers (AH26, Dentsply Maillefer; Sealapex, Kerr) can be considered. Calcium-silicate sealers (EndoSequence BC Sealer HiFlow) are strongly recommended, being the only class of sealer that actually has substantive sealing ability. However, more evidence and long-term studies are needed to prove their effectiveness.

Overdenture Abutments

Saving a few teeth to support an overdenture greatly eases an elderly patient's transition from the partly edentulous to the completely edentulous state.[71] The primary value of an overdenture abutment is providing vertical support. At least two abutments should be retained, at least one on either side of the arch, to provide a stable prosthesis (Fig 7-16). After completion of root canal treatment, the abutment tooth can be prepared to form a dome, and the access preparation can be plugged with amalgam or resin composite. The dome shape is necessary to provide a hygienic and cleansable emergence profile, at least a couple millimeters above the adjacent soft tissues; its height is only limited by the space available for the base of the prosthesis and the prosthetic teeth. A domed abutment also facilitates prosthesis delivery and adjustment; only the top of the dome should actively contact the base of the prosthesis. If sufficient tooth structure does not remain for dome preparation, a dome-shaped casting, retained by a conservative post, can be made. Overdenture abutments can also be used to enhance the stability of RPDs. If the crown of a tooth in a partly edentulous dentition breaks off close to the gumline, it can often be converted into an overdenture abutment.

Complications and corrective actions

If an overdenture abutment is lost, that part of the denture can simply be relined. The consequences of overdenture abutment loss are not severe, particularly after the patient has made a successful transition to complete dentures. If the top of the abutment has been flattened, it will be more difficult to maintain gingival health, and inflamed gingiva may be pinched; in this event, an indirect casting should be considered to provide appropriate emergence form and a rounded

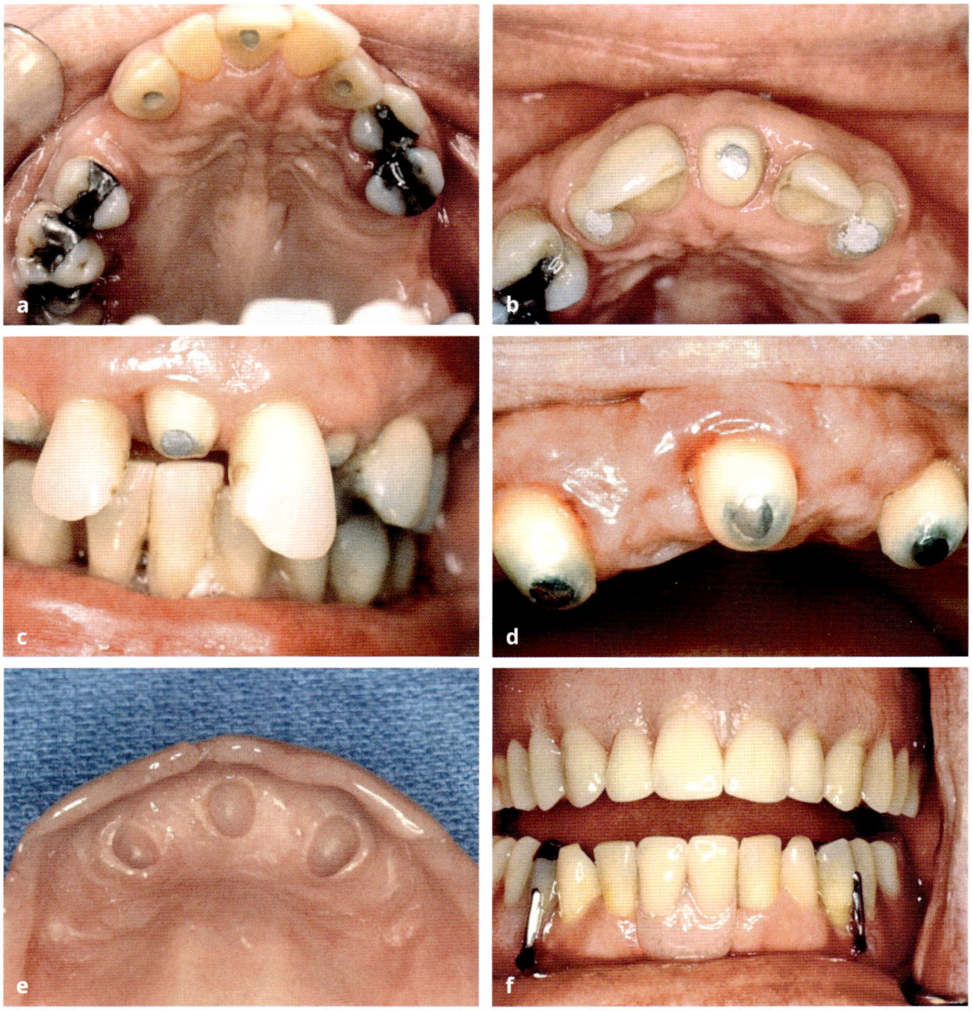

Fig 7-16 *(a)* The patient suffered from severe periodontal disease and repeated periodontal abscesses. *(b)* Three abutment teeth—left, right, and anterior—received root canal treatment and amalgam plugs; *(c and d)* these teeth received dome preparations, and the other teeth were extracted. *(e and f)* An immediate overdenture was delivered and relined in the anterior area, providing oral rehabilitation.

contour. By far the most common error concerning overdenture abutments is a failure to consider them in initial treatment planning.

Posts

It has been known for half a century that posts weaken endodontically treated teeth and are associated with more serious types of tooth fracture, vertical, as well as with root perforation.[7,10,70,72–78] In addition, post preparation and provisionalization before post cementation presents increased risk of coronal leakage.[45,79] For these reasons, posts should be avoided whenever possible. However, posts are still used with undue frequency.

As explained above, posts are rarely needed in molars, because a coronoradicular build-up provides adequate resistance and retention forms, conserves tooth structure, avoids the risk of perforation, and decreases the risk of root fracture. Posts may be needed more often in anterior teeth where minimal ferrule remains.[80] Even so, a post may have difficulty resisting the more horizontal tipping or jiggling forces that anterior teeth receive.[56] The loss of adequate ferrule or stump is irreversible. Posts may be needed in premolars when buccal or lingual walls of the tooth have been lost; a rule of thumb is to place a conservative post in each canal that is adjacent to a lost wall (see Fig 7-15).[81]

If a post is necessary, it is recommended that only minimal root structure be removed during preparation. The post should be as follows: *narrow*, < ¼ of the narrowest part of the root width; *parallel-sided*, as much as reasonably possible, to improve resistance and retention forms and to avoid a wedging effect; *passive*, so it does not stress the root when loaded; *serrated or roughened*, so it can be gripped by its cement; and *vented*, so excess cement can escape to reduce pressure during cementation and the post can be easily seated to length (ParaPost X-System Metal, Coltene; see Fig 7-12).[75,82–84] It is important that a post be fully seated and there be no void between the post and the obturation (see Fig 7-13).[85,86]

When planning for post length, it is important to retain sufficient apical obturating material: ≥ 4 mm is typically recommended. In addition, it is generally recommended that the length of a post extend below the cementoenamel junction to a length as long as the tooth crown.[75,87] If both of these criteria cannot be met, the apical 4 mm of obturation and the root should be preserved at the expense of post length. It is also important to note that 2D radiographs will not show root curvatures that turn directly away from or toward the viewer. For example, palatal roots of maxillary molars tend to curve back toward the buccal, predisposing to post perforations on their palatal aspects. Root concavities can be indicated by the presence of multiple periodontal outlines on a root, the inner lines representing the minimal root thickness. Oblique off-angle views should accompany the usual straight-on radiographic view so that an impression of 3D curvatures and root concavities may be gained.

Ideally, posts should be placed at the time of obturation, when the 3D root canal anatomy has been freshly learned and the rubber dam remains in place (see Fig 7-15).[19] Furthermore, the challenges of provisionalization are then reduced.[88] If post placement is to be delayed, it is recommended that the post space be filled with a nonsetting $Ca(OH)_2$ intracanal medicament. However, it is important that all of the $Ca(OH)_2$ is removed before cementation; irrigation, mechanical cleaning, and patience are also needed.

If a post preparation is to be made at a later appointment or made in a tooth that has previously received root canal treatment, it is recommended that rubber dam isolation be achieved and that gutta-percha first be removed using a heated instrument, an electrically heated plugger, or a Schilder plugger that has been heated in a flame. Heated pluggers can remove the bulk of the gutta-percha without the danger of perforation or deviation, a common error in post space preparation.[78] Next, it is recommended to use a Gates-Glidden drill one size smaller than the desired post; because it has rounded flutes and no shoulder, it tends to follow the natural anatomy.[78] Finally, the post space can be completed using a post drill or a Peeso reamer.

The vast majority of posts used today are prefabricated and can be placed at time of obturation. However, custom posts can have some advantages, as long as they are designed with the attributes described above. Custom posts tend to be better adapted, somewhat improving resistance and retention. Also, the custom post and core are formed in one piece, somewhat improving the delivery of occlusal stresses to the remaining tooth structure.[87]

Fiber posts have been touted for their flexibility, or low elastic modulus, bending like dentin. However, we must remember what we are asking a post to do: to resist lateral, jiggling, or tipping forces when insufficient ferrule remains. Additionally, we place posts in the centers of roots, where the root canals are, but that is the most mechanically ineffective location, at the neutral axis of the root.[50] Material at the neutral axis of a beam, column, or rod does very little to resist bending forces mechanically, because at that location, the tensile and compressive forces balance out to net zero. Thus, a flexible post will transfer more stresses to the restoration-tooth interface margins. Additionally, fiber posts that contain serrations tend to be substantially weaker and more flexible than smooth-sided alternatives of the same diameter. Hence, smooth-sided fiber posts may have relative advantage over serrated fiber posts (DT Light-Post, Bisco). Furthermore, the mechanical properties of fiber posts degrade substantially over time and insult, whereas metallic posts' mechanical properties are stable.[89]

If a post is needed due to insufficient ferrule or stump height, then a material stiffer than dentin is needed to provide increased mechanical resistance. So, if only a minimal ferrule remains, it is suggested that posts be made of titanium, stainless steel, or yellow gold, all materials with moderate moduli of elasticity. If a moderate ferrule remains, glass fiber posts may provide sufficient mechanical resistance.[90] If a substantial ferrule exists, then a post is not needed and should be avoided.[91] Even when a post is used, the height of the remaining stump remains the most important prognostic factor.[92] Ferrari et al have reported that fiber posts improved restoration survival over premolars without posts, in all cases where less than three complete walls of premolars' natural crowns remained, but comparison was not made to metallic posts.[93]

Restorations retained by metallic posts have higher survival rates than those retained by fiber posts.[94] However, anecdotally, it appears that when a fiber post fails, it may do so with less damage to the remaining tooth structure.[88,94–96]

Adhesive bonding of posts to radicular dentin—the "monobloc"—remains a concept, not a reality. Nonetheless, strong adhesive cements will achieve some bonding, improve retention, and decrease leakage.[97,98] Auto-curing resin-composite, auto-curing resin-modified glass-ionomer, and conventional glass-ionomer cements are recommended for cementing both posts and crowns in endodontically treated teeth.

Complications and corrective actions

If excessive obturation material is removed, it should be replaced. Preparation of a post space at the time of obturation greatly facilitates such adjustments.

Should an excessively wide or tapered preparation be made, the loss of tooth structure is irreversible and the prognosis irreversibly lessened, but not necessarily dramatically.[99] Restoration should be completed according to the above principles as much as possible.

If a perforation occurs during post space preparation, it can be repaired conservatively and nonsurgically by an endodontist using a microscope and a calcium silicate material (Fig 7-17). Internal perforation repair is surprisingly predictable.

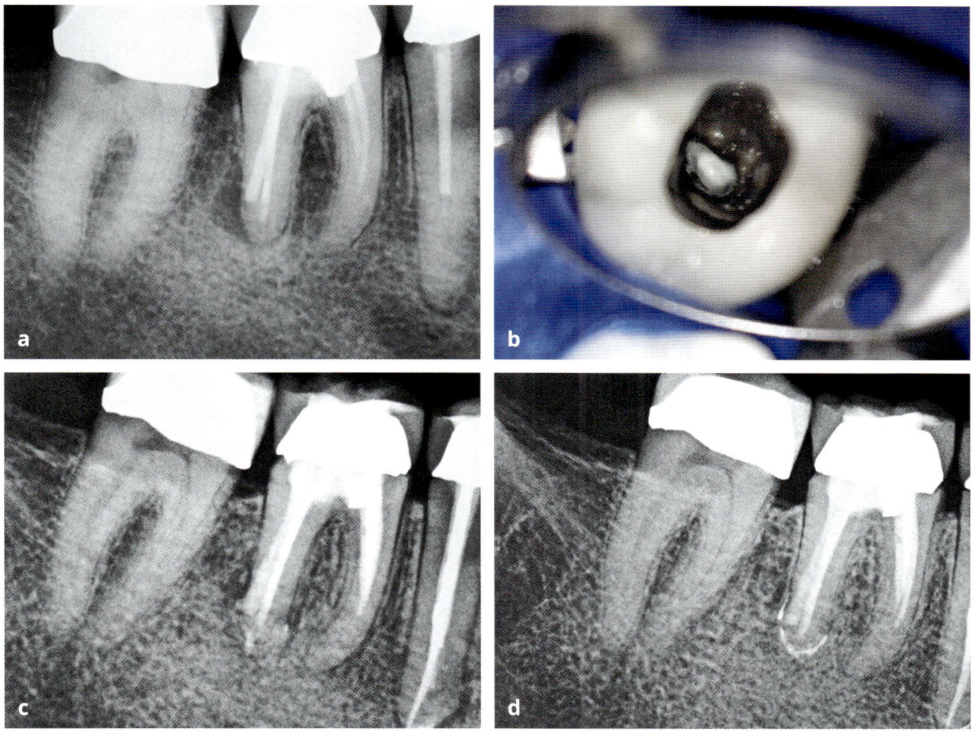

Fig 7-17 *(a)* Tooth no. 30 had an apical post preparation perforation. *(b and c)* Sufficient mechanical and visual access was obtained for post removal and the perforation was repaired using a calcium silicate material, mineral trioxide aggregate (ProRoot MTA, Tulsa/Dentsply). *(d)* Recall indicated healing and an intact lamina dura.

Post preparation perforations may not initially be recognized at the time of post space preparation; a periodontal ligament that has only been nicked by a drill may not bleed much, if at all. At that time, using a microscope for visual assessment is helpful; using an inverted paper point to check for a persistent moist spot may also be helpful. Routine radiographic follow-up evaluations may help to identify radiolucencies, which are indicators of the inflammatory or infectious sequellae of post perforations.

If a metallic post fractures or needs to be removed to facilitate nonsurgical endodontic retreatment, it can be removed by an endodontist using a microscope and ultrasonic vibration. Post extractors can also be used, but they apply substantial forces to the remaining root and therefore should only be used after considerable ultrasonic instrumentation has assailed the luting cement. Posts that are parallel or serrated or those that have been luted with tough resinous cements will be considerably more difficult to remove.

Loosening of a post may be a precursor to fracture, but loosening may not be noticed until dislodgement occurs. If a post is to be recemented, a strong auto-setting adhesive resin-composite cement is suggested (Panavia SA Cement Universal, Kuraray).

If a glass fiber post fractures, it can be carefully removed by first making a small pilot hole, then using a special tapered stainless-steel drill, and finally using a Peeso reamer (DT Light-Post Removal Kit, Bisco; UniCore Post and Drill System, Ultradent). This is possible because fiber posts have unidirectional fibers, so they splinter easily. Ultrasonic endodontic instrumentation can also assist in their disintegration.

If a root fractures vertically or obliquely, extraction, with or without replacement, is the only course of action. The risk of root fracture is increased by post placement, particularly with large, tapered, or actively engaged posts.

Coronal Coverage

Anterior endodontically treated teeth that fail generally do so through repeated horizontal tipping or jiggling forces dislodging the natural or artificial crown or causing cervical fracture, or "snap-off"; in contrast, posterior endodontically treated teeth generally fail through repeated vertical forces causing vertical tooth fracture. Hence, restorative recommendations differ.

Full-crown preparations should generally be avoided on anterior teeth in favor of multiple resin-composite restorations, a porcelain veneer, internal bleaching, or all of the above.[74] An access preparation necessarily removes tooth structure from the center of the crown. After circumferential preparation to a depth of 1 mm or more, at the level of the cementoenamel junction, little tooth structure remains.

Conversely, coronal coverage is generally recommended for the restoration of posterior endodontically treated teeth.[67,74,100,101] The purpose of the coronal coverage is to hold the cusps together to prevent vertical cracks from being driven through the grooves and fossae by opposing cusps. The most conservative option should be chosen, whether that be an onlay, a three-quarter crown, or a full crown. A preparation for a cast gold restoration is more conservative than that for a CAD/CAM all-ceramic restoration. Limited evidence has suggested that coronal coverage may not be needed in posterior teeth when the access preparation is conservative and most of the marginal ridges are intact (see Fig 7-9).[67,102]

Nonetheless, it is clear that many posterior teeth that would benefit from cuspal coverage do not receive it.[6,103]

In the past, attention was primarily focused on *retention form*, the feature of a tooth preparation that resists dislodgment of a crown in a vertical direction or along the path of placement.[53] However, *resistance form*, the feature of a tooth preparation that enhances the stability of a restoration and resists dislodgment along an axis other than the path of placement, is more relevant to preventing restorative failure of endodontically treated teeth.[53]

Complications and corrective actions

If a root fractures vertically or obliquely, extraction, with or without replacement, is the only course of action. If a posterior tooth at risk of fracture due to lack of coronal coverage is identified, it can be restored with coronal coverage, but a comprehensive endodontic evaluation should be performed first.

Conclusion

Careful diagnosis and planning greatly decrease the risk of restorative complications. Dentists should be alert to the possibility of restorative complications and work to prevent them because they generally irreversibly lower the prognosis, even if not dramatically. The onus is to demonstrate that a complication has not occurred. The most common restorative complications are related to failure to conserve precious tooth structure, failure to prevent microbial ingress, and the undue use of excessively large posts. Many restorative complications are irreversible, so their prevention is paramount.

References

1. Baba NZ, White SN, Bogen G. Restoration of endodontically treated teeth. In: Chugal N, Lin LM (eds). Endodontic Prognosis: Clinical Guide for Optimal Treatment Outcome. Cham, Switzerland: Springer, 2017:161–192.
2. White SN, Torabinejad M. From tooth retention through root canal treatment to extraction and replacement. In: Chugal N, Lin LM (eds). Endodontic Prognosis: Clinical Guide for Optimal Treatment Outcome. Cham, Switzerland: Springer, 2017:229–238.
3. Valderhaug J, Jokstad A, Ambjørnsen E, Norheim PW. Assessment of the periapical and clinical status of crowned teeth over 25 years. J Dent 1997;25:97–105.
4. Fuss Z, Lustig J, Tamse A. Prevalence of vertical root fractures in extracted endodontically treated teeth. Int Endod J 1999;32:283–286.
5. Vire DE. Failure of endodontically treated teeth: Classification and evaluation. J Endod 1991;17:338–342.
6. Eckerbom M, Magnusson T, Martinsson T. Reasons for and incidence of tooth mortality in a Swedish population. Endod Dent Traumatol 1992;8:230–234.
7. Zadik Y, Sandler V, Bechor R, Salehrabi R. Analysis of factors related to extraction of endodontically treated teeth. Oral Surg Oral Med Oral Pathol Oral Radiol Endod 2008;106:e31–e35
8. Touré B, Faye B, Kane AW, Lo CM, Niang B, Boucher Y. Analysis of reasons for extraction of endodontically treated teeth: A prospective study. J Endod 2011;37:1512–1515.
9. Torabinejad M, White SN. Endodontic treatment options after unsuccessful initial root canal treatment: Alternatives to single-tooth implants. J Am Dent Assoc 2016;147:214–220.
10. Fuss Z, Lustig J, Katz A, Tamse A. An evaluation of endodontically treated vertical root fractured teeth: Impact of operative procedures. J Endod 2001;27:46–48.

11. Jacques J. Galen's reading of Hippocratic ethics. In: van der Eijk P (ed). Greek Medicine from Hippocrates to Galen: Selected Papers. Leiden, Netherlands: Brill, 2012:259–286.
12. Sorensen JA, Martinoff JT. Endodontically treated teeth as abutments. J Prosthet Dent. 1985;53:631–636.
13. Hatzikyriakos AH, Reisis GI, Tsingos N. A 3-year postoperative clinical evaluation of posts and cores beneath existing crowns. J Prosthet Dent. 1992;67:454–458.
14. Mentink AG, Meeuwissen R, Käyser AF, Mulder J. Survival rate and failure characteristics of the all metal post and core restoration. J Oral Rehabil 1993;20:455–461.
15. Wegner PK, Freitag S, Kern M. Survival rate of endodontically treated teeth with posts after prosthetic restoration. J Endod 2006;32:928–931.
16. De Backer H, Van Maele G, Decock V, Van den Berghe L. Long-term survival of complete crowns, fixed dental prostheses, and cantilever fixed dental prostheses with posts and cores on root canal-treated teeth. Int J Prosthodont 2007;20:229–234.
17. Ng YL, Mann V, Gulabivala K. Tooth survival following non-surgical root canal treatment: A systematic review of the literature. Int Endod J 2010;43:171–189.
18. Caplan DJ, Kolker J, Rivera EM, Walton RE. Relationship between number of proximal contacts and survival of root canal treated teeth. Int Endod J 2002;35:193–199.
19. Saunders WP, Saunders EM. Coronal leakage as a cause of failure in root-canal therapy: A review. Endod Dent Traumatol 1994;10:105-108.
20. Ray HA, Trope M. Periapical status of endodontically treated teeth in relation to the technical quality of the root filling and the coronal restoration. Int Endod J 1995;28:12–18.
21. Tronstad L, Asbjørnsen K, Døving L, Pedersen I, Eriksen HM. Influence of coronal restorations on the periapical health of endodontically treated teeth. Endod Dent Traumatol 2000;16:218–221.
22. Kirkevang LL, Ørstavik D, Hörsted-Bindslev P, Wenzel A. Periapical status and quality of root fillings and coronal restorations in a Danish population. Int Endod J 2000;33:509–515.
23. Hommez GM, Coppens CR, De Moor RJ. Periapical health related to the quality of coronal restorations and root fillings. Int Endod J 2002;35:680–689.
24. Heling I, Gorfil C, Slutzky H, Kopolovic K, Zalkind M, Slutzky-Goldberg I. Endodontic failure caused by inadequate restorative procedures: Review and treatment recommendations. J Prosthet Dent 2002;87:674–678.
25. Segura-Egea JJ, Jiménez-Pinzón A, Poyato-Ferrera M, Velasco-Ortega E, Ríos-Santos JV. Periapical status and quality of root fillings and coronal restorations in an adult Spanish population. Int Endod J 2004;37:525–530.
26. Siqueira JF Jr, Rôças IN, Alves FR, Campos LC. Periradicular status related to the quality of coronal restorations and root canal fillings in a Brazilian population. Oral Surg Oral Med Oral Pathol Oral Radiol Endod 2005;100:369–374.
27. Chugal NM, Clive JM, Spångberg LS. Endodontic treatment outcome: Effect of the permanent restoration. Oral Surg Oral Med Oral Pathol Oral Radiol Endod 2007;104:576–582.
28. Kayahan MB, Malkondu O, Canpolat C, Kaptan F, Bayirli G, Kazazoglu E. Periapical health related to the type of coronal restorations and quality of root canal fillings in a Turkish subpopulation. Oral Surg Oral Med Oral Pathol Oral Radiol Endod 2008;105:e58–e62.
29. Ng YL, Mann V, Rahbaran S, Lewsey J, Gulabivala K. Outcome of primary root canal treatment: Systematic review of the literature—Part 2. Influence of clinical factors. Int Endod J 2008;41:6–31.
30. Estrela C, Leles CR, Hollanda AC, Moura MS, Pécora JD. Prevalence and risk factors of apical periodontitis in endodontically treated teeth in a selected population of Brazilian adults. Braz Dent J 2008;19:34–39.
31. Tavares PB, Bonte E, Boukpessi T, Siqueira JF Jr, Lasfargues JJ. Prevalence of apical periodontitis in root canal-treated teeth from an urban French population: Influence of the quality of root canal fillings and coronal restorations. J Endod 2009;35:810–813.
32. Gillen BM, Looney SW, Gu LS, et al. Impact of the quality of coronal restoration versus the quality of root canal fillings on success of root canal treatment: A systematic review and meta-analysis. J Endod 2011;37:895–902.
33. Evans JT, Simon JH. Evaluation of the apical seal produced by injected thermoplasticized gutta-percha in the absence of smear layer and root canal sealer. J Endod 1986;12:101–107.
34. Yared GM, Bou Dagher F. Sealing ability of the vertical condensation with different root canal sealers. J Endod 1996;22:6–8.
35. Schafer E, Zandbiglari T. Solubility of root canal sealers in water and artificial saliva. Int Endod J 2003;36:660–669.
36. Wong JG, Caputo AA, Li P, White SN. Microleakage of adhesive resinous materials in root canals. J Conserv Dent 2013;16:213–218.
37. Swanson K, Madison S. An evaluation of coronal microleakage in endodontically treated teeth. Part I. Time periods. J Endod 1987;13:56–59.
38. Torabinejad M, Ung B, Kettering JD. In vitro bacterial penetration of coronally unsealed endodontically treated teeth. J Endod 1990;16:566–569.

39. Khayat A, Lee SJ, Torabinejad M. Human saliva penetration of coronally unsealed obturated root canals. J Endod 1993;19:458–461.
40. Monsef E, Goodman X, Fayazi S, Ogawa R, Abbott B, White SN. Dentists' knowledge of root canal treatment is sub-optimal and variable: A scoping review. Endodontic Society of the Philippines Journal 2021;14:8–15.
41. Imura N, Otani SM, Campos MJ, Jardim Júnior EG, Zuolo ML. Bacterial penetration through temporary restorative materials in root-canal-treated teeth in vitro. Int Endod J 1997;30:381–385.
42. Todd MJ, Harrison JW. An evaluation of the immediate and early sealing properties of Cavit. J Endod 1979;5:362–367.
43. Yamauchi S, Shipper G, Buttke T, Yamauchi M, Trope M. Effect of orifice plugs on periapical inflammation in dogs. J Endod 2006;32:524–526.
44. Safavi KE, Dowden WE, Langeland K. Influence of delayed coronal permanent restoration on endodontic prognosis. Endod Dent Traumatol 1987;3:187–191.
45. Fox K, Gutteridge DL. An in vitro study of coronal microleakage in root-canal-treated teeth restored by the post and core technique. Int Endod J 1997;30:361–368.
46. Lynch CD, Burke FM, Ní Ríordáin R, Hannigan A. The influence of coronal restoration type on the survival of endodontically treated teeth. Eur J Prosthodont Restor Dent 2004;12:171–176.
47. Nagasiri R, Chitmongkolsuk S. Long-term survival of endodontically treated molars without crown coverage: A retrospective cohort study. J Prosthet Dent 2005;93:164–170.
48. Landys Borén D, Jonasson P, Kvist T. Long-term survival of endodontically treated teeth at a public dental specialist clinic. J Endod 2015;41:176–181.
49. Fokkinga WA, Kreulen CM, Bronkhorst EM, Creugers NH. Up to 17-year controlled clinical study on post-and-cores and covering crowns. J Dent 2007;35:778–786.
50. Sorensen JA. Preservation of tooth structure. J Calif Dent Assoc 1988;16:15–22.
51. Libman WJ, Nicholls JI. Load fatigue of teeth restored with cast posts and cores and complete crowns. Int J Prosthodont 1995;8:155–161.
52. Reeh ES, Messer HH, Douglas WH. Reduction in tooth stiffness as a result of endodontic and restorative procedures. J Endod 1989;15:512–516.
53. The Glossary of Prosthodontic Terms: Ninth Edition. J Prosthet Dent 2017;117(5 suppl):e1–e105.
54. Pereira JR, de Ornelas F, Conti PC, do Valle AL. Effect of a crown ferrule on the fracture resistance of endodontically treated teeth restored with prefabricated posts. J Prosthet Dent 2006;95:50–54.
55. Ng CC, Dumbrigue HB, Al-Bayat MI, Griggs JA, Wakefield CW. Influence of remaining coronal tooth structure location on the fracture resistance of restored endodontically treated anterior teeth. J Prosthet Dent 2006;95:290–296.
56. Mancebo JC, Jiménez-Castellanos E, Cañadas D. Effect of tooth type and ferrule on the survival of pulpless teeth restored with fiber posts: A 3-year clinical study. Am J Dent 2010;23:351–356.
57. Juloski J, Radovic I, Goracci C, Vulicevic ZR, Ferrari M. Ferrule effect: A literature review. J Endod 2012;38:11–19.
58. Ferrari M, Vichi A, Fadda GM, et al. A randomized controlled trial of endodontically treated and restored premolars. J Dent Res 2012;91(7 suppl):72S–78S.
59. Friedman S, Rotstein I, Libfeld H, Stabholz A, Heling I. Incidence of external root resorption and esthetic results in 58 bleached pulpless teeth. Endod Dent Traumatol 1988;4:23–26.
60. Rotstein I. In vitro determination and quantification of 30% hydrogen peroxide penetration through dentin and cementum during bleaching. Oral Surg Oral Med Oral Pathol 1991;72:602–606.
61. Rotstein I, Friedman S, Mor C, Katznelson J, Sommer M, Bab I. Histological characterization of bleaching-induced external root resorption in dogs. J Endod 1991;17:436–441.
62. Dragoo MR. Resin-ionomer and hybrid-ionomer cements: Part II, human clinical and histologic wound healing responses in specific periodontal lesions. Int J Periodontics Restorative Dent 1997;17:75–87.
63. Nayyar A, Walton RE, Leonard LA. An amalgam coronal-radicular dowel and core technique for endodontically treated posterior teeth. J Prosthet Dent 1980;43:511–515.
64. Hoag EP, Dwyer TG. A comparative evaluation of three post and core techniques. J Prosthet Dent 1982;47:177–181.
65. Creugers NH, Kreulen CM, Fokkinga WA, Mentink AG. A 5-year prospective clinical study on core restorations without covering crowns. Int J Prosthodont 2005;18:40–41.
66. Cho GC, Kaneko LM, Donovan TE, White SN. Diametral and compressive strength of dental core materials. J Prosthet Dent 1999;82:272–276.
67. Dammaschke T, Nykiel K, Sagheri D, Schäfer E. Influence of coronal restorations on the fracture resistance of root canal-treated premolar and molar teeth: A retrospective study. Aust Endod J 2013;39:48–56.
68. Goldstein RL, White SN. Esthetic and traumatic emergencies. In: Goldstein RL, Chu SJ, Lee EA, Stappert CFJ (eds). Ronald Goldstein's Esthetics in Dentistry, ed 3. Hoboken, NJ: Wiley, 2018:1215–1234.
69. Standlee JP, Collard EW, Caputo AA. Dentinal defects caused by some twist drills and retentive pins. J Prosthet Dent 1970;24:185–192.

70. Lovdahl PE, Nicholls JI. Pin-retained amalgam cores vs. cast-gold dowel-cores. J Prosthet Dent 1977;38:507–514.
71. Morrow RM, Rudd KD, Birmingham FD, Larkin JD. Immediate interim tooth-supported complete dentures. J Prosthet Dent 1973;30:695–700.
72. Kantor ME, Pines MS. A comparative study of restorative techniques for pulpless teeth. J Prosthet Dent 1977;38:405–412.
73. Guzy GE, Nicholls JI. In vitro comparison of intact endodontically treated teeth with and without endo-post reinforcement. J Prosthet Dent 1979;42:39–44.
74. Sorensen JA, Martinoff JT. Intracoronal reinforcement and coronal coverage: A study of endodontically treated teeth. J Prosthet Dent 1984;51:780–784.
75. Sorensen JA, Martinoff JT. Clinically significant factors in dowel design. J Prosthet Dent 1984;52:28–35.
76. Ottl P, Lauer HC. Success rates for two different types of post-and-cores. J Oral Rehabil 1998;25:752–758.
77. Morfis AS. Vertical root fractures. Oral Surg Oral Med Oral Pathol 1990;69:631–635.
78. Jamani KD, Aqrabawi J, Fayyad MA. A radiographic study of the relationship between technical quality of coronoradicular posts and periapical status in a Jordanian population. J Oral Sci 2005;47:123–128.
79. Demarchi MG, Sato EF. Leakage of interim post and cores used during laboratory fabrication of custom posts. J Endod 2002;28:328–329.
80. Sorensen JA, Engelman MJ. Ferrule design and fracture resistance of endodontically treated teeth. J Prosthet Dent 1990;63:529–536.
81. Fan P, Nicholls JI, Kois JC. Load fatigue of five restoration modalities in structurally compromised premolars. Int J Prosthodont 1995;8:213–220.
82. Standlee JP, Caputo AA, Hanson EC. Retention of endodontic dowels: Effects of cement, dowel length, diameter, and design. J Prosthet Dent 1978;39:400–405.
83. Torbjörner A, Karlsson S, Odman PA. Survival rate and failure characteristics for two post designs. J Prosthet Dent 1995;73:439–444.
84. Peutzfeldt A, Sahafi A, Asmussen E. A survey of failed post-retained restorations. Clin Oral Investig 2008;12:37–44.
85. Moshonov J, Slutzky-Goldberg I, Gottlieb A, Peretz B. The effect of the distance between post and residual gutta-percha on the clinical outcome of endodontic treatment. J Endod 2005;31:177–179.
86. Ozkurt Z, Kayahan MB, Sunay H, Kazazoğlu E, Bayirli G. The effect of the gap between the post restoration and the remaining root canal filling on the periradicular status in a Turkish subpopulation. Oral Surg Oral Med Oral Pathol Oral Radiol Endod 2010;110:131–135.
87. Standlee JP, Caputo AA, Collard EW, Pollack MH. Analysis of stress distribution by endodontic posts. Oral Surg Oral Med Oral Pathol 1972;33:952–960.
88. Willershausen B, Tekyatan H, Krummenauer F, Briseño Marroquin B. Survival rate of endodontically treated teeth in relation to conservative vs post insertion techniques—A retrospective study. Eur J Med Res 2005;10:204–208.
89. Barbizam JV, White SN. Fatigue susceptibility of an endodontic fibre post material. Int Endod J 2014;47:202–209.
90. Signore A, Benedicenti S, Kaitsas V, Barone M, Angiero F, Ravera G. Long-term survival of endodontically treated, maxillary anterior teeth restored with either tapered or parallel-sided glass-fiber posts and full-ceramic crown coverage. J Dent 2009;37:115–121.
91. Bitter K, Noetzel J, Stamm O, Vaudt J, Meyer-Lueckel H, Neumann K, Kielbassa AM. Randomized clinical trial comparing the effects of post placement on failure rate of postendodontic restorations: Preliminary results of a mean period of 32 months. J Endod 2009;35:1477–1482.
92. Creugers NH, Mentink AG, Fokkinga WA, Kreulen CM. 5-year follow-up of a prospective clinical study on various types of core restorations. Int J Prosthodont 2005;18:34–39.
93. Ferrari M, Cagidiaco MC, Grandini S, De Sanctis M, Goracci C. Post placement affects survival of endodontically treated premolars. J Dent Res 2007;86:729–734.
94. Fokkinga WA, Kreulen CM, Vallittu PK, Creugers NH. A structured analysis of in vitro failure loads and failure modes of fiber, metal, and ceramic post-and-core systems. Int J Prosthodont 2004; 17:476–482.
95. Hu S, Osada T, Shimizu T, Warita K, Kawawa T. Resistance to cyclic fatigue and fracture of structurally compromised root restored with different post and core restorations. Dent Mater J 2005;24:225–231.
96. Mannocci F, Qualtrough AJ, Worthington HV, Watson TF, Pitt Ford TR. Randomized clinical comparison of endodontically treated teeth restored with amalgam or with fiber posts and resin composite: Five-year results. Oper Dent 2005;30:9–15.
97. Standlee JP, Caputo AA. Endodontic dowel retention with resinous cements. J Prosthet Dent 1992;68: 913–917.

98. Sterzenbach G, Karajouli G, Naumann M, Peroz I, Bitter K. Fiber post placement with core build-up materials or resin cements—An evaluation of different adhesive approaches. Acta Odontol Scand 2012;70:368–376.
99. Sorensen JA, Engelman MJ. Effect of post adaptation on fracture resistance of endodontically treated teeth. J Prosthet Dent 1990;64:419–424.
100. Hansen EK, Asmussen E, Christiansen NC. In vivo fractures of endodontically treated posterior teeth restored with amalgam. Endod Dent Traumatol 1990;6:49–55.
101. Magne P, Belser UC. Porcelain versus composite inlays/onlays: Effects of mechanical loads on stress distribution, adhesion, and crown flexure. Int J Periodontics Restorative Dent 2003;23:543–555.
102. Mannocci F, Bertelli E, Sherriff M, Watson TF, Ford TR. Three-year clinical comparison of survival of endodontically treated teeth restored with either full cast coverage or with direct composite restoration. J Prosthet Dent 2002;88:297–301.
103. Scurria MS, Shugars DA, Hayden WJ, Felton DA. General dentists' patterns of restoring endodontically treated teeth. J Am Dent Assoc 1995;126:775–779.

8

Mishaps During Nonsurgical Endodontic Retreatment

MASOUD PARIROKH
MAHMOUD TORABINEJAD

Objectives

After reading this chapter, the reader should be able to:

1. Recognize common mistakes that may happen before, during, and after secondary nonsurgical endodontic treatment.
2. Describe methods and technologies that help dental practitioners prevent common mistakes regarding diagnosis and interpretation of preoperative, intraoperative, and postoperative periapical radiographs.
3. Recognize risk factors that may help treatment providers avoid further mishaps.
4. Recognize previous mishaps and determine how to manage them.
5. Identify factors that may improve or regress prognosis of nonsurgical endodontic retreatment.

Introduction

When the quality of the initial endodontic treatment and the coronal restoration is adequate,[1] initial root canal treatment usually has high success and survival rates.[2,3] It has been reported that low quality of root canal filling and inadequate restoration of initial endodontic treatment have a significant negative impact on final outcomes of the treatment.[1,4] In fact, persistent, recurrent, and secondary infections are the most prevalent causes of endodontic failure. Whenever microorganisms could not successfully be eradicated from the root canal space during initial root canal treatment or if they found a pathway to the root canal space following an endodontic treatment, the patient would experience endodontic failure.[5]

Several indications could be considered for performing a secondary nonsurgical endodontic treatment as the treatment of choice when the initial treatment has failed. Secondary nonsurgical endodontic treatment is indicated for patients who have clinical signs of initial endodontic failure such as sensitivity to percussion and palpation, swelling, presence of sinus tract, a defective leaky restoration; a temporary restoration in place for a long time following initial endodontic treatment may also be an idicator. Teeth with incomplete root canal obturation that are candidates for receiving new restorations due to esthetics can also indicate secondary nonsurgical endodontic treatment. Radiographic indications for secondary nonsurgical endodontic treatment include enlargement of periapical lesion following the initial endodontic treatment or development of a lesion following the initial root canal treatment. Teeth with an unrestorable crown, loss of periodontal tissue support, and extensive crown/root fracture, as well as patients with no motivation for keeping their natural teeth, can be considered contraindications or poor candidates, respectively, for receiving secondary nonsurgical endodontic treatment.[6]

There are several options for patients who either experience initial endodontic failure or need to change a previous restoration for esthetic reasons. For most patients, nonsurgical secondary endodontic treatment is the first choice. However, sometimes secondary *surgical* endodontic treatment and extraction, with and without replacement, are options to be considered.[6]

Two systematic reviews on cross-sectional studies have reported a high prevalence of apical periodontitis in teeth having undergone endodontic treatment.[1,7] These teeth might need to receive secondary nonsurgical endodontic treatment to resolve the pathosis; however, performing retreatment might not always be easy. The American Association of Endodontists (AAE) has recommended an endodontic case difficulty assessment form and some guidelines to help practitioners evaluate each case in need of endodontic treatment before undertaking the procedure to help clinicians decide if they are capable of carrying out the treatment procedure or if they should refer the case to an endodontist. The AAE endodontic case difficulty assessment form addresses secondary nonsurgical endodontic treatment as a highly difficult treatment modality.[8] If an initial nonsurgical endodontic treatment was complicated due to iatrogenic accidents, complex anatomy, or location at the second or third molar teeth, then the secondary nonsurgical endodontic treatment would be even more difficult.[8]

Several mishaps might happen before, during, or after secondary nonsurgical endodontic treatment. The purpose of this chapter is to share the common errors and risk factors, recommendations for preventing mishaps, and methods to manage these challenges. An increase in the interest of general dental practitioners to seek more continuing education for secondary nonsurgical endodontic treatment may indicate an increased demand for this type of treatment.[9]

Mishaps During Diagnosis and Treatment Planning

Overall, it has been reported that about one-quarter of endodontic claims may be due to errors in diagnosis and treatment planning.[10] Therefore, careful examination and radiographic evaluation have great importance in making a proper diagnosis and reasonable treatment plan.

Consultation with a patient in need of secondary nonsurgical endodontic treatment who has been referred to an endodontist is somewhat different than consultations with patients who seek an initial nonsurgical endodontic treatment. It is crucial to discuss the cause(s) of the initial treatment failure as well as treatment options for the existing situation during the initial consultation. During the first visit following the patient's clinical examination and radiographic evaluation, time should be dedicated for case presentation including describing the steps involved in the treatment as well as explaining risks and benefits of the secondary nonsurgical endodontic treatment. One of the most common mistakes is considering the time spent on case presentation as a waste because it has minimal to no economic benefit for the operator and instead could be spent for patient treating. However, explaining in detail the steps involved in the treatment plan can prevent future misunderstandings and possible claims. In addition, the patient's satisfaction has the potential to lead to further referrals.

There are several questions that should be answered before a practitioner makes the decision to offer treatment options. These questions include the following:

- Who has done the initial nonsurgical endodontic treatment?
- When did the patient receive initial nonsurgical endodontic treatment?
- Why was the patient referred?
- What is the past dental history of the patient?
- Why is the initial treatment considered inadequate?
- What is the reason for the initial nonsurgical endodontic treatment failure?

The answers to these questions are very important and can affect the treatment plan after a failed nonsurgical endodontic treatment. For example, if the quality of the initial nonsurgical endodontic treatment looks sufficient either by radiography or CBCT and the treatment had been done by a well-known operator, the practitioner may decide to offer a *surgical* secondary endodontic treatment as the first choice. However, if the patient cannot remember who performed the initial nonsurgical endodontic treatment, the first choice should be a secondary nonsurgical endodontic treatment. The reason for the patient's visit to an endodontist's office is also important. For instance, the patient's dentist may observe a periapical radiolucency in a tooth that previously received nonsurgical endodontic treatment while the patient has had no clinical symptoms. Therefore, the patient has been referred for further evaluation and possible treatment. In that case, careful evaluation, asking past dental history, observing radiographic images that have previously been taken of the patient, or even consulting with the dentist who performed the initial treatment would be beneficial. It is very important to differentiate between a periapical lesion in its healing phase or a lesion that did not exist at the time of initial nonsurgical endodontic treatment and developed afterward.

In fact, a common error is to always assume that the presence of periapical radiolucency indicates pathosis. The lesions may be in their healing phase, and if previous radiographic images or CBCT are available, it is imperative to compare these with the current images (Fig 8-1).[11]

Secondary nonsurgical endodontic treatment has been reported to be a predictable and successful procedure even when CBCT is used to evaluate the treatment outcome.[11] However, when CBCT was used to evaluate root canal retreatment outcomes, lower healing rates were found than with periapical radiography. It is well documented that detecting bone healing following root canal treatment in patients with periapical lesions might be more optimistic with radiography than with CBCT (see Fig 8-1).[12,13] In other words, the practitioner might observe a healed periapical lesion on a conventional periapical radiograph, but CBCT may show a radiolucent area around the root-canal-treated tooth. Torabinejad et al[12] emphasized that when CBCT shows a radiolucent area around roots that have undergone root canal treatment, it does not necessarily mean pathosis is present. If the periapical radiograph shows a healed lesion and the patient does not complain about clinical symptoms, further diagnostic workup is necessary to prevent overtreatment. Taking meticulous dental history, keeping the patient's documents including periapical radiographs and CBCT DICOM (Digital Imaging and Communications in Medicine) files (if available), or consulting with the practitioner who carried out the initial nonsurgical endodontic treatment can help inform a precise decision and possibly prevent further unnecessary treatments. In addition, the practitioner should notice any presence of clinical symptoms and carefully perform a clinical examination to evaluate whether the patient is in

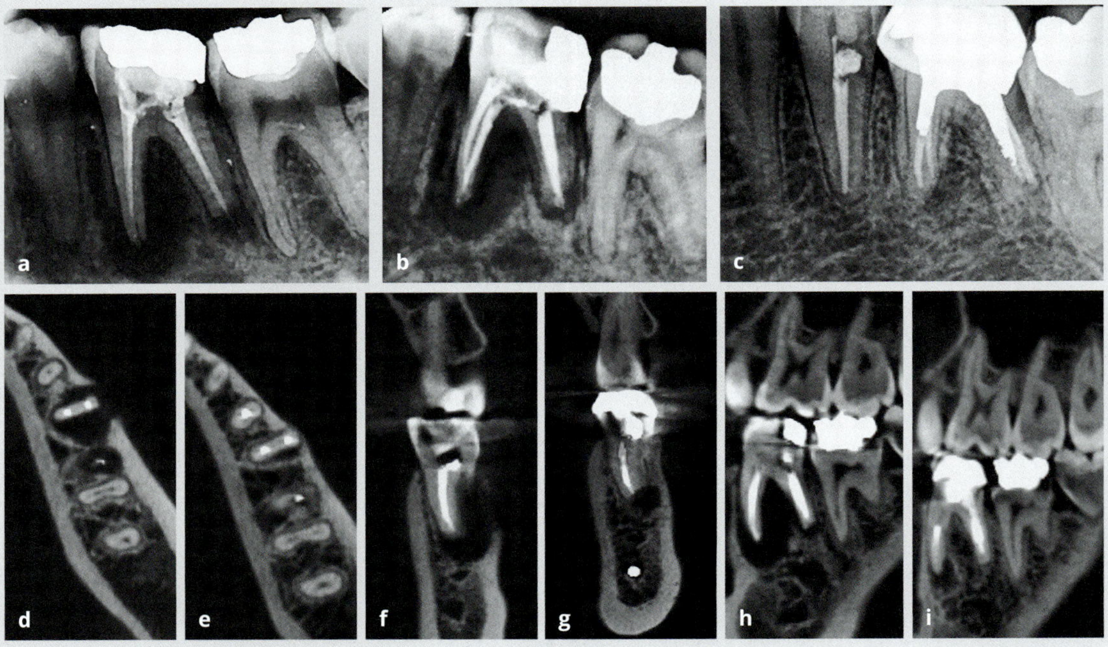

Fig 8-1 This case emphasizes the importance of documentation and of taking past dental history. *(a)* The periapical radiograph shows a periapical lesion in tooth no. 19, with incomplete obturation. *(b)* The tooth received secondary nonsurgical root canal treatment. *(c)* Five years later, the periapical radiograph shows that the periapical lesion has healed; however, the CBCT images show a different story. *(d)* Axial view immediately after secondary nonsurgical endodontic treatment shows cortical plate bone loss and radiolucency around the mesial and distal roots of tooth no. 19. *(e)* Axial view of the same tooth 5 years later shows that the cortical plate was restored, with a small radiolucent lesion around the mesial root. *(f)* A CBCT coronal view shows a large radiolucent lesion. *(g)* In contrast, the lesion has transformed into a small radiolucency 5 years later. *(h)* Sagittal view of tooth no. 19 shows a large radiolucent lesion that turned into a small radiolucent lesion 5 years later *(i)*. In this case, despite the absence of clinical symptoms and a "healed" radiolucency according to 2D radiography, the CBCT images still show a periradicular radiolucency, albeit smaller than the CBCT taken immediately following retreatment.

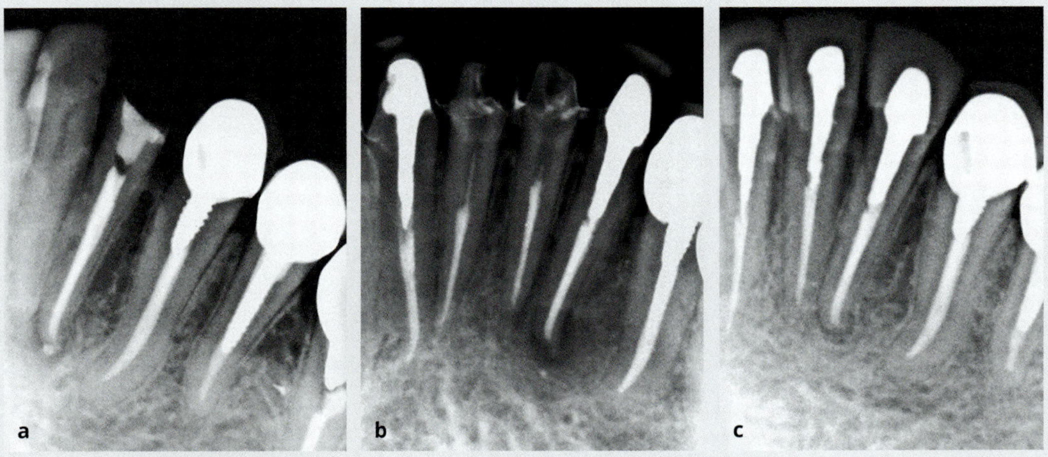

Fig 8-2 An example of the importance of a proper follow-up period after initial nonsurgical endodontic treatment. *(a)* Tooth no. 26 received root canal treatment. *(b)* Three months later, the tooth developed a radiolucent lesion without clinical symptoms. *(c)* Three years later, the lesion healed, and the tooth was asymptomatic and functional without further endodontic intervention.

the healing phase or whether the radiolucency indicates the failure of the initial nonsurgical endodontic treatment.

Another common mistake is not allowing sufficient time for a periapical lesion to heal. Sometimes, shortly after endodontic treatment, the periapical lesion increases in size, and the practitioner may consider it a sign of failure. However, after treatment and adequate follow-up time, the lesion may heal, with no need for secondary nonsurgical endodontic treatment (Fig 8-2).

Taking careful dental history; reviewing previous radiographs, CBCT images, and clinical examinations; and considering the patient's chief complaint are very important during the initial consultation. If the patient has no previous radiographs and cannot remember the treatment history, has no clinical symptoms and signs, has reasonable root canal treatment, and does not need a new restoration, they should be informed of the uncertain condition of their initial nonsurgical endodontic treatment outcome and of the necessity for follow-ups.

The practitioner should avoid jumping to a conclusion before asking the abovementioned questions and receiving enough information from the patient and from the dentist who either referred or performed the initial nonsurgical endodontic treatment. Because the endodontist is not aware of the conditions at the time of initial treatment, it is advisable for them to describe the current condition to the patient in an impartial manner. It is a mistake to alarm the patient regarding a tooth that has been treated previously by another operator and currently has no signs or symptoms of clinical failure nor presence of periapical pathosis. Patient cooperation, complexity of the root canal anatomy at the time of initial treatment, anesthesia success, and devices available at the time of initial treatment all may affect the treatment outcome. For instance, 30 years ago, a limited number of technologies were available for root canal treatment. New technologies, armamentaria, and materials such as dental operative microscope, CBCT, various types of rotary nickel-titanium instruments, advanced apex locators, and bioactive endodontic cements were not available then.[14–17] Using these newer technologies enhances the quality of endodontic treatment, increases the practitioner's self-confidence, and makes the treatment outcome more predictable.

Pitfalls during clinical and radiographic examinations

Sometimes an apparent mishap or a periapical lesion may attract a practitioner's attention so much that they forget to make further careful examinations or to ask the patient pertinent questions (Fig 8-3), a problem known as "tunnel vision." This approach has the potential for misdiagnosis. In such a case, the dentist does not pay close attention to the patient's chief complaint because the mishap seems so evident that there are no other etiologic factors for the failure or the patient's chief complaint that could account for the patient's clinical signs and symptoms.[18] In contrast, listening to the patient's chief complaint, careful examination, and undertaking sensibility tests prevent further mistakes (Fig 8-4).

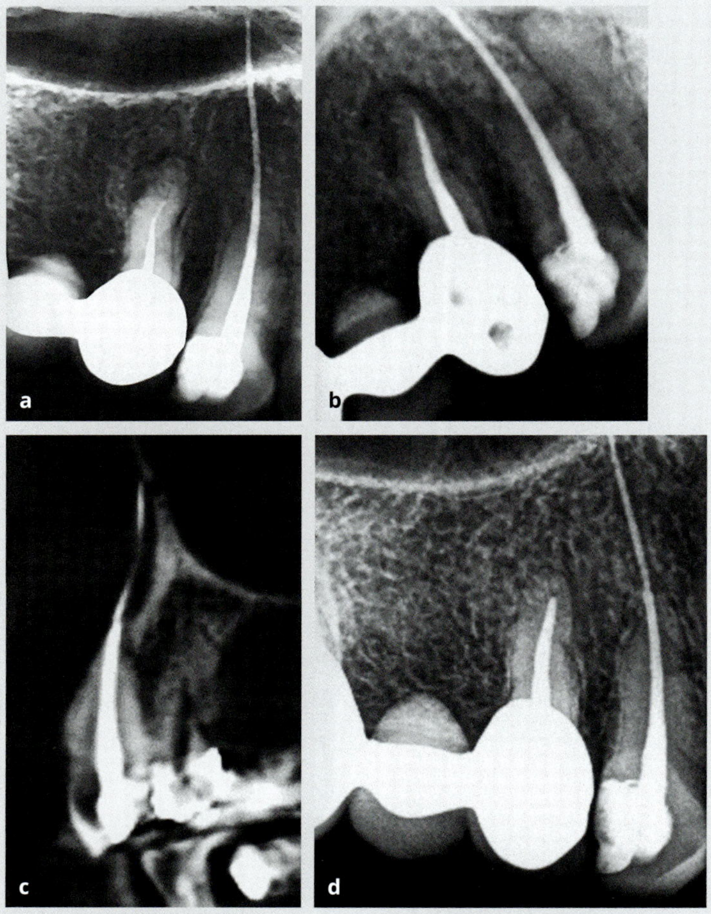

Fig 8-3 A classic case of "tunnel vision." *(a)* A patient was referred for secondary nonsurgical endodontic treatment for tooth no. 6 because of pain and diffuse swelling. *(b)* Careful examination revealed that tooth no. 5 needed secondary nonsurgical endodontic treatment. *(c)* Five years later, the patient needed CBCT for another tooth. The sagittal view showed no overfilled gutta-percha within the bone, and tooth no. 6 had no apparent periapical lesion. *(d)* After 5 years, the periapical lesion of tooth no. 5 was also healed, and the patient was symptom free.

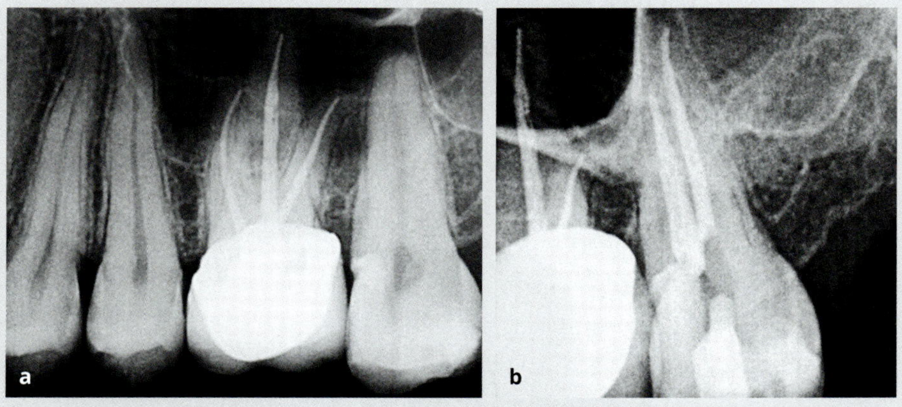

Fig 8-4 *(a)* A female patient who had received initial nonsurgical endodontic treatment 3 months earlier for tooth no. 14 was referred because she had sensitivity to hot beverages. After placing a rubber dam and using a hot bath, tooth no. 15 showed sensitivity to heat. *(b)* Following root canal treatment of tooth no. 15, the patient was symptom free.

Another common mistake is to undertake a secondary nonsurgical endodontic treatment procedure for teeth with an obvious mishap from a long time ago, even if they have no periradicular pathosis and no need for a new restoration. Regular follow-ups are actually the best course of action for these patients (Fig 8-5).[19]

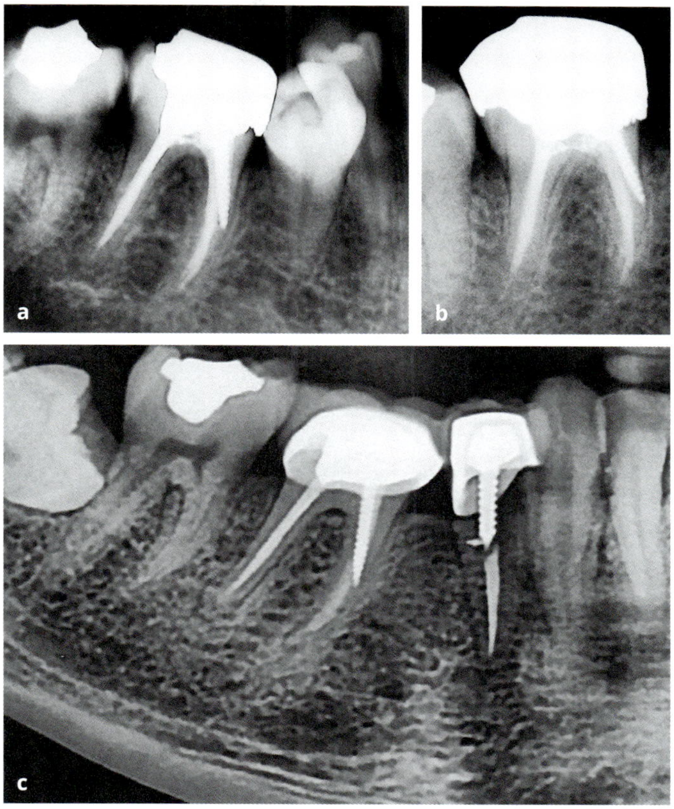

Fig 8-5 *(a)* A patient was referred for repairing post perforation in the mesial root of tooth no. 30. Because the tooth was restored 2 years earlier and had no clinical symptoms or periodontal pockets, periodic follow-ups were scheduled for the patient. *(b and c)* Seventeen and 24 years later, the tooth was still symptom free with no periodontal pockets.

A very simple way to prevent the previously mentioned errors is to follow recommendations regarding a standard clinical examination, including full attention to the patient's chief complaint, careful examination of the soft and hard tissues of the oral cavity, carrying out sensibility tests, and using radiographic aids such as periapical radiographs taken from different angles and ordering CBCT examinations in complicated cases (see chapter 1).

Proper examination and sharing possible iatrogenic mishaps and future prognosis in advance of undertaking the treatment will help prevent future misunderstandings or arguments between the patient and the practitioner. Based on the position statements of AAE[20] and the European Society of Endodontology (ESE),[21] CBCT examinations are not necessary for all patients requiring secondary nonsurgical endodontic treatment. However, in complicated cases, CBCT can be an important aid for making a proper diagnosis and treatment plan. Several investigations have reported that CBCT can significantly affect the treatment plan.[22–25] It has been demonstrated that general dental practitioners and endodontists change their opinions regarding treatment plans after examining CBCT images from the same cases.[26]

Another important factor for preventing mistakes during treatment planning is considering a multidisciplinary approach and asking a periodontist and/or a prosthodontist for their opinions and comments regarding prognosis and the cost-benefit analysis of retaining a tooth or replacing it with an implant (Fig 8-6). The patient's health history and medications are also important factors in treatment planning. For instance, secondary surgical endodontic treatment and implant options should be dismissed for patients receiving intravenous antiresorptive agents such as bisphosphonate for at least 2 years.[27,28]

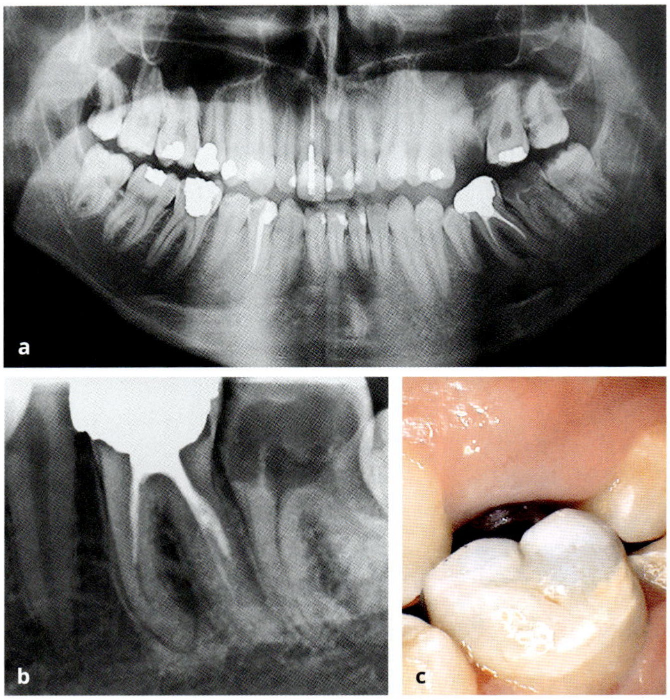

Fig 8-6 A patient requiring secondary nonsurgical endodontic treatment for tooth no. 19 was sent for a consultation with a prosthodontist due to the long-term absence of the coronal structure of the opposite tooth and the subsequent supraeruption. *(a)* Panoramic radiograph. *(b)* Periapical radiograph. *(c)* A photograph of tooth no. 19 shows its supraeruption.

Interpretation of 2D radiographs

Currently, it is well documented that detecting radiographic periradicular lesions, resorption, and mishaps is much more accurate with CBCT examinations compared to 2D periapical radiography. In fact, the percentage of false-negative and false-positive observations were much higher when 2D radiographs were compared to CBCT images.[29] To prevent misdiagnosis and error while determining treatment planning, the following conditions call for ordering CBCT and taking periapical radiographs from different horizontal angles before secondary nonsurgical endodontic treatment: suspicion of the presence of mishaps (Fig 8-7), the possibility of missed root canals not evident from periapical radiography (Fig 8-8), or if there is no apparent reason for the failure of initial nonsurgical endodontic treatment (Fig 8-9). For more information regarding the value of CBCT for diagnosis and treatment planning, see chapter 2.

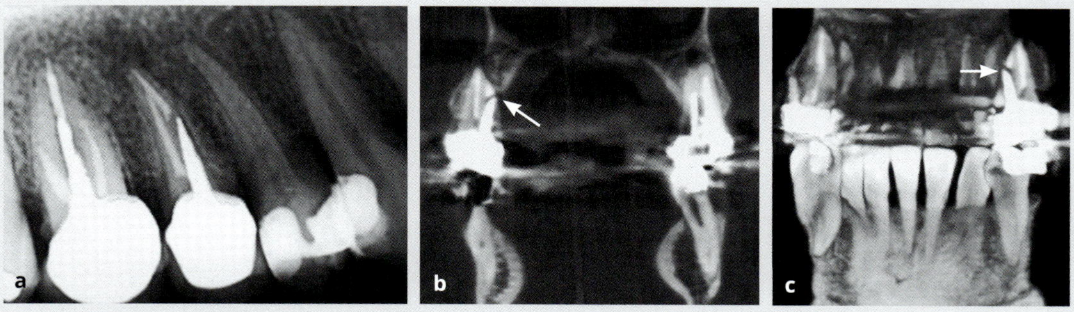

Fig 8-7 An example of a tooth suspected of having a mishap. This patient with a history of initial nonsurgical endodontic treatment on tooth no. 4 had been asymptomatic for several years; however, the tooth was sensitive to percussion, with the patient complaining of pain on chewing after receiving a post-and-core and a crown. *(a)* Periapical radiograph. *(b)* CBCT coronal view shows post perforation *(arrow)*. *(c)* Posterior view of 3D image shows post perforation *(arrow)*.

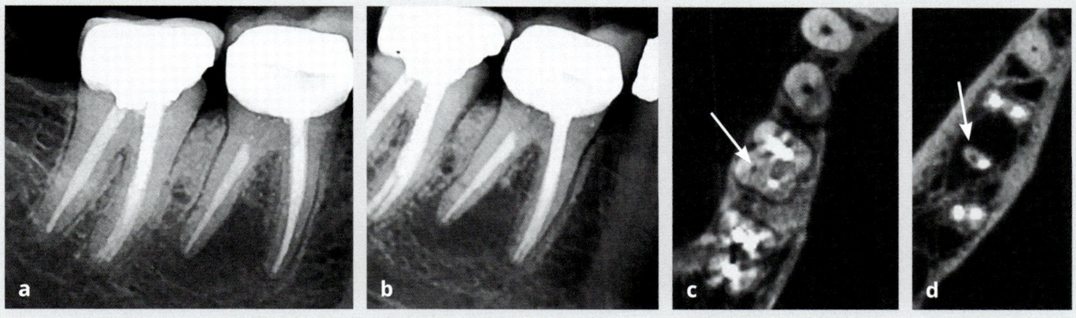

Fig 8-8 *(a and b)* Periapical radiographs with different horizontal angles of tooth no. 30 show no missed root canals. *(c and d)* Two axial views at different levels of the same tooth show that the distobuccal root canal has been overlooked *(arrows)*.

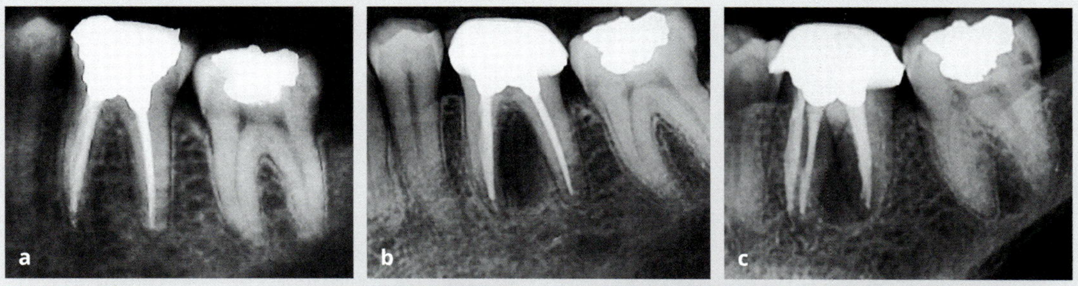

Fig 8-9 *(a)* Periapical radiograph of tooth no. 19 before crown placement. *(b and c)* Ten years later, a large radiolucency has developed between the mesial and distal roots. *(d)* Axial view of the mesial root shows strip perforation of the mesiolingual root canal *(arrow)*. *(e)* Axial view at the apical level shows no periapical lesion. *(f)* The sagittal image also shows strip perforation.

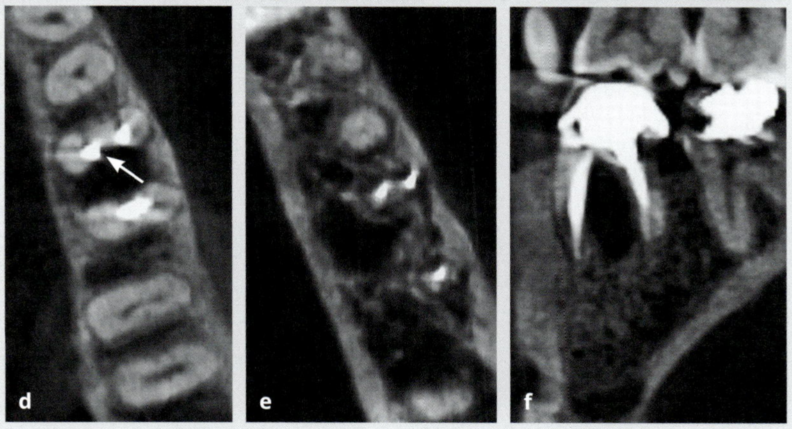

Communication with the former practitioner

Sometimes a new dentist may have to call the former dentist to gather information regarding the previously performed treatments. For instance, a dentist may perform a root canal treatment for a tooth with periapical lesion, and then the patient moves to another city. A new dentist may need information regarding the time and history of the previous treatment to make decisions about a tooth that is clinically asymptomatic despite periapical radiography showing a periapical radiolucency. This professional communication will help both dentists to satisfy their patient's need. This is a "win-win" situation that helps prevent future malpractice claims against either dentist.

Communication with patients and how to present the case without alarming them

One of the most important factors to prevent future misunderstandings and malpractice claims is the professional communication and behavior of the dental practitioner. Female dentists usually provide more patient-centered communication, which may be why malpractice claims against female practitioners are fewer than those against male practitioners.[30] An endodontist should give enough information to the patient in simple language without bias regarding limitations, risk factors, prognosis, and treatment options.[10]

It is also very important to get signed informed consent in which the treatment plan, risks, and limitations have been fully described. An investigation of endodontic claims reported that the presence of documents leads to better judgment and acceptance of the treatment outcome if there was a good reason for treatment shortcomings documented by the dentist.[30] For instance, a root canal obturation that was not at a reasonable distance from the radiographic apex has been known to be acceptable if the dentist's documentation showed that there were anatomical complications that prevented reaching the apical terminus.

Benefits and risks of the retreatment

The benefits and risks of secondary nonsurgical endodontic treatment must be made clear to the patient. A frequent misconception, particularly by patients, is to consider an implant a "forever" treatment that needs no maintenance after the treatment. It is well documented that survival rates for secondary nonsurgical endodontic treatment and dental implants are comparable[31]; however, implants need more corrective treatment after placement. A systematic review and meta-analysis reported that weighted mean prevalence of mucositis and peri-implantitis were 43% and 22%, respectively.[32] The benefits of secondary nonsurgical endodontic treatment include keeping natural teeth with high survival rates, a shorter treatment period for achieving esthetic and functional results, and fewer requirements for complementary treatments. The risks of secondary nonsurgical endodontic treatment are treatment mishaps, high risk of vertical root fracture,[33] and the potential need for further periapical surgery or replacement with an implant in cases of treatment failure. A common mistake during nonsurgical endodontic treatment is providing inadequate information regarding the risks and benefits of this procedure.

Treatment options and prognosis

One of the most critical factors during every endodontic case evaluation is to reach a proper diagnosis and prepare a reasonable treatment plan based on clinical and radiographic findings, treatment options, and patient demands. A prevalent mistake is to consider only a limited number of treatment options for cases in need of secondary nonsurgical endodontic treatment.

It is crucial to consider the treatment plan in a case-by-case manner. The treatment options should be provided based on the patient's preferences and considering economic conditions and long-term prognosis. In some cases, based on periodontal and prosthetic factors, it may be wiser to shift the treatment plan from saving a tooth to extracting it and replacing it with an implant (Fig 8-10).[34,35] However, in other cases, saving the tooth and considering a multidisciplinary approach may be the best choice for the patient. Clinicians should also evaluate their skills and armamentaria to address any mishaps that already occurred during the initial nonsurgical endodontic treatment.[6] In addition, practitioners should make their decision based on recent updates and clinical guidelines.[36] Thereby, the practitioner's treatment plan will be based on the standard of care at the time of treatment visit.

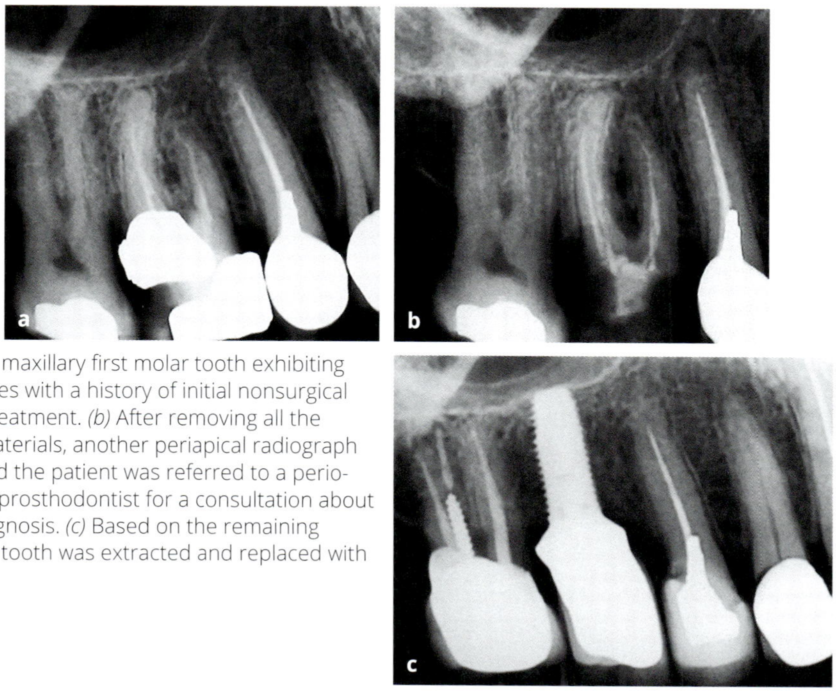

Fig 8-10 *(a)* A maxillary first molar tooth exhibiting recurrent caries with a history of initial nonsurgical endodontic treatment. *(b)* After removing all the restorative materials, another periapical radiograph was taken, and the patient was referred to a periodontist and a prosthodontist for a consultation about the tooth prognosis. *(c)* Based on the remaining structure, the tooth was extracted and replaced with an implant.

Indications and contraindications

The indications and contraindications for secondary nonsurgical root canal treatment have been described clearly.[6] However, one common error is that an asymptomatic tooth with an incomplete root canal obturation from a long time ago and no radiographic pathosis can receive a new restoration without secondary nonsurgical endodontic treatment. Most of the time, these teeth develop radiolucencies and clinical symptoms in a short time following the new restorative interventions (Fig 8-11).

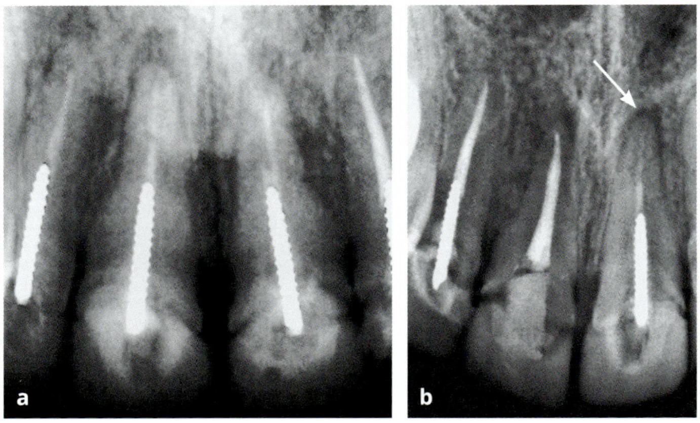

Fig 8-11 Tooth no. 9 with a history of incomplete obturation. The tooth was asymptomatic for several years; after receiving a new coronal restoration, the tooth became symptomatic in a short time. *(a)* Periapical radiograph before receiving a new crown. *(b)* Six months after crown placement, a radiolucent lesion developed *(arrow)*.

Sharing decision-making

It is essential to share all important factors that may affect the future prognosis with the patient. If the practitioner shoulders all the responsibilities regarding the diagnosis and treatment plan without sharing mishaps and challenges that are already present, a patient would have a right to dispute future outcomes, particularly if failure occurs a short time after the secondary nonsurgical endodontic treatment. One study reported that not giving enough information to the patient was one of the reasons for endodontic malpractice claims in Denmark.[30] During a comprehensive case presentation session, the practitioner should share all risk factors and challenges with the patient. The clinician should use simple words to provide the information, including the percentage of successful outcomes, the cost difference between various treatment options, the time needed for completing each treatment modality, the prognosis of the treatment, and the quality of life during and after each treatment option.[6]

Patient Preparation for Secondary Nonsurgical Endodontic Treatment

Anesthesia

Some dental practitioners and patients assume that no anesthesia is necessary for secondary nonsurgical endodontic treatment because the tooth has no dental pulp. It has been claimed that teeth requiring secondary nonsurgical endodontic intervention could be treated without anesthesia.[37] However, the inclusion criteria were limited and cannot be extended to all secondary nonsurgical endodontic cases. In fact, based on clinical experience, when patients receive anesthesia, they are much more cooperative, and the treatment is performed faster and more easily than on patients who do not receive anesthesia.[38–40]

Isolation

Secondary nonsurgical root canal retreatment might be performed due to a defective previously placed restoration (Fig 8-12), esthetic reasons (recurrent caries or tooth discoloration), or signs of initial nonsurgical endodontic treatment failure, ie, clinical signs and symptoms and/or the presence of periapical pathosis (Fig 8-13). As in initial nonsurgical root canal treatment, it is mandatory

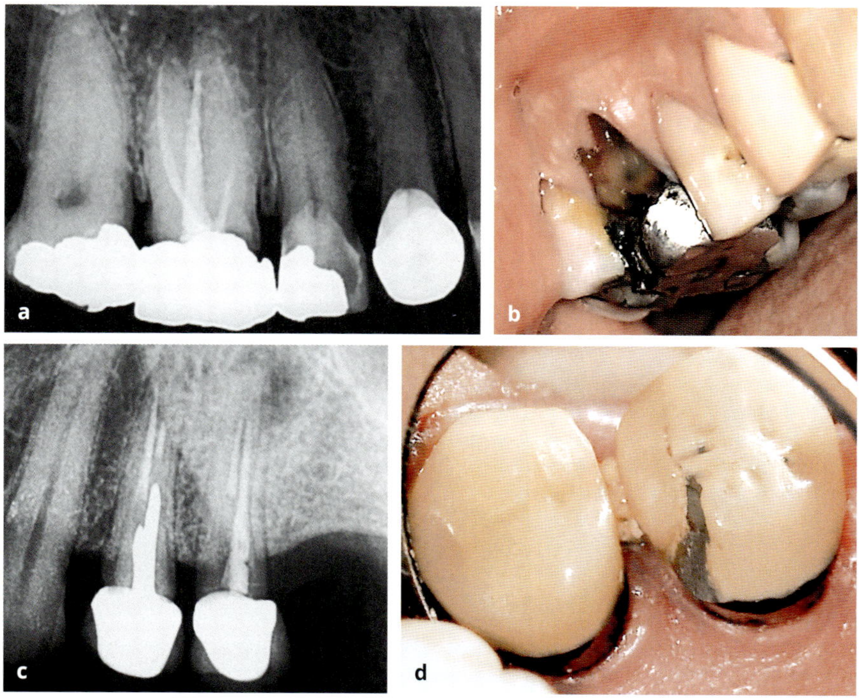

Fig 8-12 Three routine reasons for performing secondary nonsurgical endodontic treatment. *(a and b)* Recurrent caries. *(c and d)* Defective restoration of tooth no. 12 and periapical lesion of tooth no. 13.

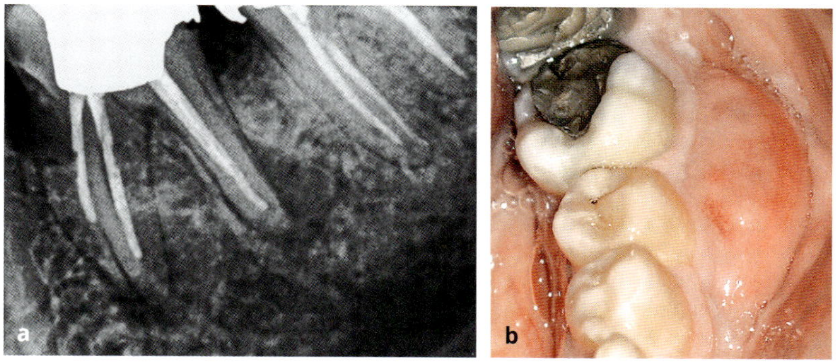

Fig 8-13 A case of initial nonsurgical endodontic treatment failure. *(a)* Periapical radiograph shows incomplete obturation and periradicular radiolucency of tooth no. 19. *(b)* Localized swelling.

to place a rubber dam before the secondary nonsurgical endodontic treatment in order to prevent further recontamination of the root canals. In most instances, the previous restoration should be removed entirely and a new restoration be placed; however, sometimes in the case of a crown with good marginal adaptation or a tooth that recently received a new restoration, the practitioner might decide to keep the restoration. A common error is to use stainless steel clamps, which might damage porcelain-fused-to-metal (PFM) crowns. In such cases, using a Kerr SoftClamp (Kerr Dental; Fig 8-14) and Cushee Rubber Dam Clamp/Cushion Blue (North America Medical Equipment) might prevent damage to the crown.

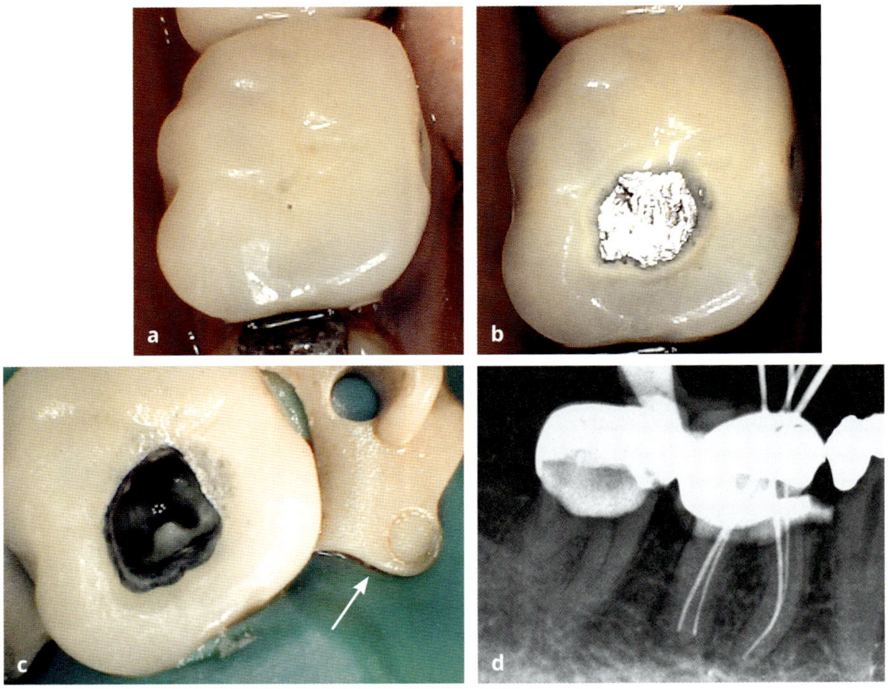

Fig 8-14 SoftClamps are very useful to prevent porcelain defects during rubber dam placement. *(a)* PFM crown before access cavity preparation. *(b)* Removing the porcelain with a round diamond bur. *(c)* Access cavity preparation with a transmetal bur and isolation with SoftClamp and rubber dam *(arrow)*. *(d)* Radiographic image of initial files after removing gutta-percha from the root canals shows that the clamp has lower radiographic density compared to stainless steel clamps.

Magnification and illumination

A common mistake for a practitioner is to undertake secondary nonsurgical root canal treatment without proper magnification and illumination. It has been demonstrated that among all the magnification tools, a dental operative microscope (DOM) is better for endodontic procedures compared to loupes and videoscopes.[41] However, a survey among general practitioners in the United States showed only 2% used a DOM in their practices.[9] No randomized clinical trials have compared the outcomes of root canal treatment procedures with or without the use of a DOM.[42] However, a retrospective study reported that employing a DOM during endodontic retreatment could significantly improve the ability to locate overlooked root canals in first maxillary molars undergoing initial nonsurgical endodontic treatment compared to those cases without using a DOM.[43] Therefore, during endodontic retreatment of teeth with possibly more than one root canal in one root, using a DOM could help the practitioner to find the overlooked root canals.

Another common mistake when magnification is not used during secondary nonsurgical endodontic treatment is missing cracks that might negatively affect future prognosis (Fig 8-15). Careful observation and use of a DOM give the practitioner more confidence and make the treatment outcome more predictable. The real advantages of using a DOM during secondary nonsurgical endodontic treatment include better illumination and magnification, removal of less tooth structure, lowering the risk of procedural accidents, and enabling better management of previous mishaps.

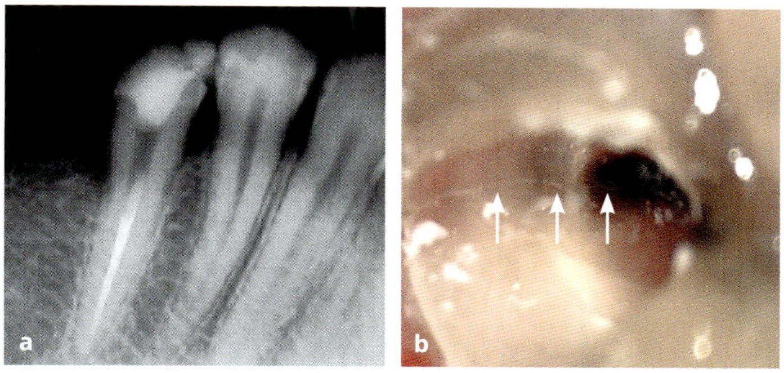

Fig 8-15 *(a and b)* An example of a crack in the distal part of a second mandibular premolar that received another nonsurgical endodontic treatment and has been prepared to receive a post and a crown *(arrows)*.

Mishaps During Access Cavity Preparation

Several factors should be considered before undertaking secondary nonsurgical endodontic treatment. These include removing all caries and previous defective restorations, observing the root canal cross section (Fig 8-16), obtaining straight-line access, determining the type of restoration, and determining the presence of posts, previous mishaps (Fig 8-17), obstacles, and calcifications (Fig 8-18). Three common errors during access preparation are *(1)* undertaking secondary nonsurgical endodontic treatment without considering the aforementioned factors, *(2)* not making a temporary restoration for isolating the tooth, and *(3)* disregarding the types of posts, such as titanium posts, that have similar radiopacity to the root canal filling materials.

Defective restorations lead to microleakage, and for that reason, all caries and defective restorations should be removed before starting nonsurgical endodontic treatment.[6] The cross section of the root canal space at the cervical level should determine the design of the access cavity. For instance, in teeth with an oval-shaped root canal, the access cavity would have an oval shape.[6] Straight-line access is mandatory to prevent breaking endodontic instruments during

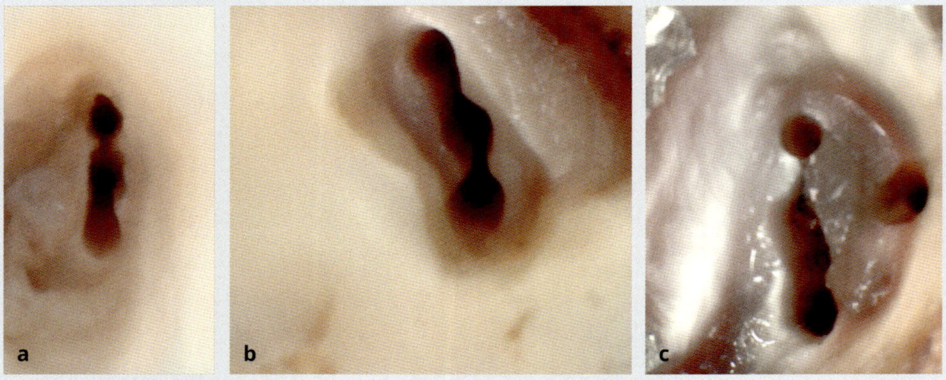

Fig 8-16 *(a to c)* Different types of root canals with oval cross sections.

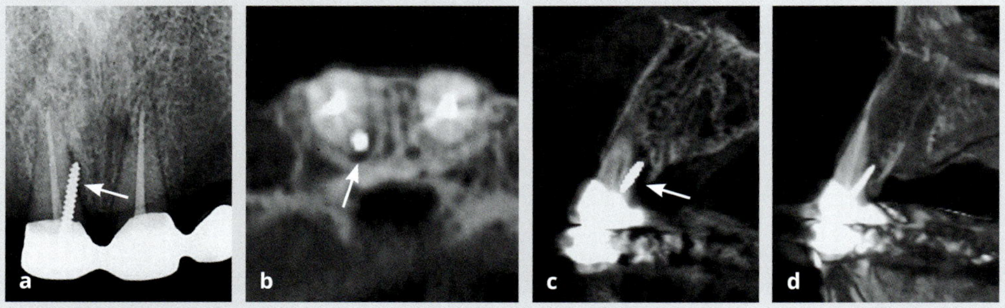

Fig 8-17 *(a)* Post perforation of tooth no. 8 *(arrow)*. *(b)* CBCT axial view shows that the post has perforated the palatal part of the root *(arrow)*. *(c)* The sagittal view and *(d)* 3D CBCT image show bone destruction around the perforated post *(arrow)*.

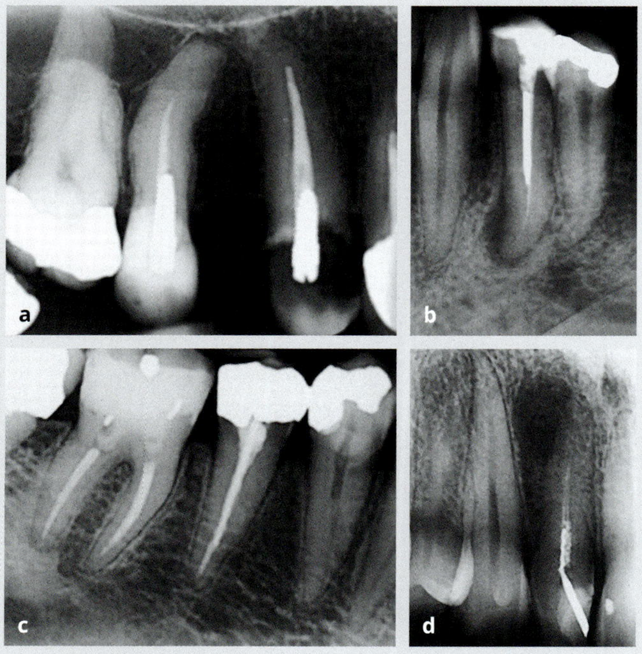

Fig 8-18 Different types of obstacles. *(a)* Ledge (tooth no. 6) and calcification (tooth no. 4). *(b to d)* Different types of separated root canal instruments: *(b)* Gates-Glidden bur, *(c)* K-file, and *(d)* Hedstrom file.

8

the removal of root canal filling materials from the root canal. One strategy for removing gutta-percha from the root canal is to use Gates-Glidden burs; however, having no straight-line access, particularly in the anterior teeth, can result in a fracture of the drill within the root canal (Fig 8-19). Another important point is to consider root depression at the mesial surface of the roots of the maxillary premolars (Fig 8-20) and the thickness of the pulp chamber floors in mandibular and maxillary molars (Fig 8-21). If a clinician ignores these variables, perforation might occur during access cavity preparation. Sometimes, after removing all caries and defective restorations, it is difficult to provide ideal isolation. Therefore, it is

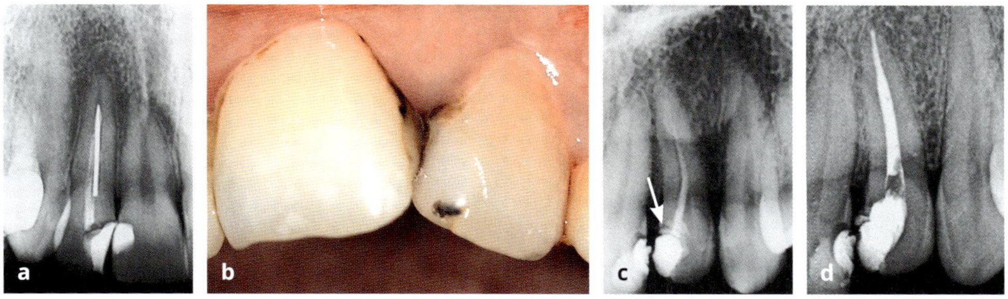

Fig 8-19 *(a)* An example of improper access cavity preparation in tooth no. 7, resulting in Gates-Glidden drill breakage during the initial nonsurgical endodontic treatment. *(b)* The buccal view of tooth no. 10 shows tooth discoloration, possibly due to improper access cavity preparation. *(c)* Periapical radiograph of the same tooth shows instrumentation during the initial nonsurgical endodontic treatment performed through pulp exposure site at the mesial cavity *(arrow)*. *(d)* Providing enough extension for the access cavity preparation during secondary nonsurgical endodontic treatment prevents further procedural accidents such as Gates-Glidden drill breakage during gutta-percha removal.

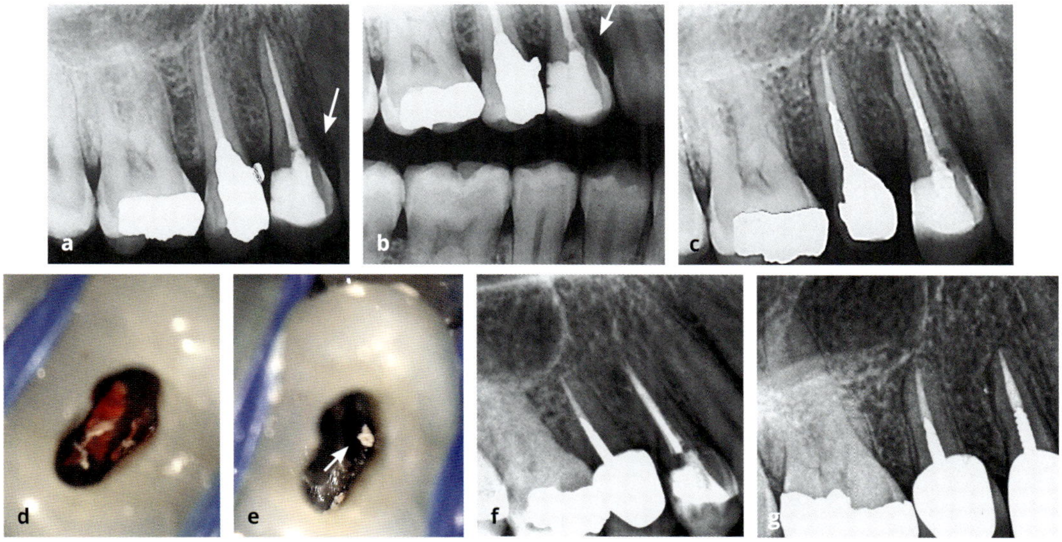

Fig 8-20 *(a to c)* Root depression of the mesial part of tooth no. 5, resulting in cervical perforation and cervical bone resorption *(arrows)*. *(d and e)* Following access cavity preparation, presence of blood and observation under a DOM confirmed root perforation *(arrow)*. *(f)* The tooth received secondary nonsurgical root canal treatment, and the perforation site was repaired, followed by placement of a post and a crown. *(g)* Fifteen months later, the tooth was symptom free.

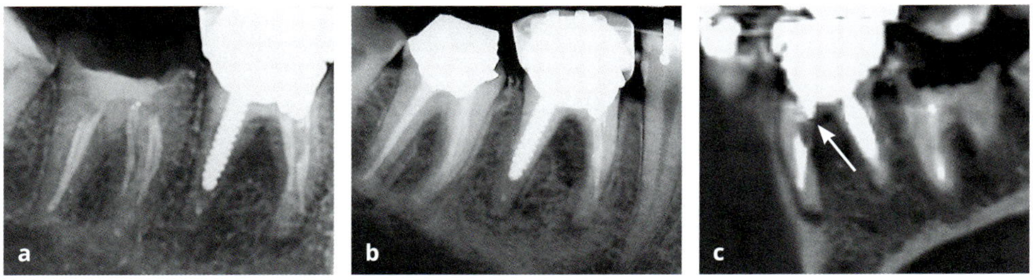

Fig 8-21 *(a and b)* Periapical radiographs of tooth no. 30 showed a radiolucent lesion at the furcation. *(c)* The sagittal view of the same tooth showed the possibility of perforation due to the low thickness of the pulp chamber floor *(arrow)*.

mandatory to place a temporary restoration to prevent further contamination and accidental swallowing or aspirating of instruments or irrigation solutions (ie, solvents, irrigants, and chelating agents) used during the procedure. If a prefabricated post is present, the practitioner should not violate the coronal part of the post during the removal of the restoration. Most parts of the restoration can be removed by burs. However, the final part of the restoration around the post can be removed using ultrasonic instruments (Fig 8-22). Another mishap might occur during access cavity preparation in teeth with PFM crowns. The porcelain might chip, and the restoration might become defective during the procedure (Fig 8-23). To prevent this, the practitioner should use a diamond round bur to begin access cavity preparation and should remove porcelain with a high-speed handpiece using copious water spray. When reaching the metal part of the restoration, a

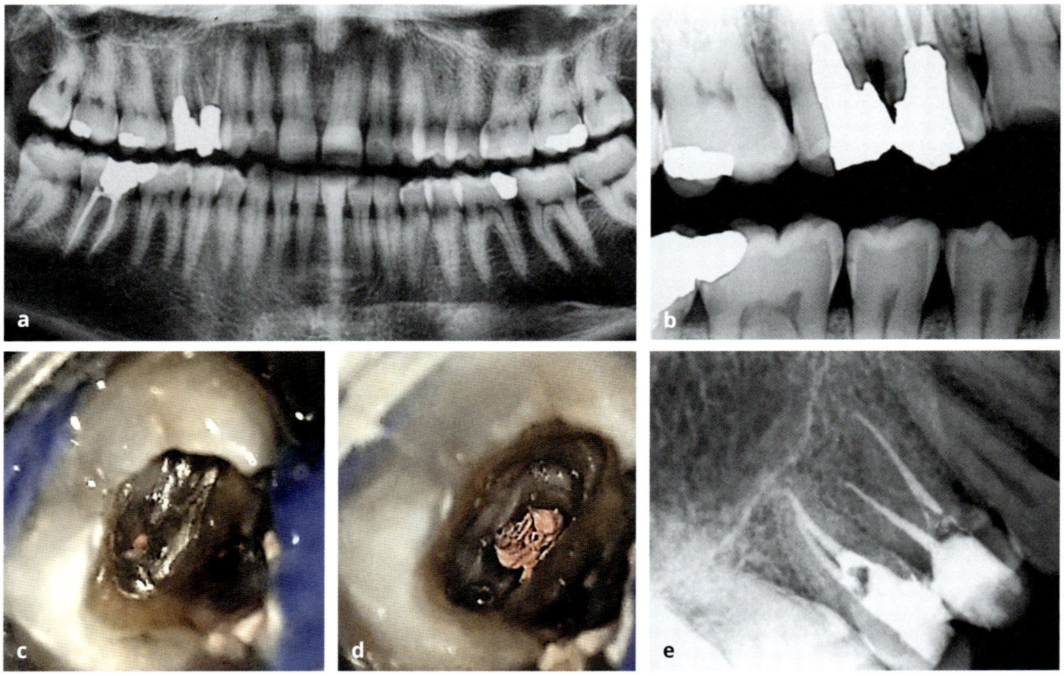

Fig 8-22 *(a and b)* Panoramic and bitewing radiographs show deep amalgam placement in teeth nos. 4 and 5. *(c)* Following careful removal of amalgam under a DOM and observing the low thickness of residual amalgam, the rest of the restoration was removed using ultrasonic vibration. *(d)* No amalgam remained. *(e)* Both teeth received secondary nonsurgical endodontic treatment.

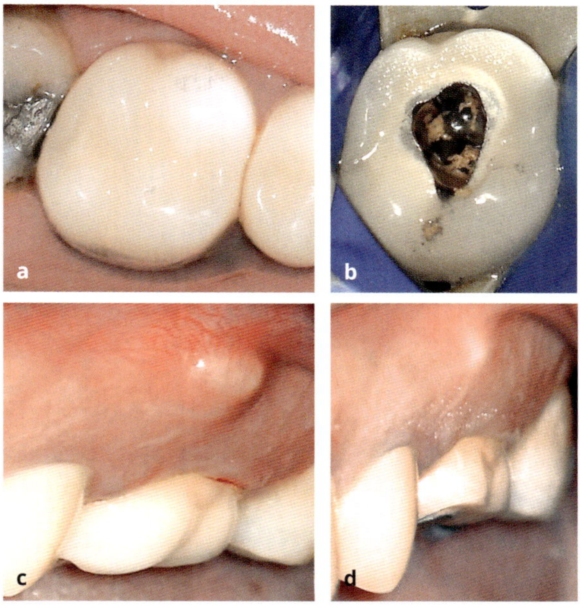

Fig 8-23 A case of porcelain chipping during access cavity preparation. *(a)* Pretreatment occlusal view of tooth no. 14. *(b)* Access cavity preparation. *(c)* Pretreatment buccal view of the same tooth. *(d)* Obvious porcelain chipping of the same tooth.

brand new transmetal (Dentsply Sirona) or diamond fissure bur with minimum vibration can be effective in penetrating the metal without chipping the porcelain (see Fig 8-14). The use of ultrasonic vibration during access cavity preparation increases the risk of porcelain chipping. Therefore, the ultrasonic tip size should be selected carefully; a large-sized ultrasonic tip would increase the risk of transmitting vibrations to the porcelain and chipping it (Fig 8-24). If, despite preventive measures, the porcelain chips, it can be repaired using composite resin.[44] Before treatment, during the examination visit or case presentation, the clinician must

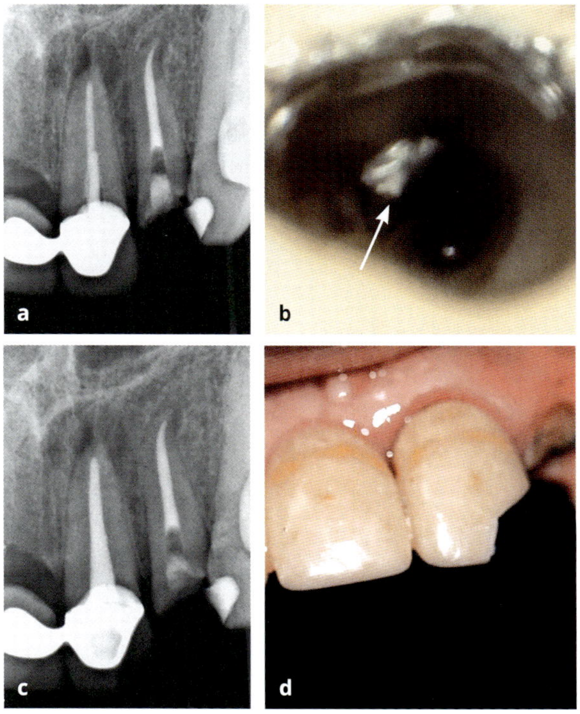

Fig 8-24 *(a)* A prefabricated post with a density similar to root canal obturation materials in tooth no. 9. *(b)* The metal structure of the post could be recognized when the access cavity was prepared through the bridge. *(c and d)* The post was removed, and secondary nonsurgical root canal treatment was performed; however, the use of an improper ultrasonic tip resulted in porcelain chipping.

inform the patient about the chance of porcelain chipping or a crown coming off during retreatment in order to prevent future claims.

The best method for managing mishaps is prevention. It has been reported that perforation occurs in 0.6% to 17.6% of cases. Several risk factors may lead to perforation, such as practitioner inexperience, tooth type, and tooth morphology.[45] In most instances, a careful review of the case before starting the secondary nonsurgical endodontic treatment procedure and consideration of all the recommendations mentioned above will prevent further mishaps.[46]

Crown removal

A common mistake is to overuse the armamentaria to forcefully remove the crown. This action may result in tooth fracture and either necessitate an unplanned crown lengthening procedure or compromise the future restoration. Sometimes the fracture might be so deep that the tooth becomes unrestorable (Fig 8-25).

If the crown could not be removed with an initial attempt using crown removal systems with gentle force, the crown should be split into two halves by a diamond fissure bur and each piece removed separately to prevent further mishaps. Crown removal must be performed after rubber dam application.

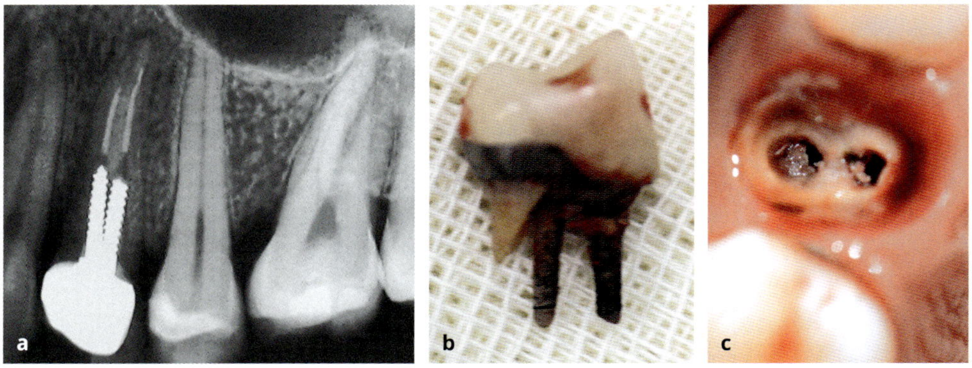

Fig 8-25 An example of a mistake that involved using forceful crown remover equipment. *(a)* Periapical radiograph of tooth no. 12 before crown removal. *(b)* Deep fracture of the tooth structure after using Automatic Crown Remover Gun Type. *(c)* The rest of the root seems unrestorable.

Post removal

When the practitioner is not familiar with root surface topography (depressions) and does not have the necessary equipment, the risk of mishaps and of failure to remove the post will increase. To avoid these mishaps, the practitioner should be familiar with the anatomy of the teeth and have the right tools to perform this task.

Another common mistake during post removal is not considering the presence of a post inside the root canal because some types of posts have radiodensity similar to root canal filling materials (ie, gutta-percha; see Fig 8-24) or the preoperative radiograph might not show them properly. To avoid this mistake, the preoperative radiographs and/or CBCT images must be carefully examined.

Another issue after post removal is the type of cements between the post and the apical root canal filling materials. In some cases, this cement is a resin glass ionomer, and its removal is very difficult.

Magnification, specific equipment, and practitioner skills are prerequisites for successful post removal. In addition, it should be kept in mind that if ultrasonic equipment is used for post removal, the temperature will rise. To prevent temperature increase during post removal, use copious water irrigant and a short cycle of ultrasonic activation; avoiding maximum power of the ultrasonic setting could prevent damage to the periodontal ligament.[47-49] Removing posts from the root canals depends on several factors. The type of post is important. Fiber posts are difficult to remove because they have the same color as dentin. Therefore, for post removal, they should be managed with different techniques than for prefabricated and casting metallic posts. Fiber post removal is a significant challenge for an endodontist. It has been reported that using different techniques for fiber post removal is associated with mishaps, such as deviation from the root canal pathway and root perforation (Fig 8-26).[50] The main reason for the difficulty of fiber post removal is the similarity in color of the fiber post and root dentin. To remove fiber posts and prevent mishaps, using a dye such as methylene blue for differentiating the post structure and dentin is helpful. In addition, a long-shank fine round bur, such as Munce Discovery Burs (CJM Engineering), in combination with magnification and ultrasonic energy can be very useful. During the removal of the fiber posts, the debris resulting from drilling the post is different than the dentinal debris (Fig 8-27). When the bur penetrates the fiber post, a specific structure of debris can be observed through DOM, which makes practitioners confident they are removing the post and not the tooth structure. Ultrasonic vibration may not be a useful tool to remove a fiber post if the previous practitioner used direct technique for cementing the post.[51] From a clinical standpoint, at the middle and apical part of the post, the bond might not be strong enough, and the ultrasonic activation would help the practitioner remove the post easily from the root canal. In such a condition, the cervical one-third of the post is very difficult to penetrate; however, the rest of the post is easier to remove.

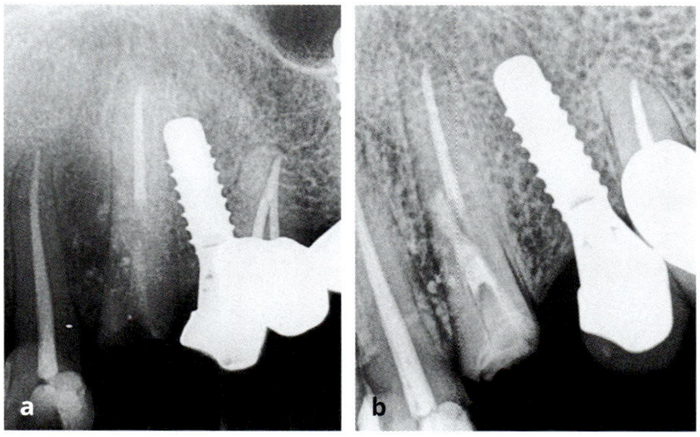

Fig 8-26 *(a)* A dentist tried to remove the fiber post without proper illumination and magnification, resulting in root perforation. *(b)* The fiber post was successfully removed under DOM magnification, using a Munce Discovery Bur and ultrasonic vibration. The perforation was repaired with CEM cement.

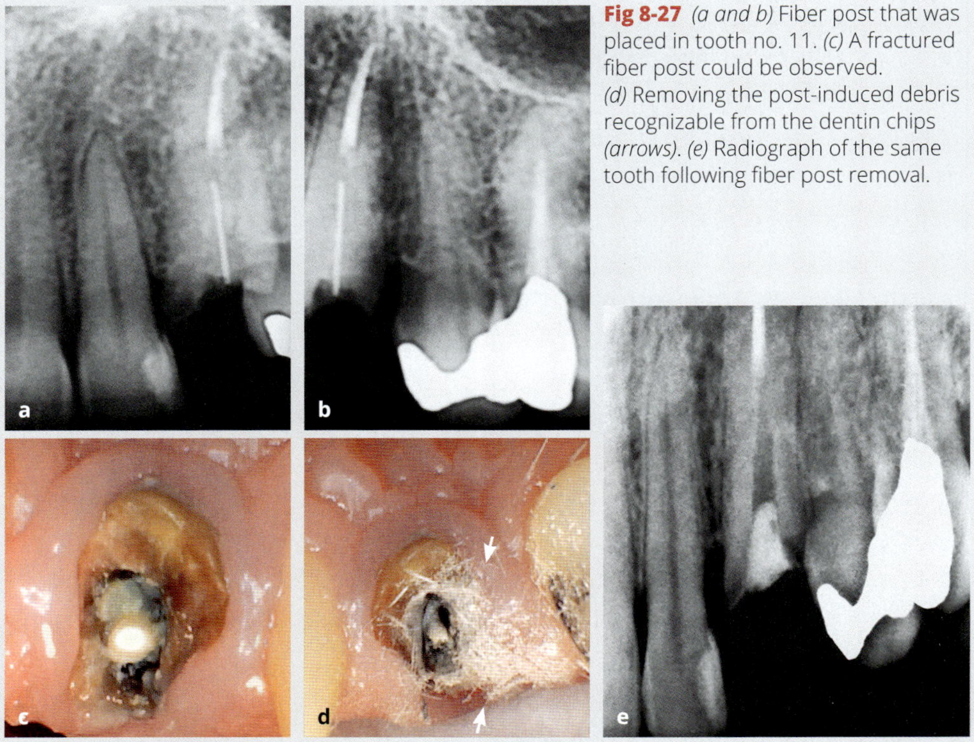

Fig 8-27 *(a and b)* Fiber post that was placed in tooth no. 11. *(c)* A fractured fiber post could be observed. *(d)* Removing the post-induced debris recognizable from the dentin chips *(arrows)*. *(e)* Radiograph of the same tooth following fiber post removal.

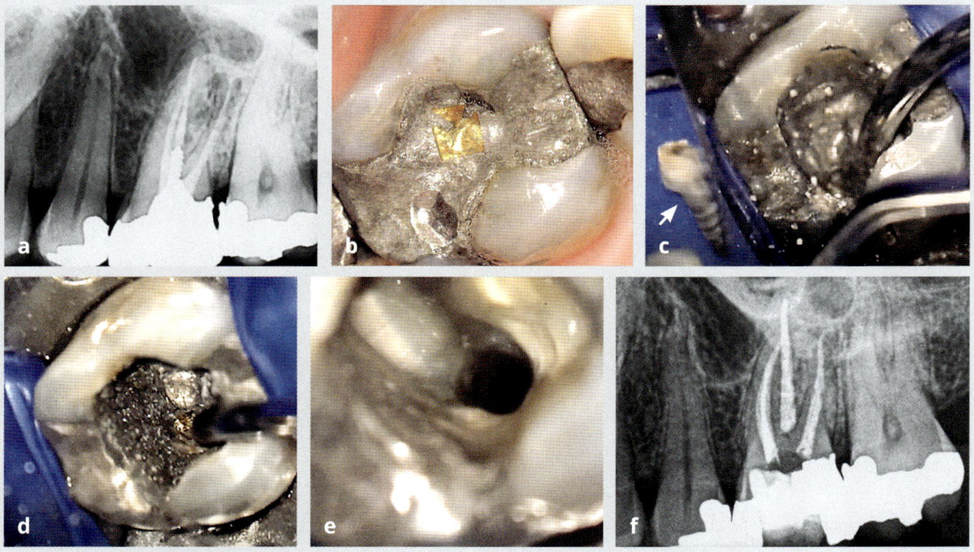

Fig 8-28 *(a and b)* Tooth no. 14 needs secondary nonsurgical endodontic treatment because the patient has recently experienced exacerbation. *(c)* During post removal, the coronal part of the post was separated from the rest of the post structure *(arrow)*. *(d)* An elongated cylindrical, active round ultrasonic tip was used to remove the rest of the post. *(e)* The post was successfully removed, and the secondary nonsurgical root canal treatment was completed. *(f)* Final radiograph after secondary endodontic treatment.

In removing prefabricated metallic posts, the practitioner should remove all the restorative materials around the post to reach the orifice of the root canal(s) and then use ultrasonic vibration to remove the post. It has been shown that if zinc phosphate has been used for the cast post cementation, a cavity prepared inside the core would decrease the traction force necessary for post removal by ultrasonic vibration.[52]

Another common error happens when a practitioner inadvertently removes the prefabricated post structure from the post cementation area of the root canal. In such a case, activating the ultrasonic tip or grasping the post with Stieglitz forceps may result in the separation of the coronal part of the post (Fig 8-28). To prevent this, when removing the restorative materials, the final part of the materials should be removed with ultrasonic activation. Moreover, constant ultrasonic movement around the post would prevent the post from thinning, which makes it prone to further separation during its removal. If the coronal part of the post is separated despite all precautions, it is important for the practitioner to decide what technique should be used to remove the remaining structure. If the post is separated just at the orifice of the root canal, an elongated cylindrical-shaped and active rounded tip of an ultrasonic scaler could be used to remove the post. However, if the post fractures below the orifice, NSK E7 Varios endodontic ultrasonic scaler tip (Nakanishi) is recommended with a DOM to remove the post from the root canal (see Fig 8-28).

Mishaps During Cleaning and Shaping

Removal of root canal filling materials

Gutta-percha is the most frequently used root canal filling material. One of the most frequent mistakes is to initially use a solvent when removing the root canal filling materials during secondary nonsurgical endodontic treatment. It has been shown that employing chloroform at this early stage results in more residual root filling materials.[53] In contrast, the root canal filling material in the cervical part of the root canal should first be removed with a Gates-Glidden drill, followed by a Hedstrom hand file. The heat generated by the drill makes the remaining gutta-percha softer and easier to penetrate with a Hedstrom hand file. If the file cannot penetrate well, then a gutta-percha solvent should be used. Another mistake is not considering the apical distance between root canal filling materials and apical foramen. In the case of overfilling, gutta-percha solvents are contraindicated (Fig 8-29); in contrast, in the case of underfilled root canals, particularly root canals with curvature, insisting on removing the filling material without a solvent might increase the risk of ledge formation, the extension of the previous ledge, or even perforation. It has also been shown that removing gutta-percha using heat might harm the periodontal ligament.[54] Therefore, relying on only heat for removing gutta-percha may also have some unwanted mishaps.

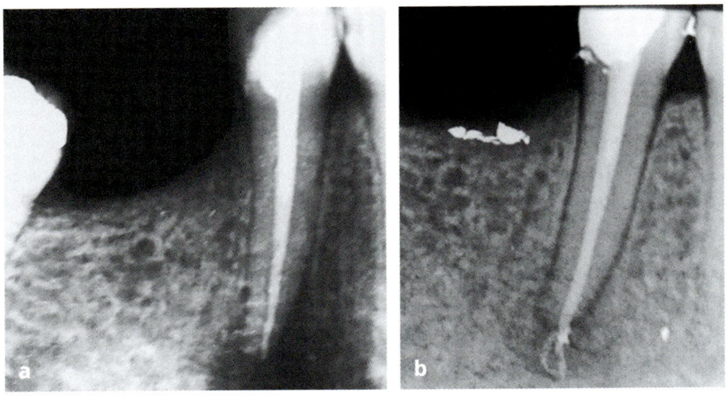

Fig 8-29 A common mistake in using a solvent when a tooth with an overfilled obturation is to be retreated. *(a)* Preoperative radiograph of tooth no. 29 shows overextended gutta-percha and a radiolucent lesion. *(b)* Overfilling due to the use of chloroform during gutta-percha removal.

Using rotary instruments for secondary nonsurgical root canal treatment is associated with more file fracture, and using rotary instruments for more than four root canals might increase the chance of broken instruments.[55] When rotary instruments are used to remove root canal filling materials, the chance of instrument fracture increases; therefore, a practitioner should use brand new instruments to prevent the chance of instrument fracture and should discard the instruments following the secondary nonsurgical endodontic treatment. For the sake of infection control, single use of hand and rotary instruments either for primary or secondary nonsurgical treatment has been suggested.[56]

The use of rotary and reciprocating instruments to remove root canal filling materials is significantly associated with higher procedural accidents, ie, ledge formation, perforation, and fractured instruments.[57–59] Using a Hedstrom hand file is a safe method to remove root canal filling materials and prevents further mishaps, particularly for practitioners with minimal experience.[57,58] A systematic review concluded that XP-endo Finisher and XP-endo Finisher R remove root canal filling material better than irrigant activation techniques.[60] It has been reported that reciprocating files could remove root canal filling materials much faster than hand and rotary instruments during endodontic retreatment.[61] However, based on a systematic review, hand instruments are the *safest* method to remove previous root canal filling materials.[59]

A practitioner should carefully evaluate the type and length of root filling materials and consider root canal curvature both before treatment and during the procedure. Moreover, overfilling materials might not always be the reason for future failure; however, insisting on removing them results in further damage to periapical tissues and increases the risk of postoperative pain and flare-up. It has been shown that overfilling is an important predictor of postoperative pain and discomfort.[62] It should be kept in mind that if overfilling happened during initial or secondary root canal treatment, the best time for removing the overfilled material would be the same visit, before setting of the root canal sealer (Fig 8-30).

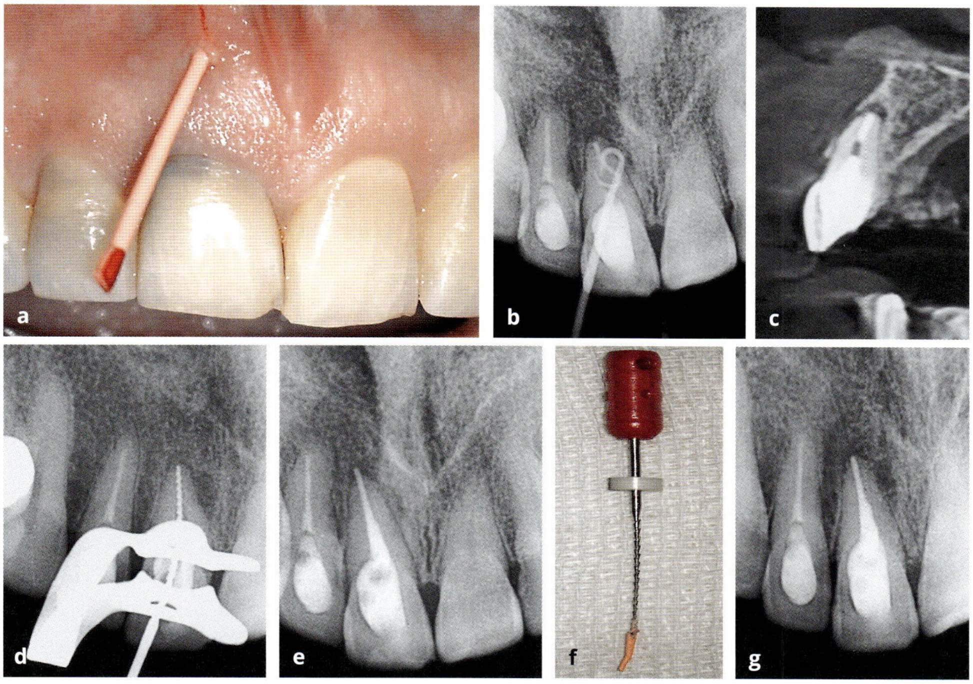

Fig 8-30 *(a)* A patient was referred due to the presence of a sinus tract at the apical part of tooth no. 8. *(b)* Periapical radiograph with tracing gutta-percha. *(c)* Sagittal view of CBCT image. *(d)* Removing root canal filling materials. *(e)* Final radiograph showed root canal overfilled. *(f)* Immediate attempt at the same visit results in removing overfilled gutta-percha. *(g)* Final radiograph with optimal root canal obturation.

In some instances, the root canal may be obturated with solid core obturators such as Thermafil (Dentsply Sirona) or GuttaCore (Dentsply Sirona). Therefore, during secondary nonsurgical endodontic treatment, the coronal part of the obturator may need to be removed during access cavity preparation, which makes the treatment very difficult.

First, careful examination of preoperative radiographs may help the endodontist recognize a solid core obturator if it has a metallic core made with stainless steel. Secondly, using magnification and careful coronal restoration removal practices during access cavity preparation can help the endodontist to differentiate between the restoration and the obturator cores. In that case, the practitioner should avoid cutting the exposed carriers during access cavity preparation and instead grasp them later with pliers such as Stieglitz forceps. If no obturator core was detected during access cavity preparation, the root canal orifice should be carefully examined. The presence of either metallic, gray, black, or white spots surrounded by gutta-percha may be an indication of a root canal filled with a solid core obturator. If the level of obturator is not above the root canal orifice, then using a solvent followed by ultrasonic vibration would help to retrieve a metallic carrier. For a plastic carrier, removing gutta-percha at the buccal and lingual side of the carrier followed by the use of System B heat plugger would be very helpful for retrieval.[63] However, care should be taken to prevent overheat generation

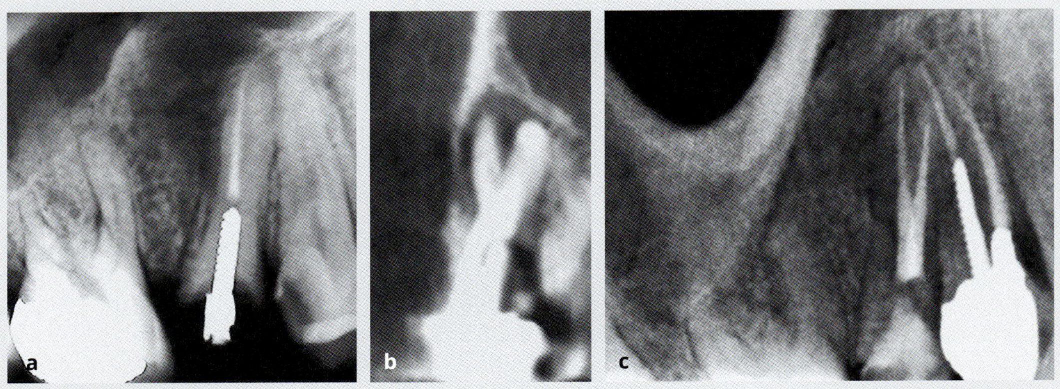

Fig 8-31 *(a)* A periapical radiograph shows the root canal obturation of tooth no. 4 was not at the center of the root but was asymmetric. *(b)* The CBCT coronal view shows that the palatal root has been missed. *(c)* The missed root canal was successfully found, prepared, and obturated during secondary nonsurgical root canal treatment.

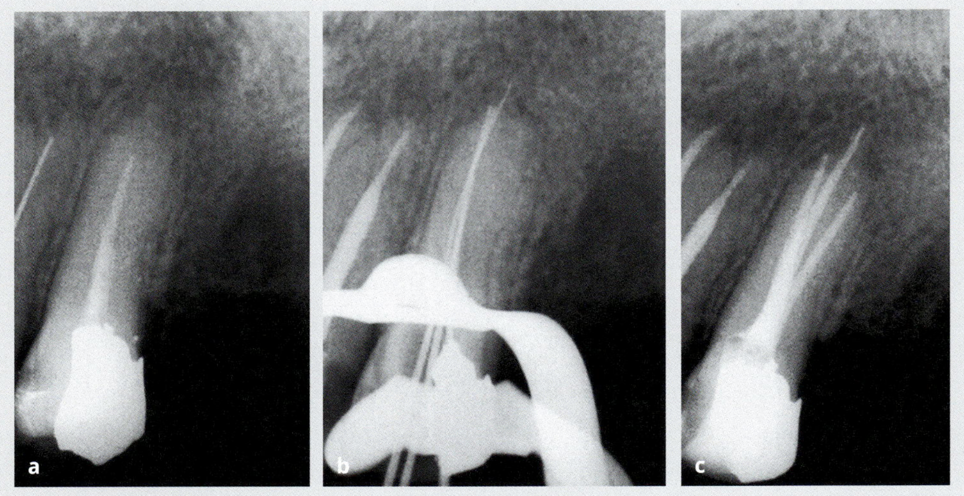

Fig 8-32 Tooth no. 13 was referred for secondary nonsurgical root canal treatment due to a defective restoration and the need for a full-coverage restoration. *(a)* Preoperative radiograph. *(b)* After removing the root canal filling material and taking the initial working radiograph, an asymmetry was noted. *(c)* Following the use of magnification and illumination, three root canals were identified.

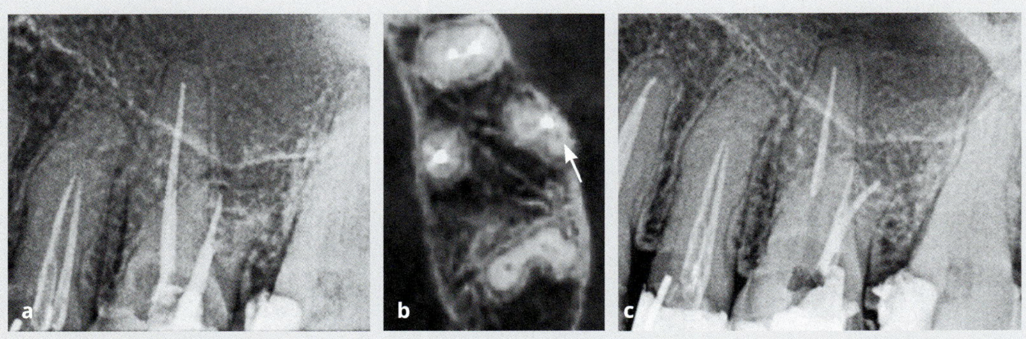

Fig 8-33 *(a)* Preoperative radiograph shows asymmetry in the buccal root of tooth no. 14. *(b)* The CBCT axial view shows that the tooth has two roots (buccal and palatal); the root canal in the buccal root has one orifice and two apical foramina *(arrow)*. *(c)* Complete obturation following the secondary nonsurgical endodontic treatment.

during the procedure because the heat may be harmful for the periodontium around the root. Another technique is to use rotary instruments for removing a plastic carrier and gutta-percha.[64] When teeth have received silver points as root canal obturation material and need secondary nonsurgical endodontic treatment, special care should be taken to not violate the coronal part of the silver point during access cavity preparation, as it may be embedded in the restorative material. After exposing the coronal part of the silver point, pliers such as Stieglitz forceps can be used to grasp the point and remove it from the root canal.[6]

Locating missed root canals

A study reported that missed root canals are found in nearly half of molar teeth undergoing secondary nonsurgical endodontic treatment.[65] A frequent pitfall for practitioners is inadequate knowledge of root canal morphology. The mesiobuccal root of maxillary molars; the distal root of mandibular molars, mandibular anterior teeth, and mandibular and maxillary premolars; and the mid-mesial canal of mandibular molars are potential candidates for a missed canal and should be examined carefully during the initial and/or secondary nonsurgical endodontic treatment.[66–70]

Practitioners should always consider anatomical variations when they are performing secondary nonsurgical endodontic treatment. Taking preoperative radiographs from different angles might help to identify a missed root canal. In general, when asymmetry is present in a preoperative periapical radiograph, the practitioner might consider the possibility of the presence of a missed root canal (Fig 8-31). During root canal retreatment, careful evaluation of diagnostic radiographs can also help detect missed root canals (Fig 8-32). In addition, CBCT is an important diagnostic tool that can help locate missed root canals (Fig 8-33). Moreover, a careful search for any missed root canal using proper magnification and illumination is mandatory to prevent future failure. Remember, teeth usually have more canals than anticipated.

Management of previous mishaps

Common mishaps that need to be addressed during nonsurgical retreatment are separated instruments, ledged canals, and perforations.

Separated instruments

Despite their unpleasant radiographic images, separated instruments do not significantly influence the final outcome.[71–74] Therefore, conservative techniques that save more root structure are always recommended (Fig 8-34). Several factors might increase the chance of failure following instrument fracture, including pulp necrosis, presence of periapical lesions, and instrument separation before proper root canal cleaning. Overall, the decision to remove a broken instrument or to leave it within the root canal should be based on the clinician's skill, the available equipment, potential risks, the condition of the root canal when the instrument

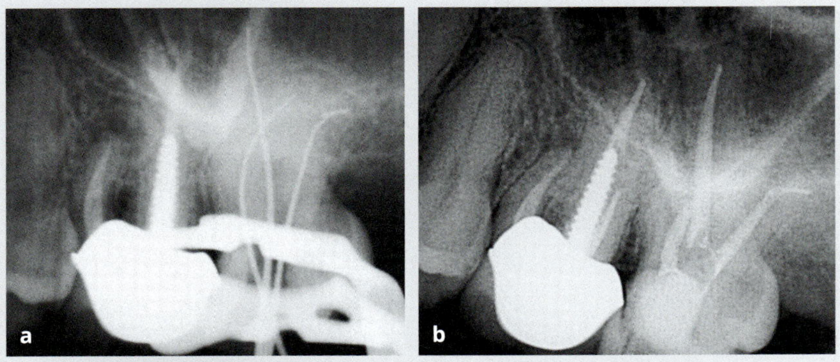

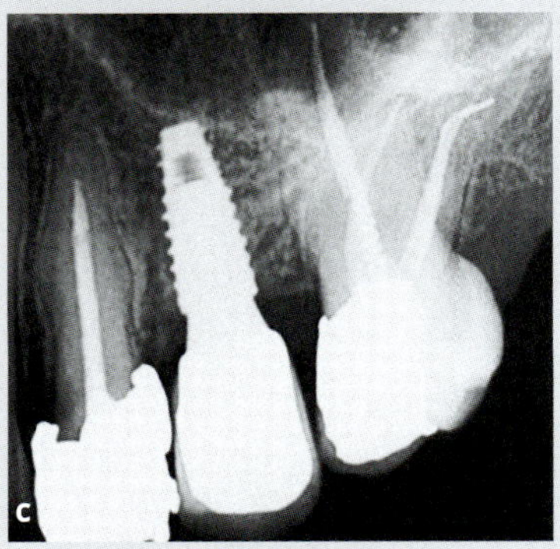

Fig 8-34 *(a)* An instrument was separated at the apical part of the distobuccal root of tooth no. 15 during root canal preparation. *(b)* Because the preoperative pulp status was vital and the instrument was broken at the final step of root canal preparation, it was decided to leave it and fill the rest of the root canal with gutta-percha and root canal sealer. *(c)* Ten years later, the patient was still symptom free, and no sign of periapical pathosis was observed in the periapical radiograph.

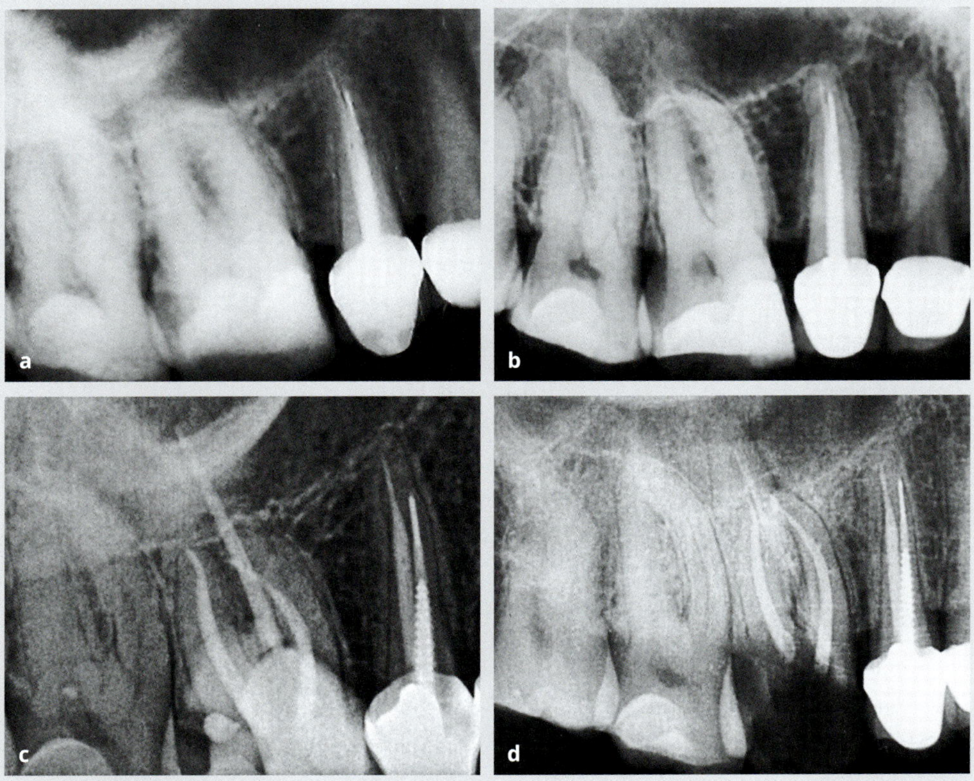

Fig 8-35 *(a)* During a routine checkup, a broken instrument was recognized in one of the root canals of tooth no. 4. Because the patient was symptom free, the instrument was not removed and he continued with regular checkups. *(b to d)* Follow-up of the patient 10, 18, and 22 years later.

fractured (ie, at the beginning or at the final step of root canal preparation), the presence or absence of periapical lesion,[75] and the vitality status of the pulp before treatment.[76] In the case of secondary nonsurgical endodontic treatment, the clinician's skill and equipment, potential risks, and the presence or absence of a periapical lesion should be considered. Ideally, it is better to remove the fractured instrument; however, sometimes a practitioner's attempt may not be successful, and more tooth structure removal may make the tooth prone to fracture. In a case with no history of previous infection, absence of periapical lesion, and no need for a new restoration, removal should not be attempted (Fig 8-35). In these cases, it is wise to inform the patient of the potential risks and benefits and to perform periodic monitoring.[77] A frequent mistake is trying to remove a broken instrument without proper magnification and illumination. In addition, it has been demonstrated that providing a staging platform and space around the broken instrument enables ultrasonic vibration to transfer energy to the separated instrument.[78] Removal of separated instruments without proper magnification and illumination is very difficult and dangerous, and the creation of a staging platform should be performed with minimal removal of tooth structures.

Ledges

In some instances, the ledge formation is obvious and can be detected in a preoperative radiograph. Every attempt should be made to bypass a ledge during retreatment. Common mistakes during ledge removal are using reaming action during root canal negotiation when reaching the ledge, forcing large files above the ledge, and using a file without precurving its tip to negotiate the existing ledge. These actions do not result in negotiation of the ledge, and they may even aggravate the situation, making it impossible to bypass the ledge.

Sharp, precurved tips and pecking motions with slight rotation are key factors for bypassing the ledges and getting back to the original root canal pathway. In addition, it is crucial to use solvents to prevent expanding the ledge. Practitioners can use precurved instruments to bypass the ledge if they are able to correctly estimate the direction of the canal extension.[79]

Another common mistake occurs when the practitioner successfully bypasses the ledge but does not take time to negotiate the ledge adequately. When this happens, in the following step, the practitioner uses either a long push-pull motion or short push-pull motion without insisting on staying apical to the defect. In such a case, the root canal pathway might be blocked, preventing renegotiation of the root canal. To prevent such a problem, the practitioner should use short pecking motions while the file tip is always kept apical to the ledge.[79]

Another common mistake is to employ forceful rotary instruments to bypass the ledge following early renegotiation of the root canal with fine files. This action might transport the root canal and lead to a perforation or result in fracturing the rotary instruments. To avoid this, it is prudent to bypass the ledge by small

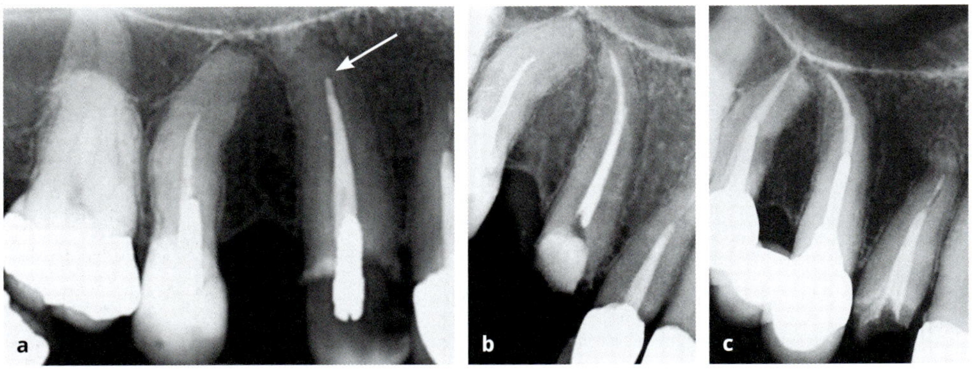

Fig 8-36 Tooth no. 6 needs a new restoration. *(a)* Preoperative radiograph shows a short, prefabricated post and a ledge that happened during initial nonsurgical endodontic treatment *(arrow)*. *(b)* After removing the post and root canal filling materials, the ledge was bypassed, and the root canal was prepared and obturated. *(c)* Five years later, the tooth was asymptomatic and functional.

hand instruments and then use rotary instruments for the final root canal preparation (Fig 8-36).

8

Perforations

Root canal perforation is one of the significant reasons for endodontic treatment failure.[80,81] Perforation repair is an important component of secondary nonsurgical endodontic treatment, and the practitioner should always follow instructions when using bioactive endodontic cements.[15,17,82–84] Several factors, such as cleaning the perforation site and using barriers in large perforations to prevent extrusion of the bioactive endodontic cement into the periodontium, can improve the final outcome (Fig 8-37).[83,84] One common mistake is not carefully reviewing the case before undertaking treatment. For instance, in maxillary premolar (two or three separate roots) and maxillary and mandibular molar teeth, the thickness of the pulp chamber floor should always be evaluated before starting treatment (see Fig 8-21).

If the previous treatment has made the furcation thin, careful removal of the restorative material should be considered. It would be more conservative if the final part of the restorative materials were removed by ultrasonic vibration to prevent further perforation.

Another common mistake is to start secondary nonsurgical endodontic treatment without considering proper management of the perforation. In the presence of an extensive root perforation, the perforation site should be repaired first before removing the root canal filling materials because of the possibility of irrigant penetration and inadvertent pushing of the root filling materials into the perforation site.

Another common mistake is to assume that different bioactive endodontic cements have similar efficacy for perforation repair.[17] The clinician should be aware of the ingredients of each material and whether the material has been successfully investigated as a perforation repair material.[17,82–85] For instance, when

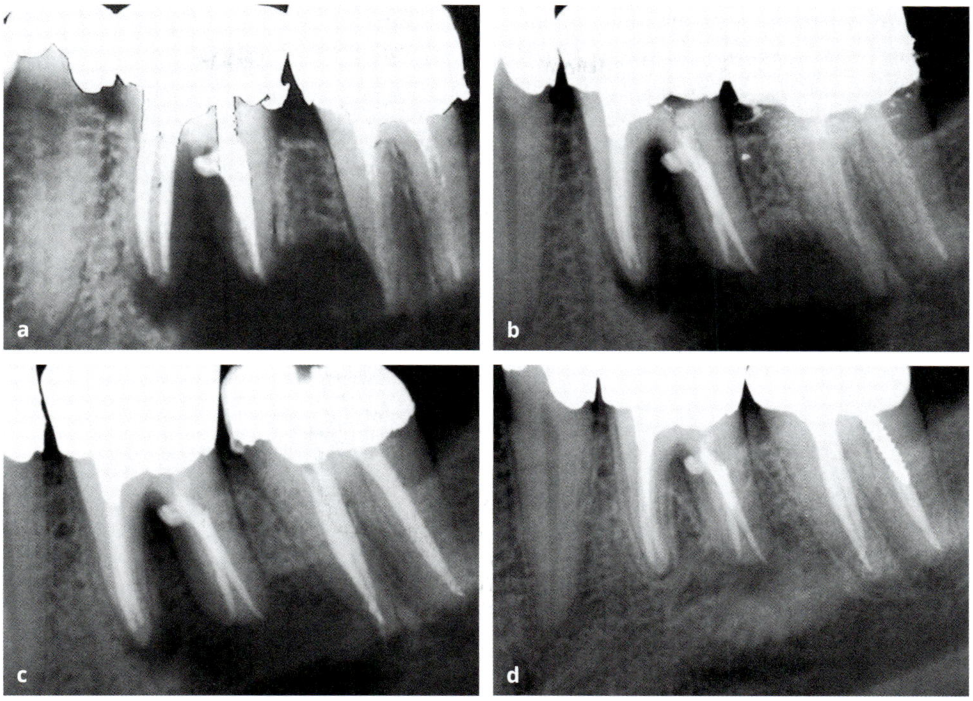

Fig 8-37 *(a)* A preoperative radiograph shows post perforation in the distobuccal root of tooth no. 19. *(b)* The post was removed, and the perforation site was cleaned and repaired with tooth-colored ProRoot MTA (Dentsply Tulsa Dental Specialties). *(c)* Tooth no. 18 also received secondary nonsurgical endodontic treatment. *(d)* Thirty months later, the radiolucent lesion was healed.

esthetic is important, a bioactive endodontic cement with no bismuth oxide is preferable.[17,84]

Root Canal Preparation

Several factors should be considered during root canal preparation when retreating a case. First, before root canal preparation, the previously prepared root canal should be carefully evaluated. If the root canal is well prepared but persistent or secondary infection has caused failure, the practitioner should mostly focus on irrigation, using passive ultrasonic irrigation, apical negative pressure, or sonic irrigation to remove the debris, smear layer, and biofilm.[86] A recent investigation raised doubts about the ability of ultrasonic activation to remove root canal filling materials, reporting that the ultrasonic activation might push the filling materials into the dentinal tubules.[87] To prevent this, other active intracanal techniques such as apical negative pressure and sonic irrigation may also be considered.

The second common mistake is failing to consider the cross section of the root canal during secondary nonsurgical endodontic treatment. It has been shown that when rotary instruments are used for the secondary nonsurgical endodontic treatment of oval root canals, the remaining debris, necrotic tissue, and initial root filling materials might significantly increase.[88–90] The XP-endo Finisher and XP-endo Finisher R systems can be used to remove root canal filling materials.[60]

Use of ultrasonic or agitating sonic devices such as EndoActivator (Dentsply Sirona) might provide a cleaner root canal surface following the removal of root canal filling materials.

Third, it has been demonstrated that in oval-shaped root canals, when a contracted access cavity design is applied, it might significantly reduce the efficacy of instruments to remove root canal filling materials.[46] To avoid this issue, it is advisable to prepare a standard access cavity in teeth with oval-shaped root canals.

Fourth, inadequate review of the case and its variables such as remaining dentin thickness is another common mistake during root canal preparation in teeth that require retreatment. If CBCT is available, the quality of previous root canal preparation and the remaining dentin thickness can be easily evaluated. Sometimes conventional periapical radiographs do not provide enough information, which may result in mishaps such as strip perforation (Fig 8-38).

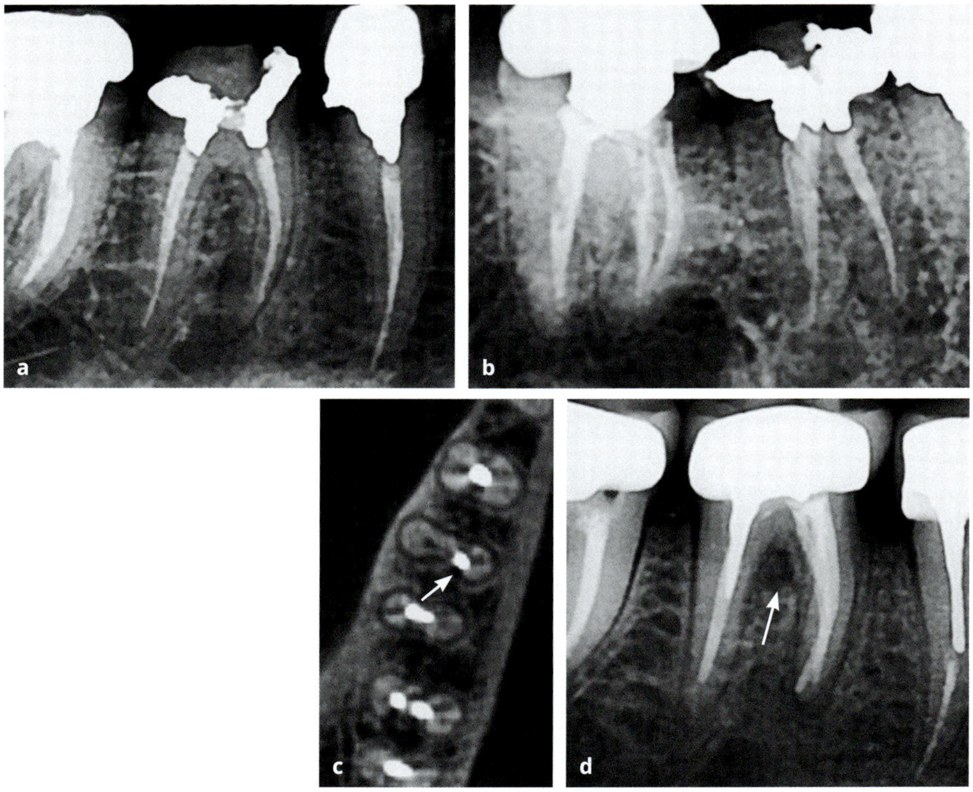

Fig 8-38 An example of ignoring 3D technology, resulting in further failure. *(a and b)* The periapical radiographs from different horizontal angles of tooth no. 30 showed the possibility of a missed root canal in the mesial root. *(c)* Axial view of the tooth shows that the mesiobuccal root canal was missed. It also shows extremely low dentin thickness between the mesiolingual root canal and periodontium *(arrow)*. The patient was informed about the possibility of strip perforation if a secondary nonsurgical endodontic treatment was undertaken. The patient did not accept the endodontist's comment and sought another clinician without giving the second clinican the comment of the first endodontist. *(d)* Several months later, the patient returned with a chief complaint of sensitivity during mastication, and a periodontal pocket with a radiolucent lesion was observed *(arrow)*.

Two other common mistakes can also happen during root canal preparation: *(1)* not removing the smear layer and *(2)* not considering the possibility of the presence of old bacterial biofilm. It has been demonstrated that removing the smear layer can significantly increase the successful outcome of secondary nonsurgical endodontic treatment.[91] The use of 5.25% sodium hypochlorite during root canal preparation and final irrigation with alternative use of the sodium hypochlorite and 17% ethylenediaminetetraacetic acid (EDTA) was shown to successfully remove root canal biofilm and smear layer.[92] Choosing the irrigant for removing the smear layer and eliminating biofilm should be based on available literature. Several irrigants such as sodium hypochlorite with low concentration, alternative use of EDTA and sodium hypochlorite, and MTAD are useful for removing the smear layer; however, if the practitioner intends to remove the biofilm, then QMix (Dentsply Tulsa Dental Specialties), Tetraclean (Ogna Laboratori Farmaceutici), and higher concentration of sodium hypochlorite (> 2%) should be considered.[93,94]

Prognosis

A common mistake is to believe that *all* secondary nonsurgical endodontic treatment procedures are associated with less successful outcomes. It is true that the overall success rate of secondary nonsurgical endodontic treatment is significantly lower than initial nonsurgical endodontic treatment[95]; however, the studies considered had cases that received secondary nonsurgical endodontic treatment by dental students and general practitioners in addition to endodontists.[3,96] The high survival rate of the teeth receiving secondary nonsurgical endodontic treatment performed by *endodontists* might persuade a clinician to render the treatment.[97] To achieve the best outcomes, practitioners should identify the cause of the previous failure and correct it.[98] Whether performing initial nonsurgical endodontic root canal therapy or secondary nonsurgical endodontic treatment, adequate root canal filling and proper restoration significantly impact the success rate, improving the health and function of teeth.[99] Therefore, if the cause of failure can be detected and managed, there will be no significant difference between the outcomes of the initial and secondary nonsurgical endodontic treatments.[6]

Another common mistake is to consider microsurgery retreatment superior to secondary nonsurgical root canal treatment. A systematic review and meta-analysis reported that the long-term outcome of endodontic retreatment is significantly higher than the surgical endodontic treatment that has provided significantly greater short-term outcomes.[3] In addition, a recent study reported no significant difference between the two treatment modalities in terms of survival rates.[100]

Another common mistake is to consider secondary nonsurgical root canal treatment completed without placing an effective final restoration. Initial or secondary nonsurgical root canal treatment can be assumed completed only after providing a proper tooth restoration.[101]

References

1. Jakovljevic A, Nikolic N, Jacimovic J, et al. Prevalence of apical periodontitis and conventional nonsurgical root canal treatment in general adult population: An updated systematic review and meta-analysis of cross-sectional studies published between 2012 and 2020. J Endod 2020;46:1371–1386.
2. Kebke S, Fransson H, Brundin M, Mota de Almeida FJ. Tooth survival following root canal treatment by general dental practitioners in a Swedish county—A 10-year follow-up study of a historical cohort. Int Endod J 2021;54:5–14.
3. Torabinejad M, Corr R, Handysides R, Shabahang S. Outcomes of non-surgical retreatment and endodontic surgery: A systematic review. J Endod 2009;35:930–937.
4. García-Guerrero C, Delgado-Rodríguez CE, Molano-González N, et al. Predicting the outcome of initial non-surgical endodontic procedures by periapical status and quality of root canal filling: A cohort study. Odontology 2020;108:697–703.
5. Siqueira JF Jr. Aetiology of root canal treatment failure: Why well-treated teeth can fail. Int Endod J 2001;34:1–10.
6. Terauchi Y, Parirokh M, Handysides R. Non-surgical retreatment. In: Torabinejad M, Fouad A, Shabahang S. Endodontics: Principles and Practice, ed 6. St Louis: Elsevier, 2021.
7. Tibúrcio-Machado CS, Michelon C, Zanatta FB, Gomes MS, Marin JA, Bier CA. The global prevalence of apical periodontitis: A systematic review and meta-analysis. Int Endod J 2021; 54:712–735.
8. American Association of Endodontists. Case Assessment Tools. https://www.aae.org/specialty/clinical-resources/treatment-planning/case-assessment-tools. Accessed 7 February 2023.
9. Savani GM, Sabbah W, Sedgley CM, Whitten B. Current trends in endodontic treatment by general dental practitioners: Report of a United States national survey. J Endod 2014;40:618–624.
10. Givol N, Rosen E, Taicher S, Tsesis I. Risk management in endodontics. J Endod 2010;36:982–984.
11. Zhang MM, Fang GF, Chen XT, Liang YH. Four-year outcome of nonsurgical root canal retreatment using cone-beam computed tomography: A prospective cohort study. J Endod 2021;47:382–390.
12. Torabinejad M, Rice DD, Maktabi O, Oyoyo U, Abramovitch K. Prevalence and size of periapical radiolucencies using cone-beam computed tomography in teeth without apparent intraoral radiographic lesions: A new periapical index with a clinical recommendation. J Endod 2018;44:389–394.
13. Antony DP, Thomas T, Nivedhitha MS. Two-dimensional periapical, panoramic radiography versus three-dimensional cone-beam computed tomography in the detection of periapical lesion after endodontic treatment: A systematic review. Cureus 2020;12:e7736.
14. Nekoofar MH, Ghandi MM, Hayes SJ, Dummer PMH. The fundamental operating principles of electronic root canal length measurement devices. Int Endod J 2006;39:595–609.
15. Parirokh M, Torabinejad M. Mineral trioxide aggregate: A comprehensive literature review—Part I: Chemical, physical, and antibacterial properties. J Endod 2010;36:16–27.
16. Patel S, Durack C, Abella F, Shemesh H, Roig M, Lemberg K. Cone beam computed tomography in Endodontics—A review. Int Endod J 2015;48:3–15.
17. Parirokh M, Torabinejad M, Dummer PMH. Mineral trioxide aggregate and other bioactive endodontic cements: An updated overview—Part I: Vital pulp therapy. Int Endod J 2018;51:177–205.
18. Kulild JC. Diagnostic testing. In: Ingle JI, Bakland LK, Baumgartner JC (eds). Ingle's Endodontics, ed 6. Hamilton, Ontario: BC Decker, 2008:532–547.
19. Roda RS, Gettleman BH, Johnson SC. Nonsurgical retreatment. In: Berman LH, Hargreaves KM (eds). Cohen's Pathways of the Pulp, ed 12. St Louis: Elsevier, 2021.
20. Special Committee to Revise the Joint AAE/AAOMR Position Statement on use of CBCT in Endodontics. AAE and AAOMR joint position statement: Use of cone beam computed tomography in endodontics 2015 update. Oral Surg Oral Med Oral Pathol Oral Radiol 2015;120:508–512.
21. Patel S, Brown J, Semper M, Abella F, Mannocci F. European Society of Endodontology position statement: Use of cone beam computed tomography in endodontics: European Society of Endodontology (ESE) developed by. Int Endod J 2019;52:1675–1678.
22. Ee J, Fayad MI, Johnson BR. Comparison of endodontic diagnosis and treatment planning decisions using cone-beam volumetric tomography versus periapical radiography. J Endod 2014;40:910–916.
23. Mota de Almeida FJ, Knutsson K, Flygare L. The impact of cone beam computed tomography on the choice of endodontic diagnosis. Int Endod J 2015;48:564–572.
24. Rodríguez G, Abella F, Durán-Sindreu F, Patel S, Roig M. Influence of cone-beam computed tomography in clinical decision making among specialists. J Endod 2017;43:194–199.
25. Bhatt M, Coil J, Chehroudi B, Esteves A, Aleksejuniene J, MacDonald D. Clinical decision-making and importance of the AAE/AAOMR position statement for CBCT examination in endodontic cases. Int Endod J 2021;54:26–37.
26. Rodríguez G, Patel S, Durán-Sindreu F, Roig M, Abella F. Influence of cone-beam computed tomography on endodontic retreatment strategies among general dental practitioners and endodontists. J Endod 2017;43:1433–1437.

27. Johnson BR, Fayad MI, Berman LH. Periradicular surgery. In: Berman LH, Hargreaves KM (eds). Cohen's Pathways of the Pulp, ed 12. St Louis: Elsevier, 2021.
28. Zamparini F, Pelliccioni GA, Spinelli A, Gissi DB, Gandolfi MG, Prati C. Root canal treatment of compromised teeth as alternative treatment for patients receiving bisphosphonates: 60-month results of a prospective clinical study. Int Endod J 2021;54:156–171.
29. Nair MK, Levin MD, Nair UP. Radiographic interpretation. In: Berman LH, Hargreaves KM (eds). Cohen's Pathways of the Pulp, ed 12. St Louis: Elsevier, 2021.
30. Bjørndal L, Reit C. Endodontic malpractice claims in Denmark 1995-2004. Int Endod J 2008;41:1059–1065.
31. Chércoles-Ruiz A, Sánchez-Torres A, Gay-Escoda C. Endodontics, endodontic retreatment, and apical surgery versus tooth extraction and implant placement: A systematic review. J Endod 2017;43:679–686.
32. Derks J, Tomasi C. Peri-implant health and disease. A systematic review of current epidemiology. J Clin Periodontol 2015;42(suppl 16):S158–S171.
33. García-Guerrero C, Parra-Junco C, Quijano-Guauque S, Molano N, Pineda GA, Marín-Zuluaga DJ. Vertical root fractures in endodontically-treated teeth: A retrospective analysis of possible risk factors. J Investig Clin Dent 2018;9:e12273.
34. Torabinejad M, White SN. Endodontic treatment options after unsuccessful root canal treatment: Alternatives to single-tooth implants. J Am Dent Assoc 2016;147:214–220.
35. Parirokh M, Zarifian A , Ghoddusi J. Choice of treatment plan based on root canal therapy versus extraction and implant placement: A mini review. Iran Endod J 2015;10:152–155.
36. Bhattacharyya S, Das DP, Bhattacharyya A, Maity AB, Das D. Clinical guideline and treatment planning decisions of single-tooth implants versus preserving natural teeth with non-surgical endodontic therapy. J Family Med Prim Care 2020;9:2654–2658.
37. Kfir A, Blau-Venezia N, Tsesis I, Goldberger T, Metzger Z. Does root canal treatment in necrotic pulp or retreatment cases with periapical lesions require anaesthesia? An in vivo clinical study. Int Endod J 2017;50:330–338.
38. Parirokh M, Abbott PV. Various strategies for pain-free root canal treatment. Iran Endod J 2014;9:1–14.
39. Abbott PV, Parirokh M. Strategies for managing pain during endodontic treatment. Aust Endod J 2018;44:99–113.
40. Parirokh M, Abbott PV. Present status and future directions—Mechanisms and management of local anaesthetic failures. Int Endod J 2022;55(suppl 4):951–994.
41. Al Shaikhly B, Harrel SK, Umorin M, Augsburger RA, Jalali P. Comparison of a dental operating microscope and high-resolution videoscope for endodontic procedures. J Endod 2020;46:688–693.
42. Del Fabbro M, Taschieri S, Lodi G, Banfi G, Weinstein RL. Magnification devices for endodontic therapy. Cochrane Database Syst Rev 2015;2015:CD005969.
43. Khalighinejad N, Aminoshariae A, Kulild JC, Williams KA, Wang J, Mickel A. The effect of the dental operating microscope on the outcome of nonsurgical root canal treatment: A retrospective case-control study. J Endod 2017;43:728–732.
44. Ahmad I. Salvaging fractured porcelain crowns with a direct composite repair technique. Pract Proced Aesthet Dent 2002;14:233–238.
45. Sarao SK, Berlin-Broner Y, Levin L. Occurrence and risk factors of dental root perforations: A systematic review. Int Dent J 2020;71:96–105.
46. Niemi TK, Marchesan MA, Lloyd A, Seltzer RJ. Effect of instrument design and access outlines on the removal of root canal obturation materials in oval-shaped canals. J Endod 2016;42:1550–1554.
47. Lipski M, Debicki M, Droździk A. Effect of different water flows on root surface temperature during ultrasonic removal of posts. Oral Surg Oral Med Oral Pathol Oral Radiol Endod 2010;110:395–400.
48. Davis S, Gluskin AH, Livingood PM, Chambers DW. Analysis of temperature rise and the use of coolants in the dissipation of ultrasonic heat buildup during post removal. J Endod 2010;36:1892–1896.
49. Lipski M, Mrozek J, Droździk A. Influence of water cooling on root surface temperature generated during post space preparation. J Endod 2010;36:713–736.
50. Haupt F, Pfitzner J, Hülsmann M. A comparative in vitro study of different techniques for removal of fiber posts from root canals. Aust Endod J 2018;44:245–250.
51. Makarewicz D, Le Bell-Rönnlöf AM, Lassila LVJ, Vallittu PK. Effect of cementation technique of individually formed fiber-reinforced composite post on bond strength and microleakage. Open Dent J 2013;7:68–75.
52. Graça IAA, Sponchiado Júnior EC, Marques AAF, de Moura Martins L, Garrido ÂDB. Assessment of a cavity to optimize ultrasonic efficiency to remove intraradicular posts. J Endod 2017;43:1350–1353.
53. Ma J, Al-Ashaw AJ, Shen Y, Gao Y, Yang Y, Zhang C, Haapasalo M. Efficacy of ProTaper Universal Rotary Retreatment system for gutta-percha removal from oval root canals: A micro-computed tomography study. J Endod 2012;38:1516–1520.
54. Livada R, Hosn K, Shiloah J, Anderson KM. Management of heat-induced bone necrosis following thermal removal of gutta-percha. Quintessence Int 2018;49:535–542.

55. Gomes MS, Vieira RM, Böttcher DE, Plotino G, Celeste RK, Rossi-Fedele G. Clinical fracture incidence of rotary and reciprocating NiTi files: A systematic review and meta-regression. Aust Endod J 2021;47:372–385.
56. Sonntag D, Peters OA. Effect of prion decontamination protocols on nickel-titanium rotary surfaces. J Endod 2007;33:442–446.
57. Rödig T, Hausdörfer T, Konietschke F, Dullin C, Hahn W, Hülsmann M. Efficacy of D-RaCe and ProTaper Universal Retreatment NiTi instruments and hand files in removing gutta-percha from curved root canals—A micro-computed tomography study. Int Endod J 2012;45:580–589.
58. Rödig T, Reicherts P, Konietschke F, Dullin C, Hahn W, Hülsmann M. Efficacy of reciprocating and rotary NiTi instruments for retreatment of curved root canals assessed by micro-CT. Int Endod J 2014;47:942–948.
59. Rossi-Fedele G, Aly Ahmed HM. Assessment of root canal filling removal effectiveness using micro-computed tomography: A systematic review. J Endod 2017;43:520–526.
60. Uzunoglu-Özyürek E, Küçükkaya Eren S, Karahan S. Contribution of XP-endo files to the root canal filling removal: A systematic review and meta-analysis of in vitro studies. Aust Endod J 2021;47:703–714.
61. Alakabani TF, Faus-Llácer V, Faus-Matoses V. Evaluation of the time required to perform three retreatment techniques with dental microscope and ultrasonic activation for removing filling material from the oval root canal. J Clin Exp Dent 2018;10:e810–e814.
62. Demenech LS, de Freitas JV, Tomazinho FSF, Baratto-Filho F, Gabardo MCL. Postoperative pain after endodontic treatment under irrigation with 8.25% sodium hypochlorite and other solutions: A randomized clinical trial. J Endod 2021;47:696–704.
63. Wolcott JF, Himel VT, Hicks ML. Thermafil retreatment using a new "System B" technique or a solvent. J Endod 1999;25:761–764.
64. Fracchia DE, Amaroli A, de Angelis N, et al. GuttaCore Pink, Thermafil and warm vertically compacted gutta-percha retreatment: Time required and quantitative evaluation by using ProTaper files. Dent Mater J 2020;39:229–235.
65. Witherspoon DE, Small JC, Regan JD. Missed canal systems are the most likely basis for endodontic retreatment of molars. Tex Dent J 2013;130:127–139.
66. Wolf TG, Kim P, Campus G, Stiebritz M, Siegrist M, Briseño-Marroquín B. 3-dimensional analysis and systematic review of root canal morphology and physiological foramen geometry of 109 mandibular first premolars by micro-computed tomography in a mixed Swiss-German population. J Endod 2020;46:801–809.
67. Martins JNR, Marques D, Silva EJNL, Caramês J, Mata A, Versiani MA. Second mesiobuccal root canal in maxillary molars—A systematic review and meta-analysis of prevalence studies using cone beam computed tomography. Arch Oral Biol 2020;113:104589.
68. Santos MC, Souza-Gabriel AE, Cruz-Filho AM, Sousa-Neto MD, Silva RG. Detection of the internal anatomy of lower anterior teeth using cone-beam computed tomography. Aust Endod J 2021;47:442–449.
69. Shen Y, Gu Y. Assessment of the presence of a second mesiobuccal canal in maxillary first molars according to the location of the main mesiobuccal canal—A micro-computed tomographic study. Clin Oral Investig 2021;25:3937–3944.
70. Wolf TG, Kozaczek C, Campus G, Paqué F, Wierichs RJ. Root canal morphology of 116 maxillary second premolars by micro-computed tomography in a mixed Swiss-German population with systematic review. J Endod 2020;46:1639–1647.
71. Ng YL, Mann V, Gulabivala K. A prospective study of the factors affecting outcomes of non-surgical root canal treatment: Part 2: Tooth survival. Int Endod J 2011;44:610–625.
72. Spili P, Parashos P, Messer HH. The impact of instrument fracture on outcome of endodontic treatment. J Endod 2005;31:845–850.
73. Panitvisai P, Parunnit P, Sathorn C, Messer HH. Impact of a retained instrument on treatment outcome: A systematic review and meta-analysis. J Endod 2010;36:775–780.
74. Fu M, Zhang Z, Hou B. Removal of broken files from root canals by using ultrasonic techniques combined with DOM: A retrospective analysis of treatment outcome. J Endod 2011;37:619–622.
75. Madarati AA, Hunter MJ, Dummer PM. Management of intracanal separated instruments. J Endod 2013;39:569–581.
76. Ungerechts C, Bårdsen A, Fristad I. Instrument fracture in root canals—Where, why, when and what? A study from a student clinic. Int Endod J 2014;47:183–190.
77. McGuigan MB, Louca C, Duncan HF. Clinical decision-making after endodontic instrument fracture. Br Dent J 2013;214:395–400.
78. Gerek M, Başer ED, Kayahan MB, Sunay H, Kaptan RF, Bayırlı G. Comparison of the force required to fracture roots vertically after ultrasonic and Masserann removal of broken instruments. Int Endod J 2012;45:429–434.

79. Jafarzadeh H, Abbott PV. Ledge formation: Review of a great challenge in endodontics. J Endod 2007;33:1155–1162.
80. Yamaguchi M, Noiri Y, Itoh Y, et al. Factors that cause endodontic failures in general practices in Japan. BMC Oral Health 2018;18:70.
81. Siew K, Lee AHC, Cheung GSP. Treatment outcome of repaired root perforation: A systematic review and meta-analysis. J Endod 2015;41:1795–1804.
82. Torabinejad M, Parirokh M. Mineral trioxide aggregate: A comprehensive literature review- Part II: Sealing ability and biocompatibility properties. J Endod 2010;36:190–202.
83. Parirokh M, Torabinejad M. Mineral trioxide aggregate: A comprehensive literature review—Part III: Clinical applications, drawbacks, and mechanism of action. J Endod 2010;36:400–412.
84. Torabinejad M, Parirokh M, Dummer PMH. Mineral trioxide aggregate and other bioactive endodontic cements: An updated overview—Part II: Other clinical applications and complications. Int Endod J 2018;51:284–317.
85. de Sousa Reis M, Scarparo RK, Steier L, de Figueiredo JAP. Periradicular inflammatory response, bone resorption, and cementum repair after sealing of furcation perforation with mineral trioxide aggregate (MTA Angelus) or Biodentine. Clin Oral Investig 2019;23:4019–4027.
86. Virdee SS, Seymour DW, Farnell D, Bhamra G, Bhakta S. Efficacy of irrigant activation techniques in removing intracanal smear layer and debris from mature permanent teeth: A systematic review and meta-analysis. Int Endod J 2018;51:605–621.
87. da Silva Machado AP, Câncio Couto de Souza AC, Lima Gonçalves T, et al. Does the ultrasonic activation of sealer hinder the root canal retreatment? Clin Oral Investig 2021;25:4401–4406.
88. Rechenberg DK, Paqué F. Impact of cross-sectional root canal shape on filled canal volume and remaining root filling material after retreatment. Int Endod J 2013;46:547–555.
89. Crozeta BM, Silva-Sousa YTC, Leoni GB, et al. Micro-computed tomography study of filling material removal from oval-shaped canals by using rotary, reciprocating, and adaptive motion systems. J Endod 2016;42:793–797.
90. Siqueira Junior JF, Rôças IDN, Marceliano-Alves MF, Pérez AR, Ricucci D. Unprepared root canal surface areas: Causes, clinical implications, and therapeutic strategies. Braz Oral Res 2018;32(suppl 1):e65.
91. Ng YL, Mann V, Gulabivala K. A prospective study of the factors affecting outcomes of nonsurgical root canal treatment: Part 1: Periapical health. Int Endod J 2011;44:583–609.
92. Tawakoli PN, Ragnarsson KT, Rechenberg DK, Mohn D, Zehnder M. Effect of endodontic irrigants on biofilm matrix polysaccharides. Int Endod J 2017;50:153–160.
93. Pappen FG, Shen Y, Qian W, Leonardo MR, Giardino L, Haapasalo M. In vitro antibacterial action of Tetraclean, MTAD and five experimental irrigation solutions. Int Endod J 2010;43:528–535.
94. Stojicic S, Shen Y, Qian W, Johnson B, Haapasalo M. Antibacterial and smear layer removal ability of a novel irrigant, QMix. Int Endod J 2012;45:363–371.
95. Goldberg F, Cantarini C, Alfie D, Macchi RL, Arias A. Relationship between unintentional canal overfilling and the long-term outcome of primary root canal treatments and nonsurgical retreatments: A retrospective radiographic assessment. Int Endod J 2020;53:19–26.
96. Ng YL, Mann V, Gulabivala K. Outcome of secondary root canal treatment: A systematic review of the literature. Int Endod J 2008;41:1026–1046.
97. Salehrabi R, Rotstein I. Epidemiologic evaluation of the outcomes of orthograde endodontic retreatment. J Endod 2010;36:790–792.
98. He J, White RK, White CA, Schweitzer JL, Woodmansey KF. Clinical and patient-centered outcomes of nonsurgical root canal retreatment in first molars using contemporary techniques. J Endod 2017;43:231–237.
99. Ng YL, Gulabivala K. Outcome of non-surgical re-treatment. Endod Topics 2011;18:3–30.
100. Haxhia E, Ibrahim M, Bhagavatula P. Root-end surgery or nonsurgical retreatment: Are there differences in long-term outcome? J Endod 2021;47:1272–1277.
101. Estrela C, Pécora JD, Estrela CRA, et al. Common operative procedural errors and clinical factors associated with root canal treatment. Braz Dent J 2017;28:179–190.

9

Errors During Surgical Endodontics

MAHMOUD TORABINEJAD
ZAHED MOHAMMADI
MASOUD PARIROKH
MOHAMMAD SABETI

Objectives

After reading this chapter, the reader should be able to:

1. Know the indications and contraindications of periapical surgery (PAS).
2. Determine the etiology of failure through examination and treatment.
3. Describe the mishaps during the following:
   a. Patient interview
      i. Addressing chief complaint
      ii. Recording medical history
      iii. Recording dental history
   b. Clinical examination
      i. Extraoral examination
      ii. Intraoral examination
      iii. Clinical tests
   c. Radiographic examination
   d. Incision and drainage
   e. Periapical surgery
      i. Flap design
      ii. Flap reflection
      iii. Flap retraction
      iv. Osteotomy
      v. Periapical curettage
      vi. Apical resection
      vii. Root-end cavity preparation
      viii. Placing root-end filling material
      ix. Flap closure
      x. Postoperative complications

When initial treatment is unsuccessful and nonsurgical retreatment does not succeed, or is not possible, surgical endodontics is needed to save a tooth. The goals of this procedure include sealing all portals of communication between the root canal system and periradicular tissues, eliminating contaminants from the periradicular tissues, providing an environment for complete regeneration of periradicular tissues, and ultimately saving natural dentition. The use of a dental operating microscope, microsurgery instruments, and new root-end filling materials has significantly changed the art and science of surgical endodontics.[1,2]

Like other medical or dental procedures, mishaps can occur during diagnosis and treatment planning as well as during the technical components of surgical endodontics. To avoid mishaps, the clinician should use a systematic approach to gather pertinent medical and dental information, perform necessary tests, and analyze the gathered information to develop a differential diagnosis, definitive diagnosis, and subsequent treatment plan. This chapter will focus on appropriate steps to obtain information during a patient interview related to their medical and dental histories, clinical and radiographic signs and symptoms, the implications of the gathered data in treatment planning for surgical endodontics, and finally the mishaps during these steps.[3–7]

Mishaps During Patient Interview

The main benefit of surgical endodontics is retention of the patient's natural dentition. However, there are situations when the teeth cannot be saved and have to be extracted. Despite recent advances in the art and science of endodontic surgery, the outcomes of this procedure can be overstated and cause misunderstanding between the patient and the clinician. Heroic efforts in saving every single tooth with surgical endodontics is counterproductive and should not be attempted. During the patient interview, steps involved in periapical surgery and its alternatives should be discussed in layman's terms and must include a candid explanation of benefits, risks, and cost. The risks of surgical endodontics, which include damage to the gingival tissue, scar tissue formation after surgery, and postoperative complications such as bruising and paresthesia, should always be discussed with the patients before performing surgical endodontics. After complete discussion, a consent form, which is an agreement between the patient and the practitioner, should be signed by the patient or their legal guardian and witnessed by a third party.[6,8] A common mistake is not providing a comprehensive explanation to the patient regarding the surgical procedures. Sometimes a patient is referred only to receive a simple opinion due to the presence of a periapical lesion around a tooth with initial or retreated endodontic treatment. A common mistake is looking at the current radiograph without examining the previous radiographs (Fig 9-1).

Mishaps during the patient interview can relate to the chief complaint, health and medical history, and dental history.

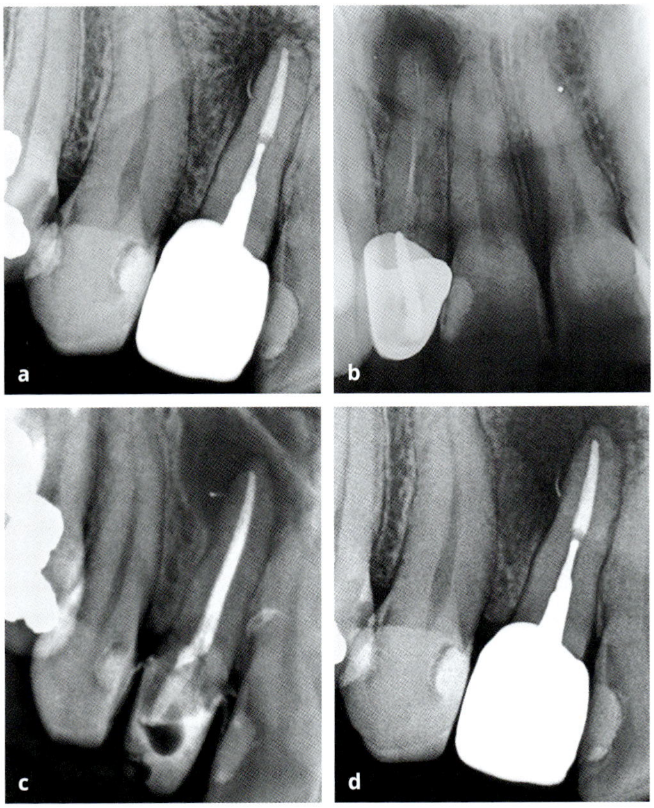

Fig 9-1 *(a)* This 37-year-old female patient was referred for evaluation of a periapical radiolucency around tooth no. 7. *(b and c)* Evaluating her dental history showed that she received nonsurgical endodontic retreatment 3 years before her visit due to the presence of a periapical radiolucency and inappropriate root canal treatment (incomplete obturation). *(d)* Compared to the periapical radiograph 6 months after treatment, the follow-up radiograph *(a)* showed healing of the periapical lesion.

9

Chief complaint

As stated in chapter 1, clinicians should listen to the chief complaint very carefully; patients usually judge the character of the provider based on the treatment outcome and how well their chief complaint is addressed. Ignoring the patient's chief complaint not only results in missing valuable diagnostic information, but it may also cause a lack of trust between the patient and the provider.

Health and medical history

The most common diseases that may influence endodontic procedures are cardiovascular disease, hematologic disorders, diabetes, cancer, kidney disease, and neurologic disorders (see chapter 1). Patients with these conditions should be carefully evaluated for periapical surgery (PAS). Because hemostasis is important during PAS, it should be avoided in patients with recent myocardial infarction (MI), unstable angina, recent coronary artery bypass surgery (within 3 months), uncontrolled or untreated hypertension, refractory arrhythmias, and uncontrolled hyperthyroidism, because these patients cannot have enough epinephrine to control hemostasis. Another group of patients that are not good candidate for surgical endodontics are those taking antithrombotic medications. These patients are high risks for excessive bleeding during a surgical endodontic procedure. Surgical endodontics should be avoided on patients with uncontrolled diabetes, kidney diseases, or white blood cell disorders, as well as patients on immune suppression medications or with radiation to head or throat more than 60 Grays or with low healing capacity. Patients on antiresorptive agents and medications known to increase the risk of osteonecrosis of the jaw (bisphosphonate, denosumab, and anti-angiogenic drugs) should be carefully evaluated when considering surgical endodontic intervention. When in doubt, consultation with the patient's physician is indicated.[6,7,9]

Dental history

Information regarding history of dental treatment is very important when considering PAS. Consulting with the previous provider(s), receiving clinical and radiographic information, and comparing your data with that of previous provider(s) can supply valuable clues regarding the cause(s) of the patient's problems and the potential success of future treatments, including PAS (see Fig 9-1). Performing PAS without knowing the previous dental history can result in serious misunderstandings among the patient, the provider, and insurance companies.

Mishaps During Clinical Examination

A clinical examination consists of careful observation and diagnostic testing of extraoral and intraoral tissues to compare them with other normal structures without apparent pathosis.[7]

Extraoral examination

A careful extraoral examination of a patient may reveal the cause of intraoral pathosis. Lack of attention to this part of treatment can result in misdiagnosis and mistreatment of the patient (Fig 9-2).

Intraoral examination

Intraoral examination consists of testing the soft and hard tissues of the oral cavity. During hard tissue examination of the oral cavity, the presence or absence of hard tissue abnormalities such as exostosis should be examined. The teeth should be examined with a mirror and an explorer for discolorations, fractures, abrasions, erosions, caries, failing restorations, or other abnormalities. Abnormal findings can affect flap design and surgical approach to the offending tooth. The soft tissue examination includes a careful visual evaluation and digital evaluation of the lips, oral mucosa, cheeks, tongue, periodontium, palate, and muscles of mastication. The alveolar mucosa and gingiva are examined for the presence of inflammation, ulceration, discoloration, swelling, dehiscence, fenestration, and sinus tract formation. An important part of soft tissue examination is determination of periodontal biotypes. Lack of attention to soft tissue examination, especially to the type of periodontal biotypes, can result in poor esthetic outcomes and an unsatisfied patient. There are several ways to detect different gingival biotypes, including the following: *(1)* direct measurement (spreader and rubber stop), *(2)* probe transparency, *(3)* ultrasonic devices, and *(4)* CBCT.[10]

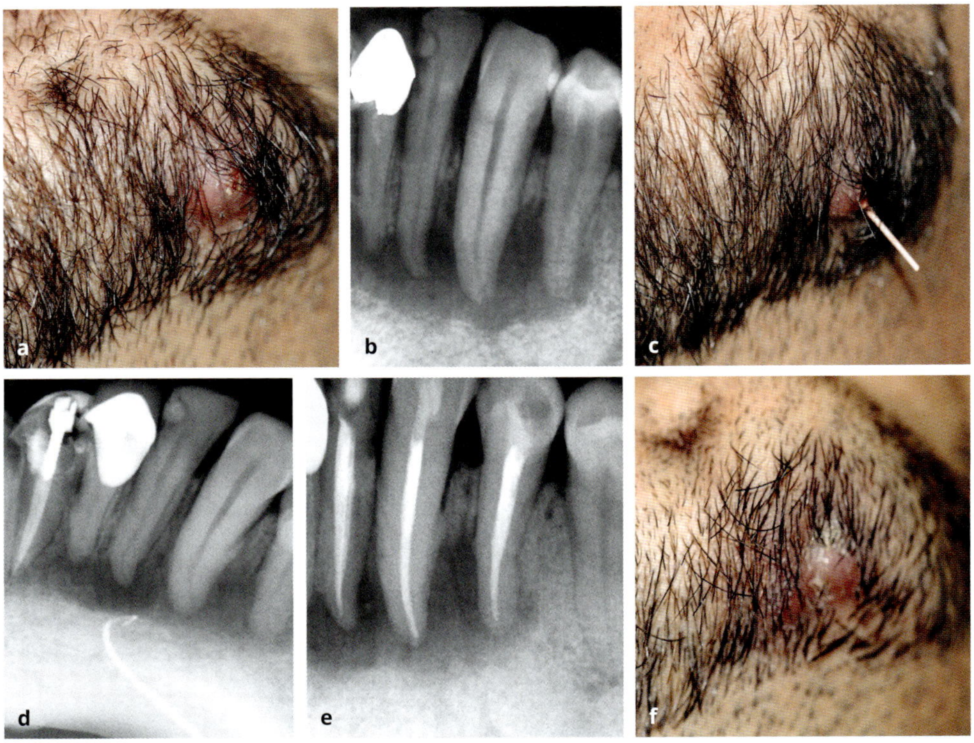

Fig 9-2 *(a)* An extraoral fistula that was treated surgically a number of times because its origin from a chronic periapical lesion from mandibular anterior teeth was not recognized. *(b)* A periapical radiograph showing the presence of pathosis in mandibular anterior and first premolar teeth. *(c and d)* Tracing of the extraoral fistula with gutta-percha cone revealed a periapical lesion as the source of infection. *(e and f)* One week after nonsurgical root canal treatment, the extraoral fistula was closed.

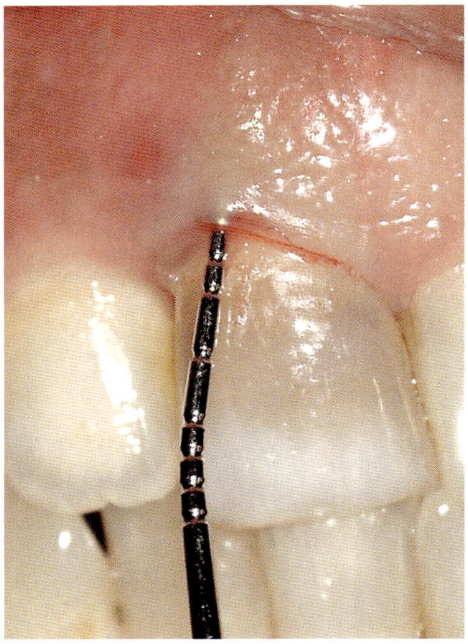

Fig 9-3 A thin gingival biotype can be detected when a periodontal probe is visible through the sulcus.

The easiest and least invasive method is the probe transparency method (Fig 9-3). A common mistake is not using proper magnification and illumination during clinical examination. Sometimes it is possible to recognize a vertical root fracture by using a dental operative microscope during examination (Fig 9-4).

Clinical tests

As stated in chapter 1, clinical tests include a number of methods to determine the presence or absence of pathologic conditions in the dentition. These tests include percussion, palpation, probing, vitality tests, and radiographic examination. A common mistake while performing clinical tests is the exclusion of control teeth for comparison.[11] A control tooth provides vital information for the clinician to compare the patient's baseline responses. A common mistake during a percussion test is the assumption that the tenderness

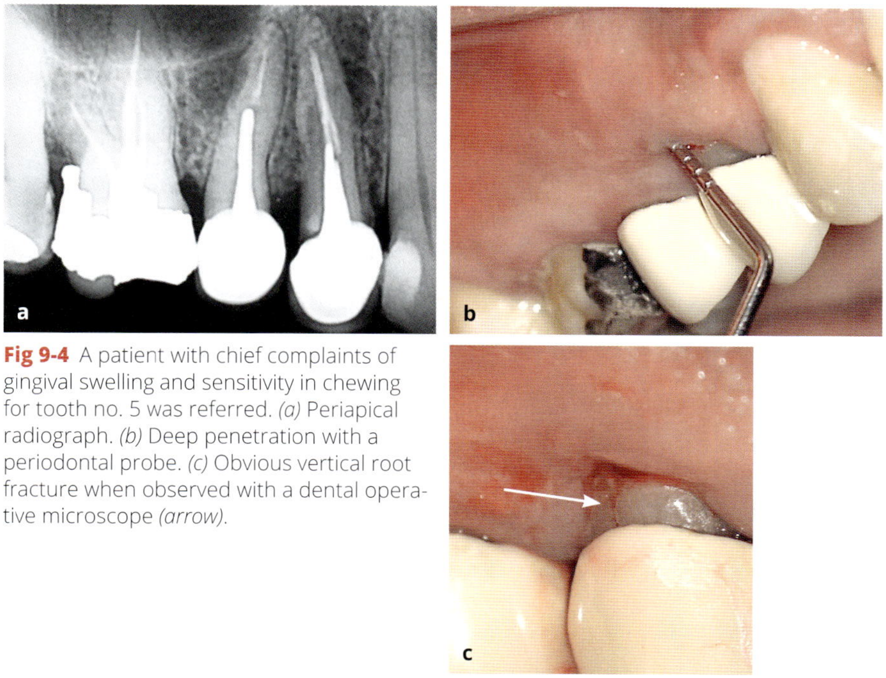

Fig 9-4 A patient with chief complaints of gingival swelling and sensitivity in chewing for tooth no. 5 was referred. *(a)* Periapical radiograph. *(b)* Deep penetration with a periodontal probe. *(c)* Obvious vertical root fracture when observed with a dental operative microscope *(arrow)*.

of a tooth to percussion is due to the presence of periapical inflammation and disregarding periodontal inflammation. A painful response to palpation usually indicates presence of periapical inflammation in a tooth with pulpal and/or periapical disease.[11] The cold test is the most reliable method to determine the presence or absence of vital tissue in a tooth. Probing is an important clinical test but unfortunately is the least used test for diagnosis and treatment planning. Periapical and periodontal lesions destroy periradicular tissues and may mimic each other. Probing is a diagnostic tool that can accurately differentiate between these two entities, and it determines the type of treatment and the flap design during surgical endodontics. Like periodontal probing, the mobility test is underused and overlooked in many cases and often not correctly recorded. A common mishap is a false assumption that all teeth with severe mobility, regardless of their etiology, have a poor prognosis and need extraction. Severe mobility as a result of periapical disease can be treated successfully with PAS.[7,11]

Mishaps During Radiographic Examination

A conventional periapical radiograph is a 2D image of a 3D object captured using radiographic film or digital sensors. 2D methods reproduce the 3D anatomy as a 2D image. Therefore, critical information of the 3D anatomy of the tooth/teeth and adjacent structures is obscured, and even with paralleling techniques, distortion and superimposition of dental structures in periapical views are unavoidable.[12–14]

The role of CBCT in planning for periapical microsurgery has been well documented.[13] It presents 3D geometric accuracy and is more sensitive in detecting any change in density of bony structures compared to conventional radiographs (see chapter 2). Therefore, by using CBCT, the accuracy for the diagnosis of the periapical status is increased significantly.[12,15,16] The different spatial views of CBCT images eliminate the superimposition of anatomical structures, especially in the mandibular premolars and molars (Fig 9-5).[17]

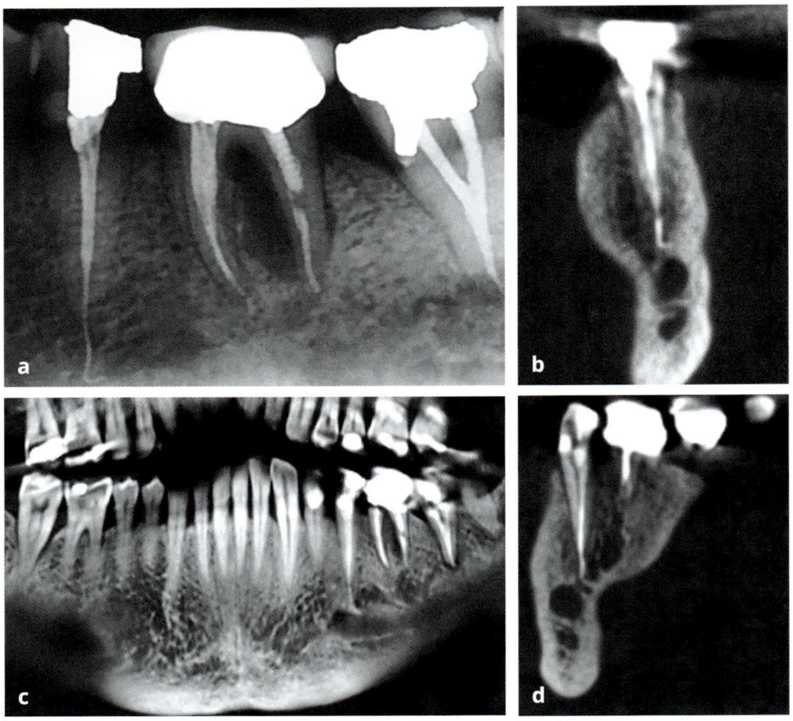

Fig 9-5 CBCT is an important technology for detecting anatomical landmarks. *(a)* Tooth no. 20 has persistent pain following root canal treatment. Overextension of the root canal filling materials may be the reason for the persistent pain. *(b)* Coronal, *(c)* panoramic, and *(d)* sagittal images provided information regarding the distance between the overextended materials and the mandibular canal and mental foramen.

In the maxillary molars and premolars, the roots overlap with anatomical structures such as the maxillary sinus and the zygomatic process. CBCT enables 3D visualization of periapical tissues without superimposition of the overlying zygomatic process, alveolar bone, or adjacent roots. In the posterior region of the mandible, the roots of the premolars and molars are in close proximity to the mental foramen and mandibular canal as well as in presence of mental foramina.[18,19]

Another mistake may happen when a dentist ignores suspicious signs of radiolucency around a root. Careful radiographic examination may lead them to order CBCT to rule out possible causes of failure of initial endodontic treatment that may not be obvious in 2D radiographs (Fig 9-6).

Ray et al[20] recommended using surgical guides for a more conservative and safe approach during PAS. Rigolone et al[21] showed that when conducting apical

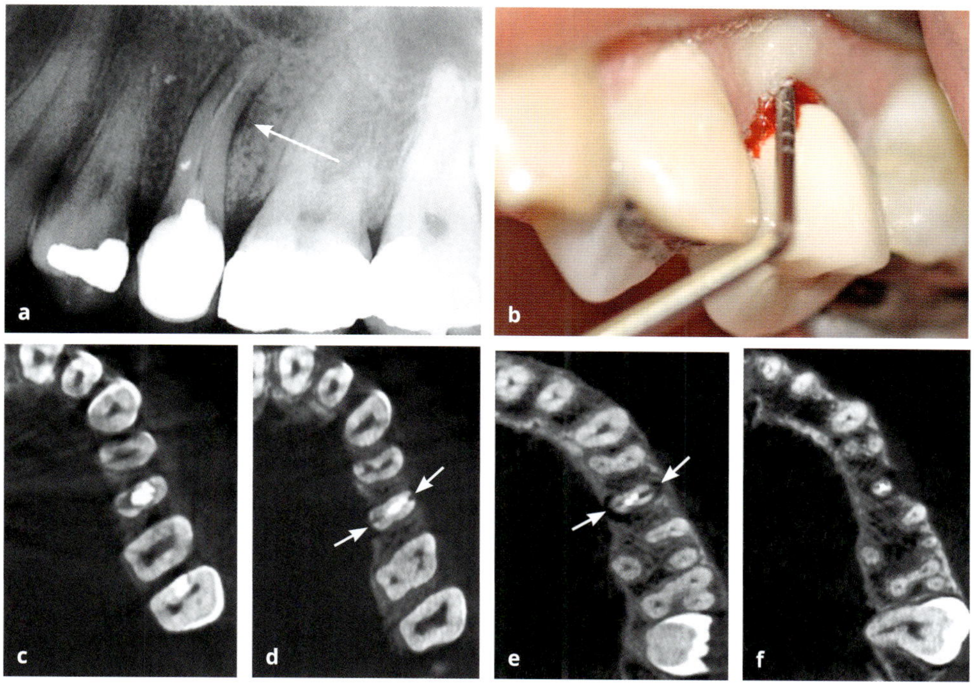

Fig 9-6 A patient was referred with a history of initial root canal treatment in tooth no. 13. *(a)* Periapical radiograph shows a lateral widening of the PDL *(arrow)*. *(b)* Clinical examination revealed a deep pocket at the buccal and palatal sides of tooth no. 13. *(c to f)* Axial CBCT images at different levels showed a vertical fracture line *(arrows)*.

microsurgery in palatal roots of maxillary first molars, CBCT plays an important role in measuring the distance between the cortical plate and the palatal root apex.

CBCT can be used to determine other factors, such as the thickness of the cortical plate, the cancellous bone pattern, fenestrations, the shape of the maxilla and mandible, and the inclination of the roots of teeth planned for periapical surgery.[20–22] However, several variables can affect the accuracy and resolution of CBCT images (Fig 9-7), including voxel size, thickness of prepared slices, kilovoltage, and field of view (see chapter 2).[23–25]

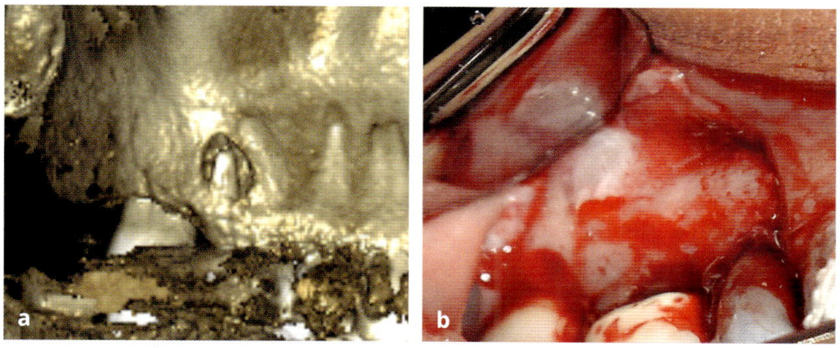

Fig 9-7 *(a)* A 3D reconstruction CBCT image shows bone loss around the distobuccal root of tooth no. 3 with no cortical bone. *(b)* The same patient, following flap reflection, shows cortical bone over the root.

Using CBCT, an endodontist can diagnose root morphology, the number of root canals, convergence or divergence of roots, and missed (and thereby untreated) root canals that are not usually recognized even by taking several 2D radiographs with different horizontal or vertical angles (Fig 9-8).[20,22] Bornstein et al, using CBCT, showed that the Schneiderian membrane close to the roots of maxillary teeth with apical lesions appears significantly thicker compared to those teeth without apical lesions.[26] It has been shown that CBCT is a more reliable technology for assessing anatomical landmarks compared to 2D radiographic images.[27]

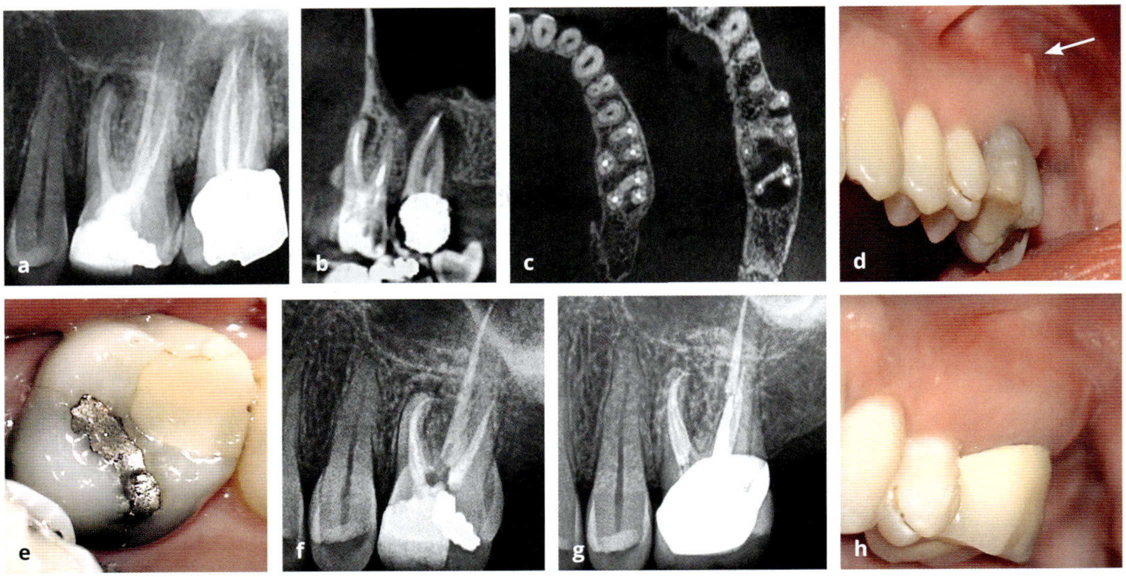

Fig 9-8 *(a)* A patient with a chief complaint of persistent infection on the left side of the upper jaw. Teeth nos. 14 and 15 showed periapical lesions and a history of root canal treatment. *(b)* The CBCT sagittal image shows that tooth no. 15 had a larger periapical lesion. *(c)* The CBCT axial image shows missed second mesiobuccal root canals in both teeth. *(d)* The patient decided to have tooth no. 15 extracted because she thought it was the culprit; however, 3 weeks after extraction, a sinus tract appeared again *(arrow)*. *(e and f)* Tooth no. 14 received a secondary nonsurgical endodontic treatment, and the missed second mesiobuccal root canal was found. *(g and h)* The 6-month follow-up shows that the periapical lesion was healed, and the patient was satisfied with no recurrent infection.

Surgical Endodontic Procedures

Surgical endodontic procedures consist of incision and drainage, periapical surgery, and adjunctive surgery procedures such as tooth replantation and tooth transplantation.

Incision and Drainage

Mishaps can happen during incision and drainage (I&D) as a result of lack of anesthesia and/or making incisions improperly. Obtaining adequate anesthesia is essential for performing any surgical procedure. Due to the presence of severe inflammation in the soft and hard tissues in acute apical abscesses, it may be difficult to accomplish this task, and the operator may need to use regional block anesthetic techniques such as Gow-Gates, Vazirani-Akinosi blocks, second division block, and infraorbital block to obtain profound anesthesia. When severe percussion sensitivity exists, intraosseous and intraligamental injections are helpful to obtain effective anesthesia. In some cases, nitrous oxide/oxygen sedation or intravenous (IV) sedation are needed to perform I&D. Spraying ethyl chloride solution and numbing the soft tissue surface is another method to make this procedure less painful and more comfortable.[28] A common mistake during I&D is performing this procedure without adequate anesthesia and thereby hurting the patient.

After obtaining adequate anesthesia, a vertical incision should be made using a no. 11 or 15 scalpel (Fig 9-9). The advantage of a vertical incision is that it is parallel to the major blood vessels and nerves and leaves very little scarring. Another mistake during I&D is placing a horizontal incision, which results in an unsightly scar after healing.[29] Placing a vertical incision during I&D has less potential for scar tissue formation.

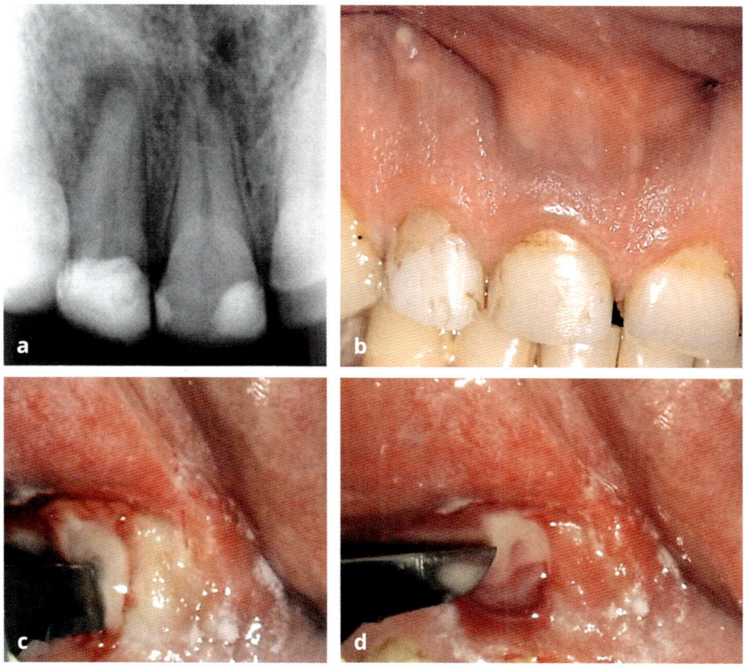

Fig 9-9 *(a)* The periapical radiograph shows tooth no. 7 has a periapical radiolucency; however, the abscess formed over tooth no. 8. *(b)* Tooth no. 8 has had type III mobility and no response to the sensitivity tests. After preparing the access cavity for tooth no. 8, a small volume of pus was detected. *(c and d)* Soft tissue drainage by vertical incision was performed, followed by placing a rubber dam drain.

Hematologic screening is indicated for patients with bleeding disorders. Anatomical landmarks like the mental foramen, maxillary sinus, incisive foramen, and an inferior alveolar canal near the apical abscess should be approached carefully during incision and drainage. Lack of attention to these landmarks during history taking and I&D can result in severe bleeding and paresthesia for the patient.[29]

After making the incision and obtaining drainage, a rubber dam drain should be placed and sutured to one of the edges of the incision to maintain drainage. Placing a rubber dam drain without suturing can result in early removal of the drain and its possible displacement into the soft or hard tissues near the incision line. The drain should be removed within 2 to 3 days by the clinician to avoid discomfort and secondary infection.[29]

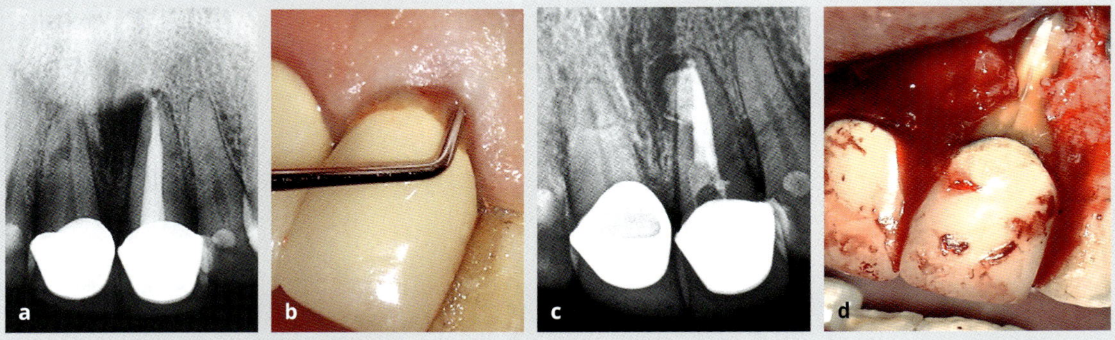

Fig 9-10 This 53-year-old female patient was referred with a chief complaint of swelling and pus drainage from the gingival sulcus of tooth no. 9. *(a)* Periapical radiograph showed a radiolucency around the apical part of tooth no. 9, which had received previous root canal treatment. *(b)* Drainage of pus from gingival sulcus and deep gingival pocket had been confirmed, and nonsurgical retreatment had been performed. *(c)* Following root canal obturation, extrusion of root canal sealer, similar to a cement trail, as well as persistent infection 1 week following the treatment made the treatment provider suspicious about the presence of a vertical root fracture. *(d)* Exploratory surgery confirmed a vertical root fracture.

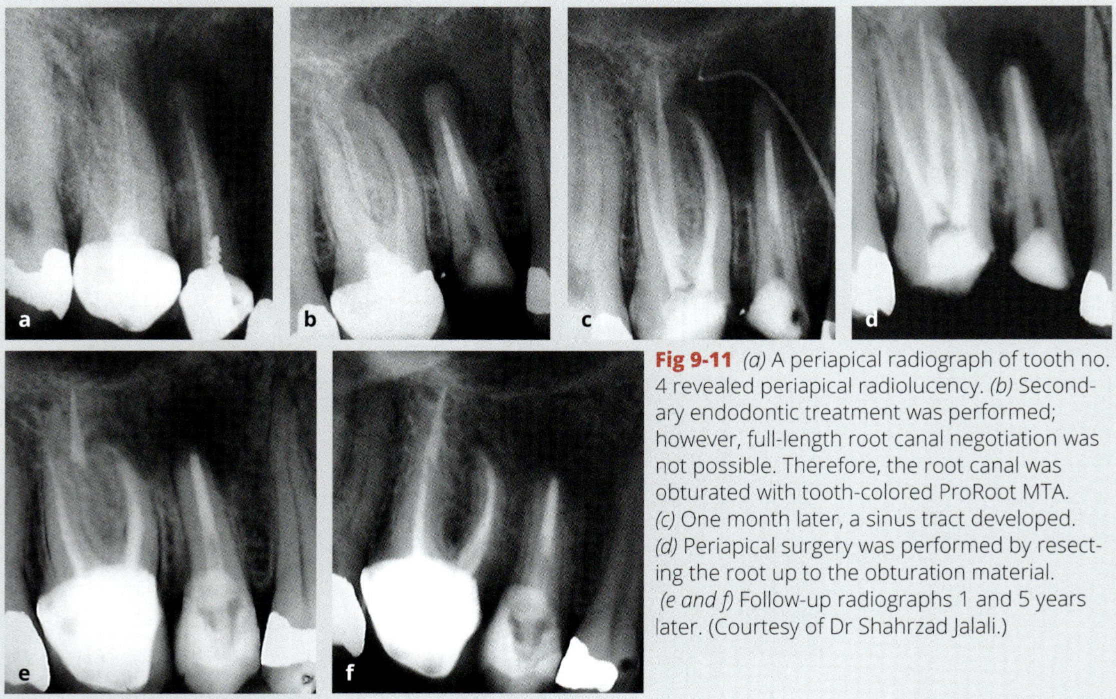

Fig 9-11 *(a)* A periapical radiograph of tooth no. 4 revealed periapical radiolucency. *(b)* Secondary endodontic treatment was performed; however, full-length root canal negotiation was not possible. Therefore, the root canal was obturated with tooth-colored ProRoot MTA. *(c)* One month later, a sinus tract developed. *(d)* Periapical surgery was performed by resecting the root up to the obturation material. *(e and f)* Follow-up radiographs 1 and 5 years later. (Courtesy of Dr Shahrzad Jalali.)

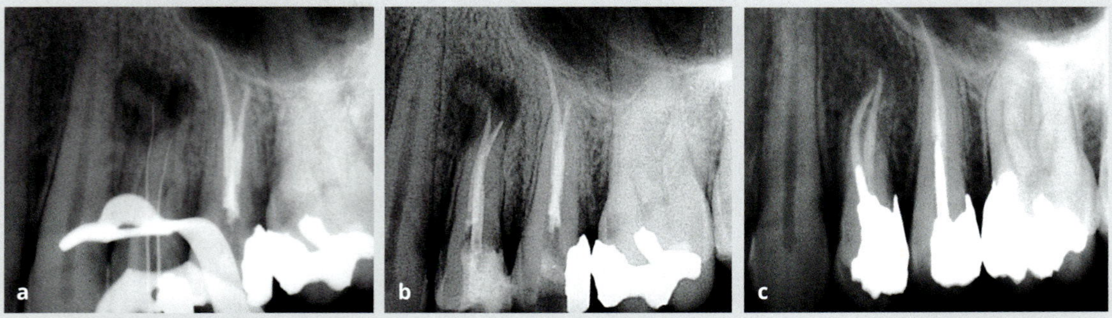

Fig 9-12 *(a)* Tooth no. 12 with severe apical curvature and periapical lesion due to pulp necrosis. *(b)* Full-length root canal negotiation was not successful. Therefore, the root canal was obturated to the length that endodontic instruments could negotiate. *(c)* Periapical lesion was healed without any other intervention 1 year later.

Periapical Surgery

Mishaps can happen when PAS is indicated or contraindicated.

Mishaps when PAS is indicated

The main indications for PAS are failing root canal treatments, procedural accidents, irretrievable materials in the root canal or periapical tissues, anatomical complexity of the root canal system that prevents complete cleaning, shaping and obturation of the root canal system through the coronal access, persistent symptomatic cases despite receiving nonsurgical root canal retreatment (Fig 9-10) or symptomatic cases for which it is not possible to do orthograde nonsurgical endodontic treatment, adjunctive surgeries, and exploratory surgery.[30]

Incomplete root canal treatment

When the quality of previous root canal treatment can be improved nonsurgically, surgical endodontics should not be performed. In teeth with short roots or with no possibility of full length root canal negotiation, it would be better to fill the root canal space with a bioactive endodontic cement such as ProRoot MTA in order to make the surgery easier, with more conservative root-end resection (Fig 9-11).

A common mistake is to plan an immediate periapical surgery following endodontic treatment in teeth with a periapical lesion if the practitioner could not fully negotiate the root canal and reach the apical foramen. In that case, the surgery can be postponed until the clinical or radiographic evaluations indicate the surgery is mandatory to overcome the treatment failure (Fig 9-12).

Procedural accidents

Procedural mishaps during nonsurgical endodontic treatment include ledge formation, root perforation, separated instruments, and underfilled or overfilled canals. Most of these accidents can be corrected nonsurgically (Fig 9-13). Treating these mishaps indiscriminately with surgery is a potential mistake for those who have neither the knowledge nor the skill to handle them (Fig 9-14).

Irretrievable filling materials

Many filling materials within the root canals and sometimes beyond the root canals can be removed with an orthograde approach. Treating these mishaps surgically, without any nonsurgical attempt, is a mistake for those who have neither the knowledge nor the skill to handle them.

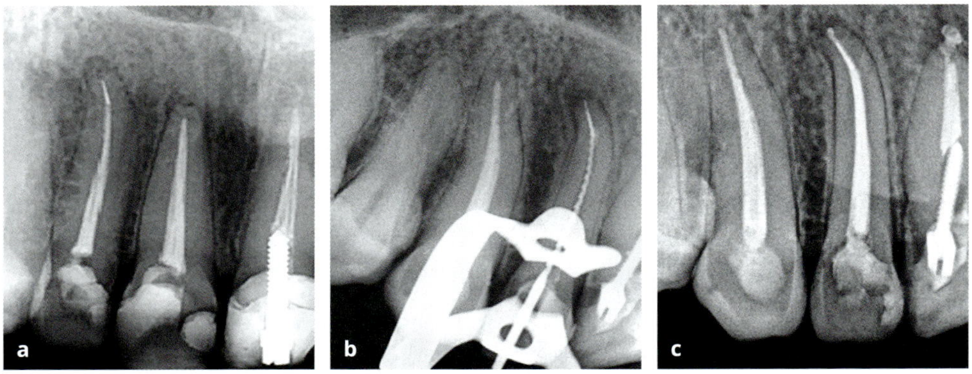

Fig 9-13 Tooth no. 7 was symptomatic and sensitive to palpation and percussion. *(a)* Periapical radiograph shows a broken instrument at the apical third of the root canal. *(b)* The broken instrument was successfully bypassed during nonsurgical secondary endodontic treatment. *(c)* Final radiograph shows full root canal length negotiation and obturation.

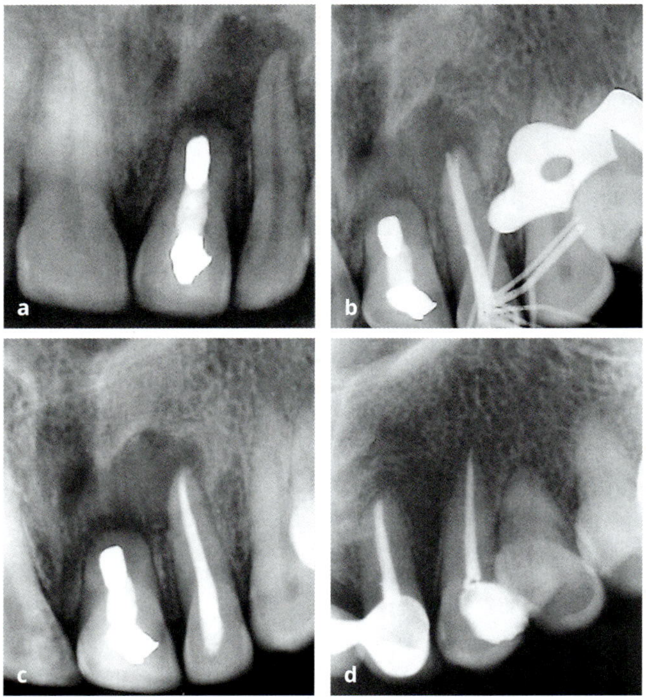

Fig 9-14 *(a)* A patient was referred with a history of a traumatic accident and initial root canal treatment followed by periapical surgery for tooth no. 9 due to the failure of the treatment. His dentist started endodontic treatment for tooth no. 10 because the tooth had no response to the pulp sensibility test. During the treatment, apical perforation occurred. The patient was referred for further management and periapical surgery if needed. *(b and c)* The root canal was cleaned, shaped, and obturated with gutta-percha and root canal sealer. *(d)* The 16-year follow-up shows that tooth no. 10 is asymptomatic, with no periapical lesion.

Symptomatic cases

Most symptomatic cases respond to nonsurgical retreatment and result in relief from pain and discomfort. Surgically treating all symptomatic cases after nonsurgical treatment is a mistake. However, when nonsurgical retreatment is not possible and symptoms persist, surgical endodontics should be considered to relieve pressure and to reduce pain and discomfort for the patient (Fig 9-15).

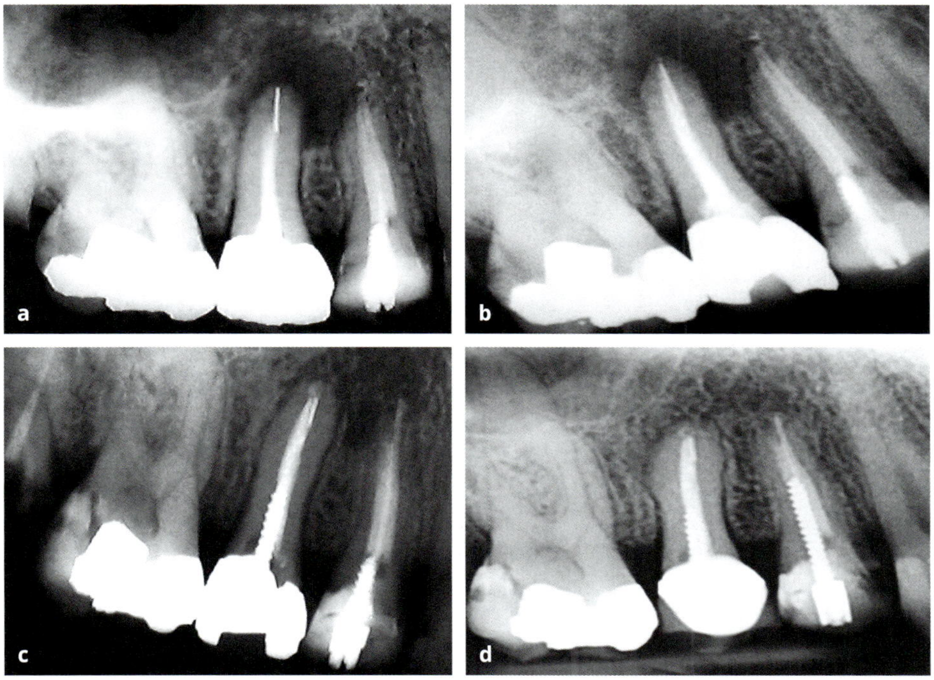

Fig 9-15 *(a)* Tooth no. 4 with periapical lesion and a broken instrument inside the root canal. *(b)* Secondary endodontic treatment was performed, and the broken instrument was bypassed. *(c)* Despite the treatment, the tooth was symptomatic, and the periapical radiolucency became larger. *(d)* A radiograph taken 10 years after periapical surgery shows complete healing and an asymptomatic tooth.

Adjunctive surgeries

Adjunctive surgical endodontic procedures include repair of perforations, repair of resorptive defects, root resection, hemisection, crown lengthening, and tooth replantation and transplantation.[29] Unfortunately, many clinicians are unaware of these surgical options and resort to extraction and implant placement (Fig 9-16).

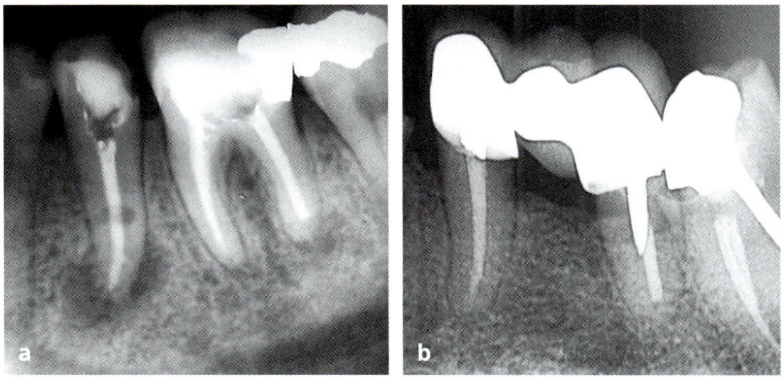

Fig 9-16 *(a and b)* Periapical radiographs of teeth nos. 19 and 20 following root canal treatment and 17 years later. Tooth no. 19 received hemisection due to a deep mesiolingual cusp fracture, and the distal root served as a posterior abutment for a bridge.

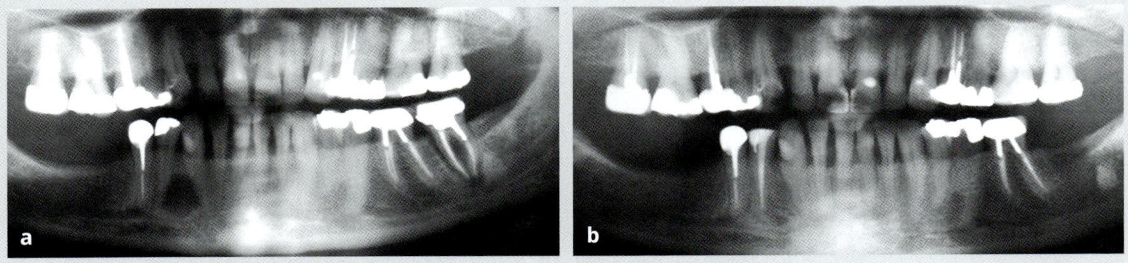

Fig 9-17 Radiolucency associated with nonvital pulp. *(a)* Panoramic view shows large radiolucency between teeth nos. 27 and 28. Tooth no. 28 had no response to pulp sensibility tests. *(b)* Panoramic radiograph of the same patient 3 years later shows no sign of radiolucency.

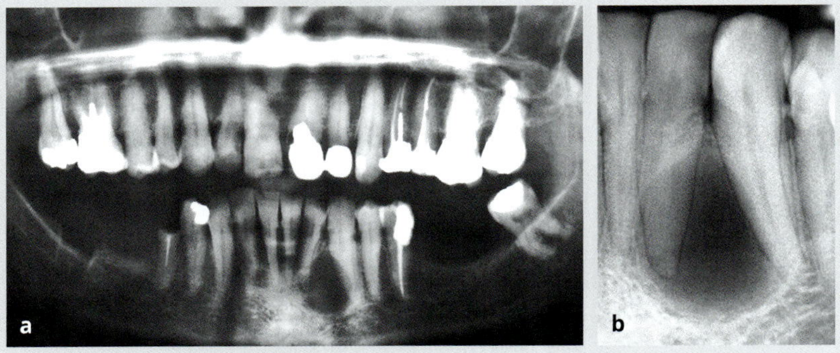

Fig 9-18 *(a)* Panoramic radiograph shows large radiolucency between teeth nos. 22 and 23. *(b)* The periapical radiograph of the same patient. Both teeth had positive responses to pulp sensibility tests. Therefore, pulp pathosis was not assumed as the origin of the developing radiolucent lesion.

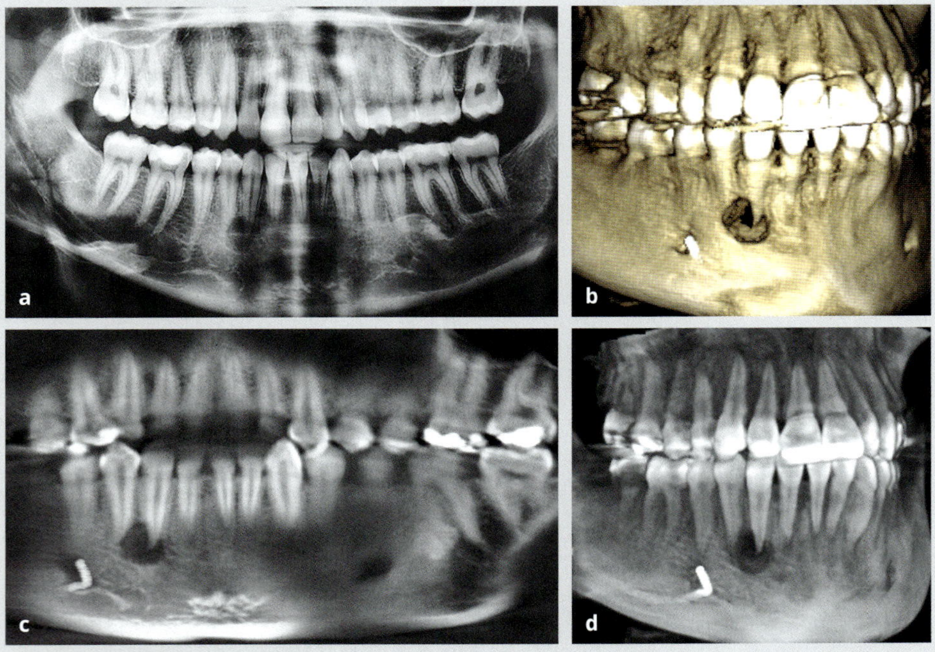

Fig 9-19 *(a)* Panoramic view shows a large radiolucent lesion between teeth nos. 27 and 28. *(b to d)* Different CBCT views show bone destruction. Teeth nos. 27 and 28 had positive responses to pulp sensibility tests. Because the patient had a history of malignancy, periapical surgery and further histopathologic evaluation should be performed.

Exploratory surgery

Most periapical lesions are caused by infection of root canal systems and can be treated nonsurgically or surgically. There are some periradicular radiolucencies that are not caused by root canal infection but mimic periapical lesions of endodontic origin. Suspicious lesions should be biopsied, and the tissues should be examined histologically to avoid dire consequences (Figs 9-17 to 9-20).

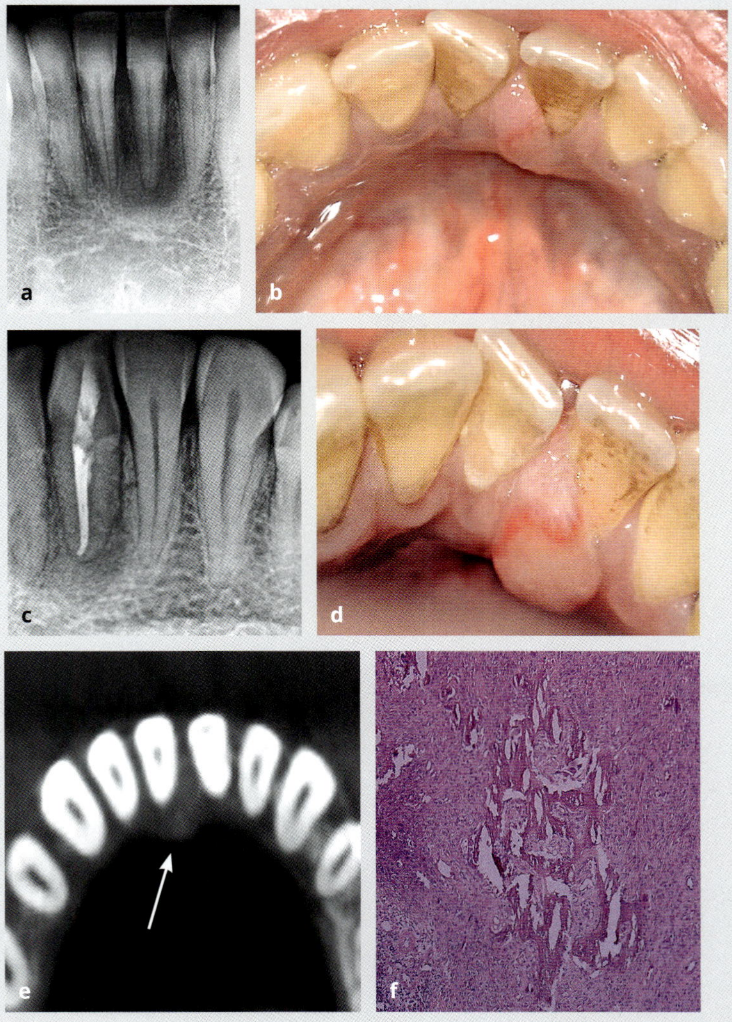

Fig 9-20 This 32-year-old female patient was referred with *(a)* periapical rarefaction of tooth no. 24 and *(b)* lingual swelling between teeth nos. 24 and 25. *(c)* Tooth no. 24 had no response to pulp sensibility tests. Therefore, following scaling, root canal treatment was performed. *(d)* One month later, the lingual swelling showed progressive enlargement. *(e)* Axial view of CBCT shows soft tissue enlargement. *(f)* Excisional biopsy was performed, and the histologic diagnosis was a peripheral ossifying fibroma. (Courtesy of Drs M. Mahmoudi and S. Amanpour.)

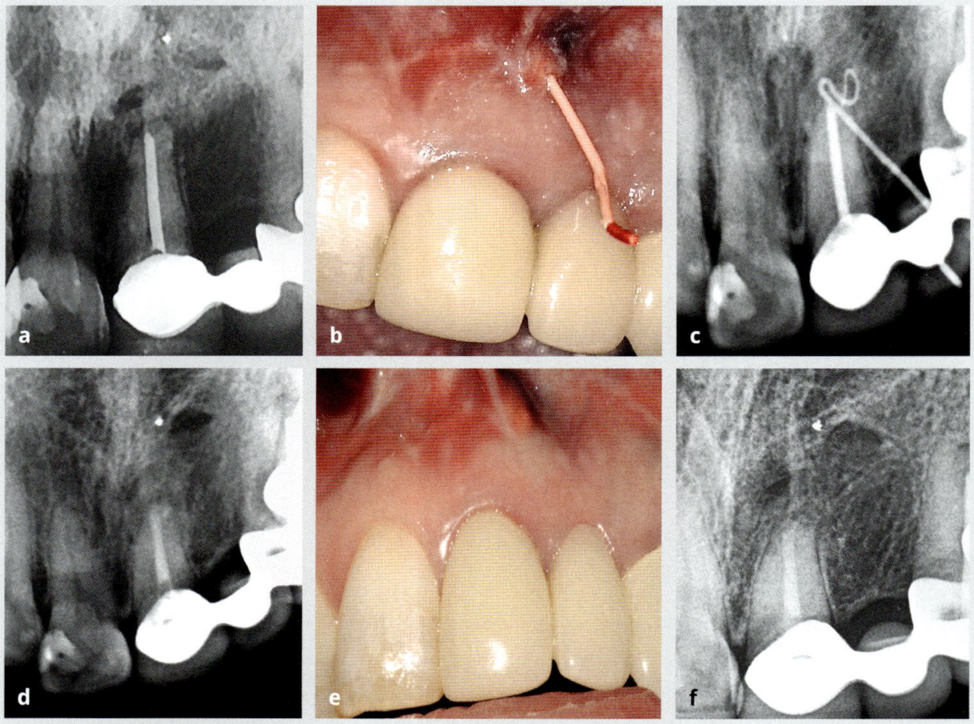

Fig 9-21 An example of contraindication for periapical surgery. *(a)* A patient who previously received periapical surgery has been referred due to the presence of a sinus tract at the apical level of tooth no. 9. The quality of root canal obturation was not reasonable and no root-end filling was detected. *(b and c)* Tracing the sinus tract showed that despite no periapical radiolucency, tooth no. 9 was the reason for infection. *(d)* Because the patient recently received the restoration, an access cavity was made through the bridge, and secondary endodontic treatment was performed. The root canal space was obturated with tooth-colored ProRoot MTA. *(e)* One week later, the sinus tract was healed. *(f)* No recurrent infection was reported up to 5 years following the secondary endodontic treatment.

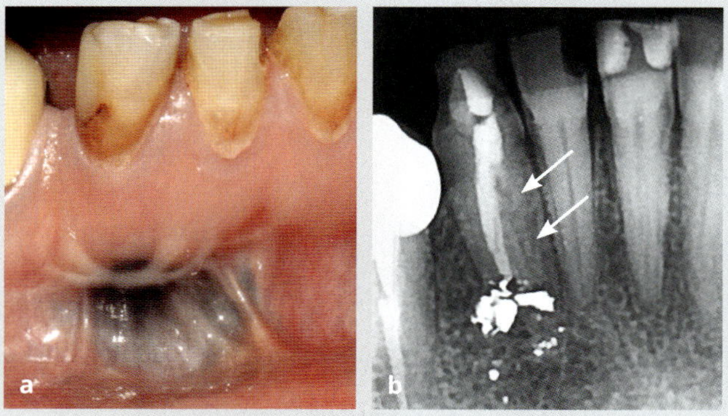

Fig 9-22 Another example of contraindication for periapical surgery. *(a)* A patient with a history of previous periapical surgery for tooth no. 26 had a chief complaint of gingival discoloration. *(b)* Periapical radiograph shows missed root canal *(arrows)* with no amalgam at the right place as root-end filling material.

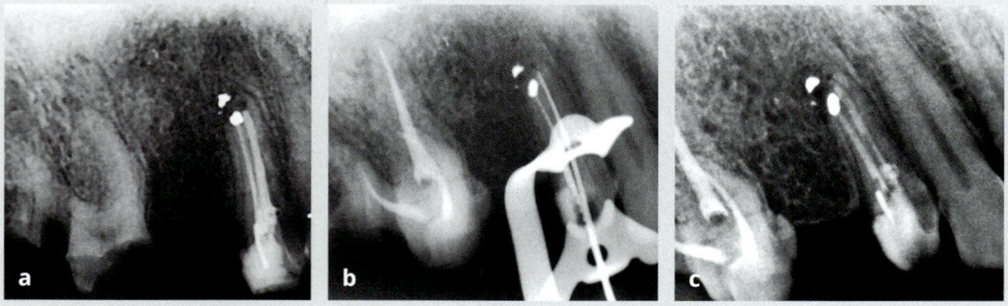

Fig 9-23 Tooth no. 5, with a history of endodontic surgery, was symptomatic. *(a)* Amalgam as the root-end filling material had been dislodged. *(b)* Secondary nonsurgical endodontic treatment had been performed to provide an apical seal. *(c)* The root canal space was obturated with ProRoot MTA.

History of previous PAS

When a history of previous PAS is present, the quality of the root canal obturation and root-end filling should be evaluated. In cases with low-quality root canal filling or root-end fillings, secondary nonsurgical treatment is recommended (Figs 9-21 to 9-23).

Mishaps when PAS is contraindicated

The main contraindications for PAS are medical or systemic complications, indiscriminate use of periapical surgery, anatomical factors, and an unidentified cause of treatment failure.

Medical or systemic complications

Patients with serious systemic diseases such as blood disorders, terminal diseases, uncontrolled diabetes, severe heart diseases, and compromised immune systems should not be treated with PAS (Fig 9-24). When in doubt, the practitioner should consult with the patient's physician.

a

M.C.H.C		31.36	gr/dl	30-36
Neutrophils.		62	%	
Lymphocytes		30	%	Child:25-65 ; Adult:25-45
Monocyte.		6	%	
Eosinophils		2	%	
Platelet Count		34	*1000/µl	140- 450
Platelets →	*L	50	x10³/ µl	plt on slide;140-450
Rdw		15.5	%	11 - 13.5

b

WBC →	78.10	+	[10^3/uL]
RBC	4.75		[10^6/uL]
HGB	13.7		[g/dL]
HCT	44.2		[%]
MCV	93.1		[fL]
MCH	28.8		[pg]
MCHC	31.0		[g/dL]
PLT	180		[10^3/uL]
RDW-SD	52.4	+	[fL]
RDW-CV	15.4	+	[%]
PDW	9.7		[fL]
MPV	9.3		[fL]
P-LCR	19.0		[%]
PCT	0.17		[%]
NRBC	0.00		[10^3/uL]
NEUT	3.23	*	[10^3/uL]
LYMPH →	74.26	*	[10^3/uL]
MONO	0.38	*	[10^3/uL]
EO	0.13		[10^3/uL]
BASO	0.10	*	[10^3/uL]

Fig 9-24 *(a)* The blood test of a patient showed a low platelet count *(arrow)*. *(b)* The number of white blood cells in this patient was abnormally high *(arrows)*. The diagnosis of acute lymphocytic leukemia was confirmed by a bone marrow biopsy.

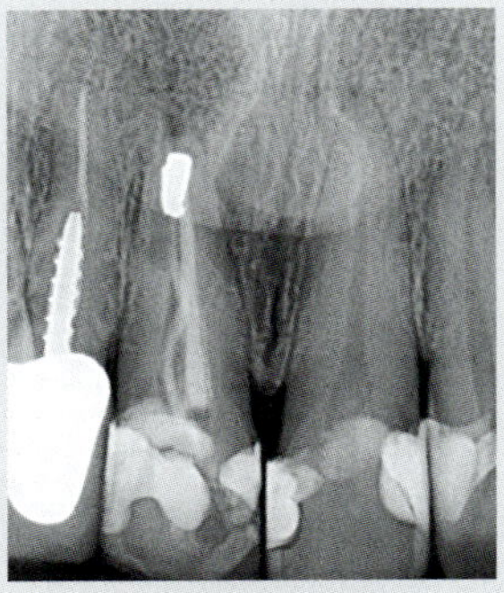

Fig 9-25 A periapical radiograph showed unnecessary surgery on a central incisor that could have been treated nonsurgically.

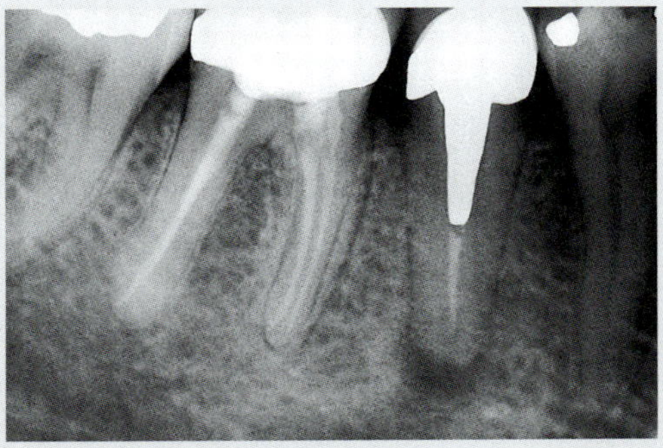

Fig 9-26 A periapical radiograph showing the presence of a periapical lesion at the apex of the second mandibular premolar adjacent to the mental foramen.

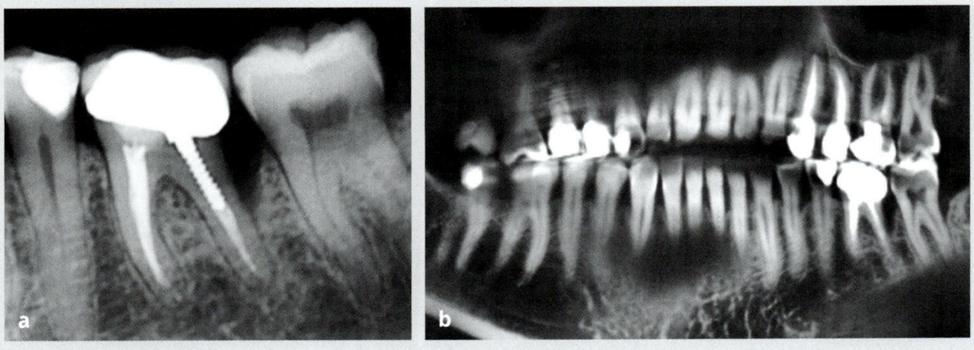

Fig 9-27 This patient was referred with a chief complaint of dull pain on the left side of the mandible. *(a)* Bone loss at the distal level of tooth no. 19 was observed in the periapical radiograph. *(b)* Panoramic CBCT view of the patient showed similar bone loss for teeth nos. 18 and 19. The patient was referred to a periodontist, and the periodontal reason for bone loss at the distal part of the teeth was confirmed.

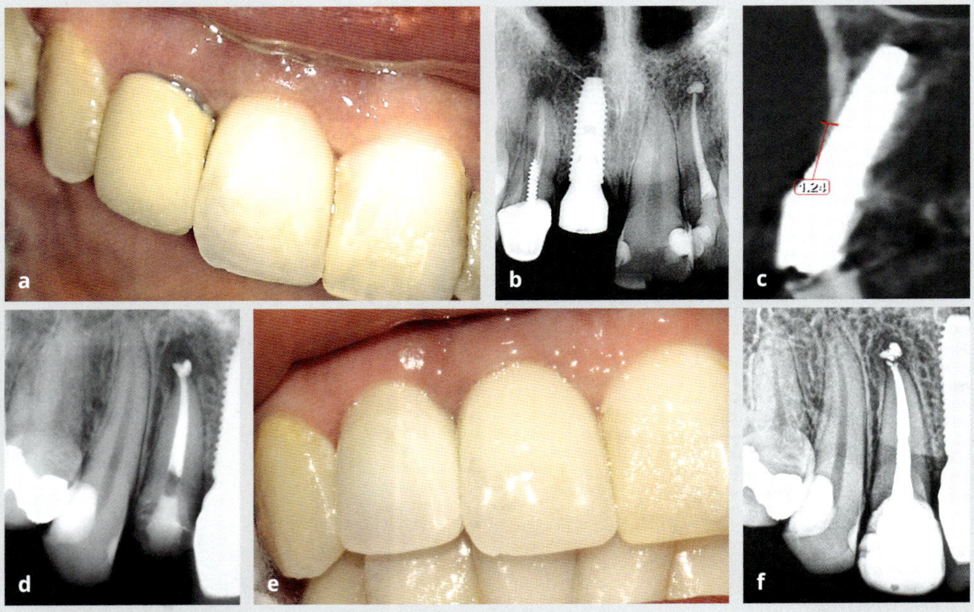

Fig 9-28 *(a)* A patient was referred due to a history of swelling and sensitivity to percussion in tooth no. 7. *(b)* Periapical lesion and low-quality root canal obturation were detected for tooth no. 7. The patient insisted on periapical surgery despite recession of the gingiva. *(c)* Following consultation with a periodontist, the treatment plan of surgery was rejected because the implant success could be compromised due to the lack of at least 1.5 mm of cortical bone over the buccal aspect of the implant. *(d)* Secondary endodontic treatment was performed. *(e)* New restoration. *(f)* Periapical radiograph 1 year later.

Indiscriminate use of surgery

Indiscriminate use of PAS for cases that can be handled nonsurgically is unethical and should be avoided (Fig 9-25). Periapical surgery is not an alternative treatment option if nonsurgical treatment is feasible and could probably result in successful outcomes. Sadly, a lack of skill in performing nonsurgical endodontics or a desire for financial gain can sometimes result in clinicians performing unnecessary surgical procedures.

Anatomical factors

When the apex or apices of teeth are close to anatomical landmarks such as the mental foramen or nasopalatine foramen, alternative treatments such as tooth replantation or extraction with or without replacement should be discussed with the patient (Fig 9-26). Lack of attention to these important anatomical landmarks can result in clinical and legal complications.

Unidentified cause of treatment failure

When there is no identifiable reason for why a previous procedure failed, surgical attempts should be avoided. Consultation with other specialists is advised (Fig 9-27).

Presence of an adjacent implant

Sometimes, particularly in the esthetic zone, an adjacent implant may influence the treatment plan. Periapical surgery may compromise esthetics or osseous integration of the implant; therefore, nonsurgical endodontic treatment should be considered if a surgical approach could compromise the implant (Fig 9-28). Periodontists believe that at least 1.5 mm of bone should cover the buccal aspect of an implant if a periapical surgery is going to be carried out for the adjacent tooth.

Mishaps during various phases of PAS

The steps involved in PAS include the following: *(1)* local anesthesia, *(2)* magnification, *(3)* flap design, *(4)* flap reflection, *(5)* flap retraction, *(6)* osteotomy, *(7)* periapical curettage, *(8)* biopsy, *(9)* hemostasis, *(10)* apical resection, *(11)* root-end cavity preparation, *(12)* selecting root-end filling materials, *(13)* mixing root-end filling materials, *(14)* placing root-end filling materials, *(15)* flap closure, *(16)* postoperative instructions, and *(17)* managing any postoperative complications.

Local anesthesia

Local anesthesia (LA) is essential for almost any dental procedure. During injection of LA, some unwanted complications—ranging from mild discomfort to severe complications and, in rare cases, death—may occur. Local anesthetics are weak bases that inhibit sodium ion inflow and thereby neuronal depolarization. Amide local anesthetic solutions are more common than ester ones.[31] Under no circumstance should any surgical procedure be performed without profound anesthesia.

In addition, clinicians should avoid injecting into the deeper subperiosteal tissue over the basal bone. This action produces vasodilation and increased bleeding during surgery.

Systemic complication

Taking thorough and careful medical history is critical for preventing serious systemic complications. Systemic complications following LA may occur as reactions to LA solutions or to vasoconstrictor. Possible causes of systemic complications include intravascular injection, excessive dosage, and rapid absorption.[31,32]

Unwanted intravascular injection of LA can cause toxicity, the magnitude of which depends on the LA dose, the vascularity of the injection site, the presence of vasoconstrictor (the vasoconstrictor decreases the systemic absorption of the LA), and the chemical properties of the drug. The central nervous system (CNS) and the myocardium are the two major sites of anesthetic-induced toxicity.

Besides LA, vasoconstrictor drugs may cause systemic reactions. However, this is still controversial. A study showed that dental surgery using LA caused significant increases in systolic blood pressure (BP) and heart rate (HR), and the increase in systolic BP was greater in middle-aged and older patients.[33]

It seems that after inferior alveolar nerve block (IANB) and intraosseous (IO) injection, even comparatively small amounts of epinephrine can induce measurable tachycardia.

Two other studies have revealed that after periodontal ligament or intraosseous X-Tip injection in mandibular molars, a dose-dependent tachycardia occurred.[34,35]

On the other hand, other clinical trials reported that the rise in BP and HR following injection of lidocaine with epinephrine was not clinically important.[36,37]

Although the results of existing studies are controversial, an increase in the amount of epinephrine during an infiltration or block injection that has the potential to cause an elevated heart rate should be avoided. Slow-speed injection, particularly during intraosseous injection, may prevent cardiovascular change during treatment. If a patient is not responding to local anesthetic, the patient should be dismissed, and the cause and alternative treatments should be explored.

Allergic reaction

Reports of adverse reactions to local anesthetics are usually attributed to a reaction to epinephrine, vasovagal syncope, or overdose toxicity. A common mistake by patients and some clinicians is to misinterpret these adverse reactions as an allergy to local anesthetic rather than a reaction to epinephrine (Fig 9-29). The amide local anesthetics appear to have little immunogenicity and therefore have an extremely low rate of true allergic reactions. Sulfite, which prevents oxidation of epinephrine in the anesthetic cartridge, may also cause allergic reactions.[38,39]

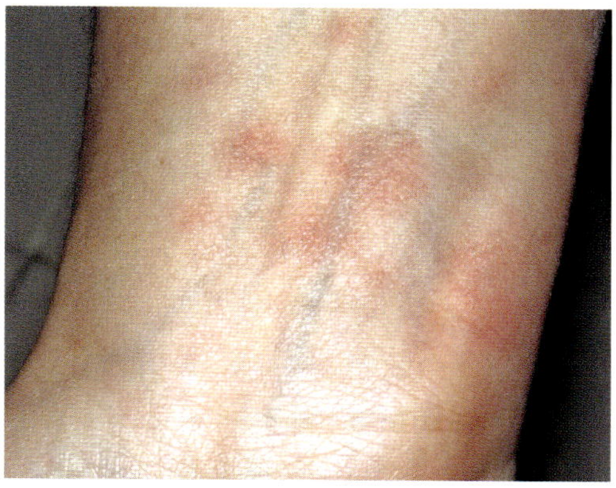

Fig 9-29 Allergic reaction to 2% lidocaine with 1:80,000 epinephrine.

Toxicity

Because of raising plasma concentration, accidental injection of the LA drugs into the blood stream may cause systemic toxicity.[38] The extent of systemic absorption depends on the LA dose, the vascularity of the injection site, the presence of vasoconstrictor in the local anesthetic, and the chemical properties of the local anesthetic. The CNS and the cardiovascular system are involved owing to the systemic toxicity of the LA.[38,40]

All local anesthetics have the potential to cause toxicity in the CNS as well as the cardiovascular system. CNS toxicity is manifested as anxiety, restlessness, tremor, and respiratory failure that may cause death. Cardiovascular toxicity is manifested as arteriole vasodilation and hypotension.[39] To avoid these mishaps, the clinician should use as little local anesthetic as possible, aspirate the syringe before injection, and use epinephrine-containing LA cartridges.[39]

Magnification and illumination

Magnification is considered one of the methods of enhancing the quality of PAS. A common mistake is not using proper magnification and illumination during PAS. A surgical operative microscope should be considered during osteotomy, root-end resection, root-end preparation, and placement of root-end filling material. However, magnification during most flap preparations, reflection, and suturing has limited advantages.[41]

Another common mistake is to use high magnification during the periapical surgery. Magnification more than 30× has minimal advantage because this action makes the procedure very difficult. Employing high magnification is more time consuming, causes more eye fatigue, results in constant changes of the field of view, focus, and clarification due to the patient's slight movements, and provides a limited amount of light—and therefore illumination—and a limited field of view.[41]

Flap design

A *flap* is defined as a loosened section of soft tissue separated from the surrounding tissues except at its base, and its purpose is to facilitate surgical access to the root apex. Adequate flap design is a fundamental prerequisite to manage the apical surgery and achieve predictable clinical results.[25] For a successful flap design, clinicians should evaluate the size of the periapical lesion, the number of teeth involved in the surgery, the length of the involved tooth or root, the proximity to vital structures, any shallow vestibules, muscle attachment, frenum pull, and the amount of bone loss in the area.

Adequate flap design, especially in the esthetic zone, is crucial for sufficient esthetic results; failing to take into account the soft tissue considerations may negate all other aspects of the treatment outcome, resulting in esthetic failure.[42] To avoid mishaps during this phase of PAS, tissue typing (thin or thick) is very important. Thin biotypes are prone to having esthetic issues (see Fig 9-3). A common mistake is misjudgment of the gingival sulcus depth when a submarginal flap is to be employed. Teeth with full crown restorations and in need of periapical surgery may be good candidates for a submarginal flap, such as Ochsenbein-Luebke flap. In that case, the depth of gingival sulcus should not be close to the horizontal part of the flap. Otherwise, gingival margin necrosis may occur and create an esthetic mishap. To prevent further complications, the practitioner should measure gingival sulcus depth and the attached gingiva width before the procedure. If the gingival sulcus depth is more than 3 mm or if the width of the attached gingiva is low, another flap design should be employed.

Flap procedures may lead to several complications,[42–44] including attachment loss and recession of the gingival margin, flap necrosis, flap tearing, tissue dehiscence, delayed healing, periodontal defect, scarring, hemorrhage, and nerve injury (Fig 9-30). A common mishap during apical surgery is raising a smaller flap than what is needed to complete surgical endodontics. Small flaps hinder the ability of the operator to perform the task at hand. Remember, large flaps heal as well as small flaps.

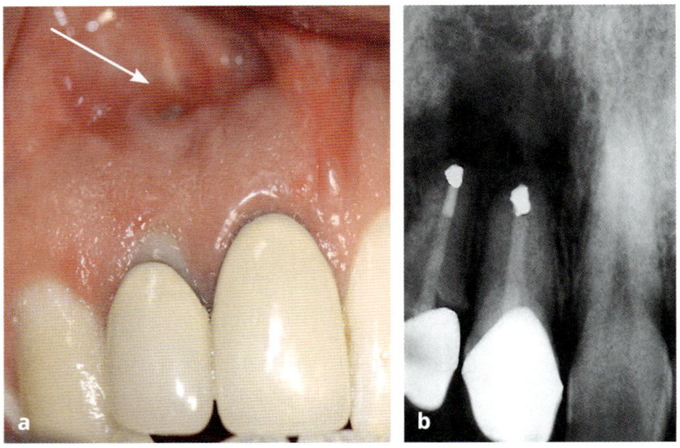

Fig 9-30 Mishap following periapical surgery. *(a)* Tooth no. 7 has had apical fenestration *(arrow)* and recession of the gingival margin following periapical surgery. *(b)* Periapical radiograph of the same patient.

9

Flap reflection

After making the incision, to gain access to the root apex, a flap should be reflected adequately, precisely, and gently. During flap reflection, the periosteum should be completely separated from the underlying cortical plate with a proper periosteal elevator.[45] Small tags of periosteum retained on the bone surface bleed, become caught in the bur during bone removal, and obscure and prevent identification of small anatomical landmarks. Inadequate flap reflection complicates various aspects of the apical surgery.[44,45] Inadequate vertical incisions prevent proper flap reflection. The reflection should be carried out to a level that would permit free movements of the mesial and distal pedicle flaps. After a complete flap retraction, a small groove can be prepared in the bone with a small round bur as a rest for the retractor. This action will prevent trauma to the flap during surgery.[46]

Flap retraction

Flap retraction is the process of holding in position the reflected soft tissues. Proper retraction depends on adequate extension of the flap incisions and proper reflection of the mucoperiosteum. Retractors should be used carefully without excessive force on the flap tissue.[40,44]

The vertical incision extension should facilitate the positioning of the retractor on solid bone during surgery. Insufficient vertical incisions may cause the retractor to traumatize the mucosal tissue of the flap and may jeopardize the blood supply of the involved tissues. To provide sufficient visibility, the retractor should be placed on solid bone apical to the periapical lesion. Inadvertent placing of the retractor on the soft tissue of the flap base results in delayed healing.[40,44,46]

Selecting an incorrect flap retractor is a common mistake clinicians can make. Appropriate selection of retractors is important, because retractors that are too small provide limited benefit and allow the flap to obscure the operating field, while retractors that are too large may traumatize the soft tissues. Furthermore, when the tissue is retracted, it is important to remember to irrigate the flapped tissues with sterile saline to prevent desiccation-related damages. Sterile water should not be used as an irrigant. It is hypotonic to the cells and can delay healing.[41,46,47]

Osteotomy

Depending on factors needed for healing, wounds may heal as repair or regeneration.[48] The surrounding periodontal tissues are essential for the postsurgical bony healing process.[49] A conservative osteotomy compared to a large osteotomy will better preserve critical local resources and facilitate improved conditions for the periapical wound healing process.[48] With small periapical bony defects following conservative osteotomy, resident osteoblasts, periodontal ligament (PDL) cells, and cementoblasts are capable of restoring the damaged periapical tissues. However, if the size of the osseous defect is too large, osseous regeneration of the wound will not occur, and the defect might heal by fibrous connective tissue repair.[48,49] Imprecise osteotomy is another mishap that can be avoided by using CBCT and targeted PAS.[12,18–20]

Another risk factor that may adversely affect the results of osteotomy during endodontic surgery is excessive heat generation.[50,51] Overheating may interrupt the blood flow or cause decreased osteoclastic and osteoblastic activity, dehydration, and desiccation, which can result in osteocytic degeneration and osteonecrosis.[50,51] According to Augustin et al,[52] drill design, drilling technique, and bone characteristics all influence the amount of heat generated during osteotomy. To minimize the possibility of overheating, round burs in a high-speed handpiece with light brushing motions using copious amounts of irrigation are recommended. There is no scientific evidence that shows that slow-speed handpieces are better than high-speed ones for osteotomy in terms of lower heat generation during osteotomy.[53] A possible mishap during osteotomy or root-end resection is displacement of the bur into the adjacent vital structures such as a mandibular canal or the maxillary sinus (Fig 9-31). To avoid this mishap, the operator must check the security of the resecting bur in the handpiece before starting the root resection.

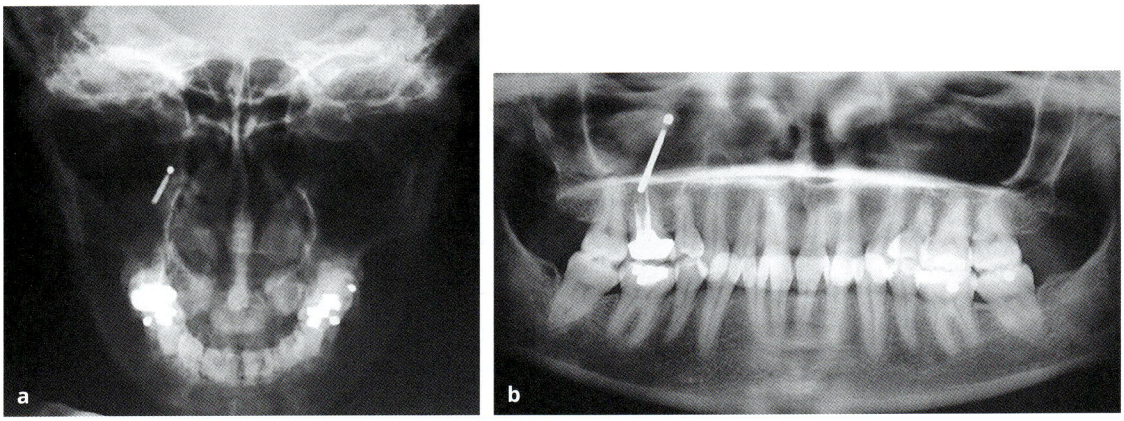

Fig 9-31 A mishap during periapical surgery. *(a and b)* A round bur was accidentally displaced into the maxillary sinus during periapical surgery.

Another common mistake is to use conventional methods and armamentaria in cases that are in close proximity to vital structures such as nerve bundles, sinus membranes, and blood vessels. In those cases, using Piezosurgery is very useful to prevent further mishaps.[41]

Periapical curettage

In order to remove the pathologic tissues and/or foreign materials (especially gutta-percha and sealer) around the root apex, curettage is usually needed. By curetting, visibility of the surgical area can also be increased. When the origin of the lesion is what is extruding into the periapical tissues, removing this cause and sealing the apex usually resolves the patient's problems. Therefore, removal of the entire lesion is not necessary and could lead to producing large osteotomies and thereby damaging normal structures. Remember, complete curettage requires larger osteotomy, which probably delays the healing process. Therefore, in most cases, very large and complete curettage is not necessary.[54] In addition, complete curettage may compromise vital structures and result in complications such as maxillary sinus perforation and paresthesia close to the mental foramen or infra-alveolar canal.

Another mishap during curettage is attempting to remove the lesion without adequate unroofing and using the front surface of a spoon excavator. To avoid this mishap, conduct satisfactory periapical curettage via adequate unroofing and initially using the back of the spoon excavator to detach the lesion from the surrounding hard tissues before removing it with the front part of the spoon excavator.

Biopsy

Periapical lesions of pulpal origin are the most common pathologic processes found during endodontic surgery. According to the existing literature, most of these lesions are either granulomas or cysts.[55–58] The prevalence of periapical granulomas ranges from 45% to 94%, and the prevalence of cysts ranges from 6% to 44%.[55–58] The existence of these wide ranges is due to the criteria used for diagnosis. Because there are other lesions that may not be of pulpal origin, any tissues removed from the periapical region during periapical surgery must be examined histologically.[59–61] A mishap can happen if not all the tissues removed during periapical surgery are biopsied and/or examined histologically.

Hemostasis

Hemostasis is defined as the process of bleeding control[29] and is achieved primarily via vasoconstrictors present in local anesthetics or other medications or materials used during periapical surgery. Many hemostatic agents have been advocated for use during PAS.[29] Their mechanism of action, ability to control bleeding, and effect on healing vary considerably. They generally assist coagulation by inducing rapid development of a blood clot.[62] The hemostatic agents most commonly used during periapical surgery are epinephrine pellets, ferric sulfate, calcium sulfate, collagen-based materials, Surgicel, Gelfoam, aluminum chloride, and HemCon.[29]

A common mistake regarding the hemostasis is expecting immediate hemostasis after the use of any of these materials. Bleeding is controlled well if adequate time is allowed for the hemostatic agents to work.

Apical resection

Despite advances in root canal disinfection, some areas of the complex root canal system, such as isthmuses that contain microorganisms, remain untouched.[63] Therefore, the incidence of isthmuses, which is age related, should be kept in mind when performing endodontic surgery. In the age group below 20 years, canals are usually oval-shaped without isthmuses. In the age group of 20 to 40 years old, the deposition of secondary dentin in the mesiodistal direction results in the formation of two canals with an isthmus.[64] The incidence of an isthmus in the apical 4 to 6 mm of the mesiobuccal root of the mandibular first molar in the age groups of 20–39 years, 40–59 years, and > 60 years is 50%, 41%, and 24%, respectively. It has been shown that both mesial and distal roots of mandibular first molars may have isthmus communications; however, the former roots have a higher prevalence of the isthmus.[65] Another problem during root-end resection is missing canals. Missing canal(s) is a serious complication because it can result in the failure of treatment.[66] Inadequate root resection can result in missing canals or other complexities such as isthmuses. To avoid these mishaps, the resected root surface should be beveled adequately to observe the entire apical aspect of the root. Inadequate root resection can easily happen if the root is cut at 90 degrees and not properly examined for the presence of root complexities and lingual canals in the mandibular and maxillary molars and premolars. In addition, examination of the root morphology in advance of periapical surgery by using CBCT would help the practitioner to recognize root anatomy as well as the direction and distance of the lingual root from the cortical bone.

Root-end cavity preparation

Root-end cavity preparation is performed by cutting a Class I cavity with a 3 to 5 mm depth. Mishaps can happen during this procedure if the preparation is not made parallel with the long axis of the root and within the root canal system. Inadequate visualization can lead to deviation of the path of the preparation from the root canal and possibly to root perforation. In order to decrease these possibilities, ultrasonic tips are very useful.[67,68] According to Wuchenich et al,[67] root-end cavities prepared using ultrasonic tips can be made with adequate depth and are parallel with the root canal walls and therefore provide better retention for root-end filling materials (Fig 9-32). In addition, the ultrasonic tips follow the direction of the canals more closely than burs do.[67] Scanning electron microscopic (SEM) examination of the cavity walls shows cleaner surfaces for root-end cavities prepared by ultrasonic tips than those made with burs.[67] However, making root-end cavity preparations with ultrasonic tips has the potential to create cracks in the root.[69] Common mistakes during root-end cavity preparation are using tips with improper angles, applying too much force, and providing inadequate irrigation. Peters et al[68] revealed that preparation using diamond-coated ultrasonic tips is easier and faster, but the tips should be used cautiously to avoid overpreparation or perforation of the root end. It should be kept in mind that with magnification, the practitioner may not always recognize cracks following root-end preparation with ultrasonic tips.[69]

Selecting and placing root-end filling materials

A common mistake during PAS is root-end resection without placing a root-end filling material. To prevent egress of microorganisms from the root canal system into the periapical tissues, resected roots should be prepared for root-end cavity and filled with a root-end filling material. Several materials have been proposed

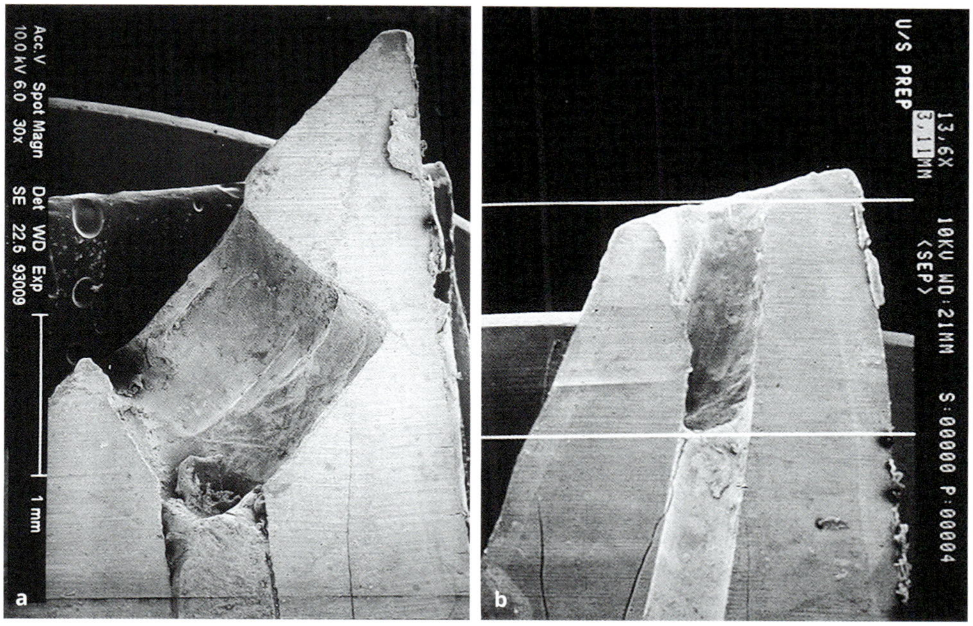

Fig 9-32 *(a)* A root-end cavity prepared with a bur. *(b)* A root-end cavity prepared with an ultrasonic tip.

for root-end filling.[70–72] Currently, mineral trioxide aggregate (MTA), commercially available as ProRoot MTA, is the gold standard (Fig 9-33). It is the most investigated material for various endodontic uses.[73–77]

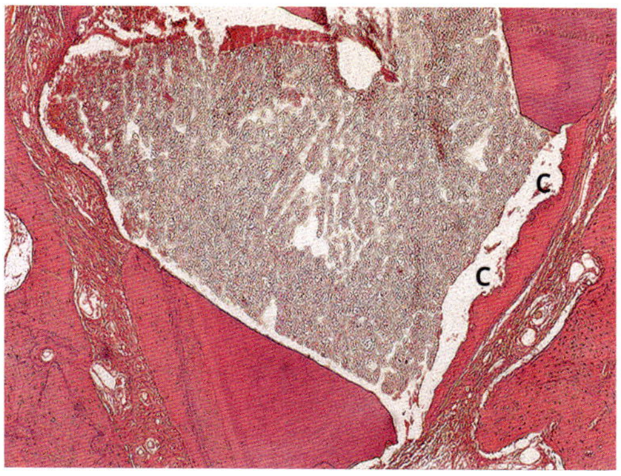

Fig 9-33 Histologic section of a dog tooth surgically treated with MTA as root-end filling material showing complete regeneration of periapical tissues and formation of cementum over MTA (C).

ProRoot MTA is a bioactive material with excellent biocompatibility and sealing ability and is not sensitive to humidity.[76] Powder-to-liquid ratio and porosity might affect the mechanical properties of dental cements. ProRoot MTA is mixed according to the manufacturer's instructions that recommend a powder-to-water ratio of 3:1. Each package of ProRoot MTA includes 0.5 g of ProRoot MTA powder and a small distilled water ampoule. ProRoot MTA powder should be thoroughly mixed with this distilled water either manually or ultrasonically.[77] The hydration reaction of MTA results in the formation of hydrated compounds whose strength increases with time.[71] Furthermore, the hydration process is a complex phenomenon that, if modified, might influence the biologic, chemical, and physical properties of the resulting product.[78,79] Fridland and Rosado[80,81] studied the effect of various water-to-powder ratios of ProRoot MTA on its solubility and porosity. They reported that an increased water-to-powder ratio resulted in higher solubility, porosity, and release of calcium hydroxide.

Despite its advantages, ProRoot MTA has a long setting time and can be washed off if proper precautions are not taken during its placement and condensation.[73] A common mistake while using ProRoot MTA as a root-end filling material is preparing it with too much liquid. The dryer the material, the easier it is to be handled.

Because most bioactive endodontic cements are hydrophilic, another common mistake is not completely drying the root-end cavity and thereby placing ProRoot MTA into a wet root-end cavity. Placing ProRoot MTA into a very wet root-end cavity may increase the water-to-powder ratio and affect the physical properties of the material.

Because of the drawbacks of MTA as a root-end filling material, several calcium silicate–based materials have been proposed as alternatives.[82,83] Most of these materials have not been investigated enough to confirm the accuracy of the manufactures' claims. Biodentine is one of these calcium silicate–based cements and is based on a powder component that contains tricalcium silicate, dicalcium silicate, calcium carbonate, zirconium oxide, calcium oxide, and iron oxide. The other component of this material is a liquid compound of calcium chloride, which accelerates setting, and a water-soluble polymer, which affords correct fluidity.[83]

Flap closure

After placing the root-end filling material and irrigating the surgical site to remove the debris created during surgery, the flap should be closed correctly. The surgical site should be closed only after careful visual and radiographic inspection of the area. A common mistake during this phase of surgery is placing the sutures before taking a radiograph to make sure the PAS has been properly conducted. Slight undermining of the unreflected soft tissue adjacent to the flap facilitates the placement of sutures. The flap is repositioned and gently compressed with a piece of chilled, sterile, moist cotton gauze to express excess blood and tissue fluids.[29,84] Silk suture has been commonly used; however, due to the braided structure of the material, monofilament structure sutures are recommended.[85–87]

Resorbable suture material can be used if the patient may not be available for suture removal; however, it should be kept in mind that resorbable sutures have different resorption rates and may stay longer or, if lost too early, lead to improper healing.

The suturing technique should be evaluated on the basis of its ability to accomplish wound closure and flap stabilization at least for several days. Usually, the sutures should provide a passive fixation mechanism and avoid stretching the tissue, tissue tearing, and compromised circulation.[29,84,88]

Surgical bleeding should be controlled prior to suture placement to prevent formation of a hematoma under the flap and ensuing culture medium formation for bacterial growth and infection.[29,88] Another common mistake during flap closure is placing too many stitches or too tight of stitches to close the wound. Place as few as possible tension-free stitches to avoid delayed would healing.

Postoperative instructions

All patients who undergo PAS should receive both oral and written postoperative instructions. Patients should be informed of the possibility of postoperative swelling and discomfort. To reduce these postoperative issues, the patient should be advised to use an ice pack (20 minutes on, 5 minutes off) on the outside of the face for a few hours following periapical surgery.[29,89] Mild analgesics such as ibuprofen should be prescribed for relief of postoperative pain. Some oozing of blood is expected after PAS. To reduce minor bleeding, the patient should place a moistened gauze pad over the area and apply finger pressure for 15 minutes. The patient should be warned against lifting their lips and checking the surgical site. This may dislodge and untie the sutures. Twenty-four hours after surgery, the patient can use warm salt water after each meal. Gentle brushing is also recommended 24 hours after the surgery.[29,89–91] Drinking lots of fluids and eating soft foods that contain high levels of protein are recommended. Patients who smoke should refrain from smoking for at least three days after the surgery. Excessive bleeding, pain, swelling, or a high temperature should be reported to the practitioner immediately. Sutures should be removed 4 to 7 days after PAS.[29,88] Providing inaccurate postoperative information to the patient may result in alarming the patient unnecessarily. Another mistake is not providing an emergency phone number for patients who have periapical surgery. Providing a contact number may relieve patients' anxiety because they know their treatment provider is available in case of an emergency.

Postoperative complications

Trismus

Any spasm of muscle is defined as *trismus*, which in the mastication muscles results in difficulty in mouth opening. Some local anesthetic techniques such as inferior alveolar nerve blocks and posterior maxillary infiltration injections may lead to trismus development. Trismus is caused by trauma from the injection needle to muscles or blood vessels with subsequent hematoma development.[92,93] Aspiration before injection can prevent this issue. Trismus has an acute phase (muscle spasm and limitation of jaw motion) and possibly a chronic phase (hypomobility, which would occur as a result of fibrosis and scar tissue development). Preventive measures to avoid trismus include decreasing the depth of injections and especially avoiding multiple mandibular block injections. Treatment protocols to manage trismus include heat application; prescribing analgesics, antibiotics, and muscle relaxants; physiotherapy; and reassuring the patient. In certain cases, when chronic hypomobility develops, surgical intervention may be indicated.[92,93]

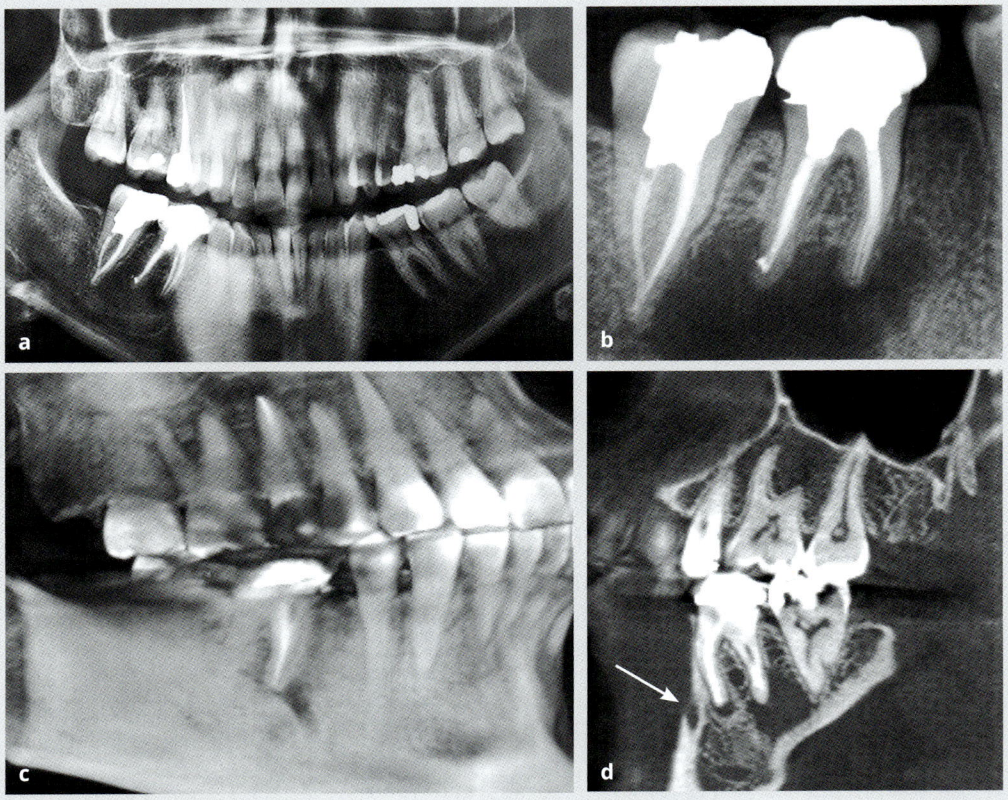

Fig 9-34 *(a)* Panoramic view of tooth no. 30 showed possible proximity to the mental foramen. *(b)* However, the periapical radiograph showed an important anatomical landmark close to tooth no. 30. *(c)* 3D CBCT view shows a very close relationship of the mesial root of tooth no. 30 to the mental foramen. *(d)* The sagittal view also shows close proximity of the mental foramen to the mesial root *(arrow)*. (Courtesy of Dr Iman Samadi.)

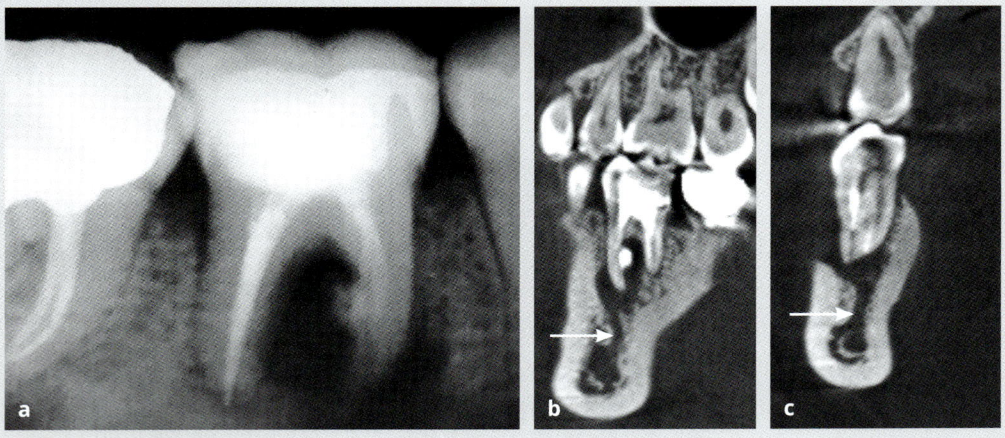

Fig 9-35 *(a)* Tooth no. 30 needs periapical surgery due to the mishap in the mesial root. *(b and c)* Sagittal and coronal CBCT views show a branch of the mandibular canal to the periapical area of tooth no. 30 *(arrows)*. (Courtesy of Dr Ali Eslambol Nassaj.)

Paresthesia

Paresthesia is defined as a burning or prickling sensation or partial numbness caused by neural injury. Patients describe it as warmth, cold, burning, aching, prickling, tingling, pins and needles, numbness, and formication (itching in the absence of stimuli).[94,95]

In the field of dentistry, causes of paresthesia are classified as systemic or local factors.[96] Some of the more important systemic factors include multiple sclerosis, sarcoidosis, metastasis, viral and bacterial infections, leukemia, and lymphoma. Local factors include traumatic injuries, such as mandibular fractures, expanding compressive lesions (benign or malignant neoplasia and cysts), impacted teeth, local infections (osteomyelitis and periapical and peri-implant infections), iatrogenic lesions after tooth extractions, anesthetic injection, and endodontic treatment (overfilling and apical surgery).

Neurosurgical procedures may be indicated in persistent cases that do not respond to conservative treatment.[97,98] Surgery should be performed within a few days following injury to avoid Wallerian degeneration (a process in which the axon distal to a site of injury degenerates).[96]

It should be kept in mind that the indications and clinical effectiveness of surgical techniques are variable and poorly documented. In addition, complete recovery of normal sensation following these surgical procedures is not always possible.[99] It should also be taken into consideration that in many cases, the altered sensation originally occurred as a result of trauma during the endodontic treatment and an additional corrective surgical procedure may introduce an additional trauma and inflammation, thus adversely affecting the patient's state.[97,98]

A mistake made by some clinicians is to not inform the patient regarding the possibility of paresthesia after PAS. To avoid legal issues, a patient should be informed before their PAS and must sign an informed consent. In addition, CBCT is a useful aid to recognize the possibility of involving nerve bundles during periapical surgery (Figs 9-34 and 9-35).

Swelling and hematoma

Hematoma is defined as leakage of blood from blood vessels and its aggregation outside the blood vessels due to injury or any surgical procedure. If an artery is damaged, it may produce rapid bleeding with significant hematoma formation and rapidly developing extensive intraoral or extraoral swelling.[100,101] This most commonly occurs in the tuberosity area, if one of the terminal branches of the maxillary artery is damaged.[100] It has been reported that during a mandibular block, failure to obtain anesthesia may be associated with hematoma formation in the pterygomandibular space as well as the dilution and inactivation of the LA by blood.[101] Hematoma formation may result in trismus or infection. The patient should be observed for any signs of recurrent bleeding or secondary infection of the hematoma. At the first indication of infection, antibiotic therapy should be initiated.[102,103] To avoid misunderstanding, the patient should be informed of the possibility of minor swelling, hematoma, and discoloration of gingival tissues as well as adjacent facial tissues (ecchymosis) before performing PAS (Fig 9-36).

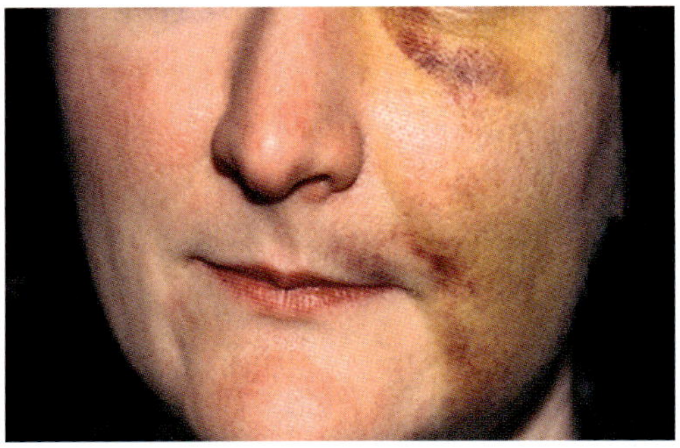

Fig 9-36 Ecchymosis following periapical surgery in the mandibular molar region 1 week after the surgery.

Tissue healing

Another mistake is to consider soft tissue healing as unreasonable in the short term following surgery. In most instances, soft tissue regeneration will take place if the principles of flap design, reflection, retraction, and suturing have been followed (Fig 9-37).

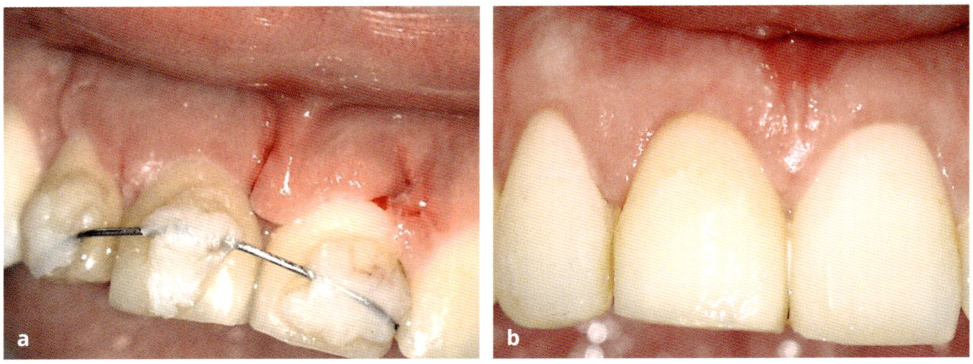

Fig 9-37 Sometimes a flap may not heal reasonably well in a short period following periapical surgery; however, if the principles of flap design, handling, and closure have been followed, the flap will heal eventually. *(a)* Following suture removal. *(b)* One year later.

Recession

Gingival recession (GR) is defined as an apical shift of the gingival margin that causes exposure of the root surface of a tooth. It is characterized by the loss of the periodontal connective tissue fibers along the root cementum as well as concomitant loss of alveolar bone (see Fig 9-30). GR can be caused by periodontal disease, inflammation, improper flossing, aggressive tooth brushing, incorrect occlusal relationships, and prominent roots. GR can appear as localized or generalized and can occur with or without loss of attached tissue.[104]

Possible causes of GR resulting from endodontic surgery include incorrect repositioning of the flap, compromised blood circulation of the flap through excessive retraction or poor flap design, and flap contraction.[104] To reduce the chances of recession after PAS, it is essential to preserve tissues attached to the root surface and to reposition flaps in a tension-free manner. Thin gingival biotype is a risk factor of postsurgical recession development.[105,106]

On the other hand, thick gingival biotype is less susceptible to recession and more prone to formation of infrabony defects and deeper pockets following endodontic surgery.[43] The type of incision (flap) is also an important predictive factor for gingival recession. Intrasulcular flaps are more susceptible to GR compared to submarginal flaps.[43] A common mistake is not considering a specific suturing technique when an intrasulcular flap is used for a tooth with a full crown in the esthetic zone. It has been shown that the vertical mattress suturing technique may prevent gingival recession following surgery.[29]

To avoid misunderstanding, the patient should be informed of the possibility of gingival recession before PAS.

References

1. Akcay H, Arslan H, Akcay M, Mese M, Sahin NN. Evaluation of the bond strength of root-end placed mineral trioxide aggregate and Biodentine in the absence/presence of blood contamination. Eur J Dent 2016;10:370–375.
2. Kadić S, Baraba A, Miletić I, et al. Push-out bond strength of three different calcium silicate-based root-end filling materials after ultrasonic retrograde cavity preparation. Clin Oral Investig 2018;22: 1559–1565.
3. Simel DL, Rennie D. The clinical examination. An agenda to make it more rational. JAMA 1997;277: 572–574.
4. Sackett DL. A primer on the precision and accuracy of the clinical examination. JAMA 1992;267:2638–2644.
5. Culica D, Rohrer J, Ward M, et al. Medical check-ups: Who does not get them. Am J Public Health 2002;92:88–91.
6. Bickley LS (ed). Bates' Guide to Physical Examination and History Taking. Philadelphia: Lippincott Williams & Wilkins, 2017.
7. Berman L, Hargreaves K. Cohen's Pathways of the Pulp, ed 12. St Louis: Elsevier, 2021.
8. Weller SC, Vickers B, Bernard HR, et al. Open-ended interview questions and saturation. PLoS One 2018;13:e0198606.
9. Lichstein PR. The medical interview. In: Walker HK, Hall WD, Hurst JW (eds). Clinical Methods: The History, Physical, and Laboratory Examinations, ed 3. Boston: Butterworths, 1990.
10. Rathee M, Rao PL, Bhoria M. Prevalence of gingival biotypes among young dentate North Indian population: A biometric approach. Int J Clin Pediatr Dent 2016;9:104–108.
11. Gutmann JL, Lovdahl PE. Problem Solving in Endodontics: Prevention, Identification and Management, ed 5. St Louis: Mosby, 2010.
12. De Paula-Silva FW, Wu MK, Leonardo MR, da Silva LA, Wesselink PR. Accuracy of periapical radiography and cone-beam computed tomography scans in diagnosing apical periodontitis using histopathological findings as a gold standard. J Endod 2009;35:1009–1012.
13. Shah P, Chong BS. 3D imaging, 3D printing and 3D virtual planning in endodontics. Clin Oral Investig 2018;22:6411–6454.
14. Corbella S, Del Fabbro M, Tamse A, Rosen E, Tsesis I, Taschieri S. Cone beam computed tomography for the diagnosis of vertical root fractures: A systematic review of the literature and meta-analysis. Oral Surg Oral Med Oral Pathol Oral Radiol 2014;118:593–602.
15. Patel S, Dawood A, Whaites E, Pitt FT. New dimensions in endodontic imaging: Part 1. Conventional and alternative radiographic systems. Int Endod J 2009;42:447–462.
16. Patel S. New dimensions in endodontic imaging: Part 2. Cone beam computed tomography. Int Endod J 2009;42:463–475.

17. Cotton TP, Geisler TM, Holden DT, Schwartz SA, Schindler WG. Endodontic applications of cone-beam volumetric tomography. J Endod 2007;33:1121–1132.
18. Ramis-Alario A, Tarazona-Alvarez B, Cervera-Ballester J, et al. Comparison of diagnostic accuracy between periapical and panoramic radiographs and cone beam computed tomography in measuring the periapical area of teeth scheduled for periapical surgery. A cross-sectional study. J Clin Exp Dent 2019;11:e732–e738.
19. Tsai P, Torabinejad M, Rice D, Azevedo B. Accuracy of cone-beam computed tomography and periapical radiography in detecting small periapical lesions. J Endod 2012;38:965–970.
20. Ray JJ, Giacomino CM, Wealleans JA, Sherydan RR. Targeted endodontic microsurgery: Digital workflow options. J Endod 2020;46:863–871.
21. Rigolone M, Pasqualini D, Bianchi L, Berutti E, Bianchi SD. Vestibular surgical access to the palatine root of the superior first molar: "Low-dose cone-beam" CT analysis of the pathway and its anatomic variations. J Endod 2003;29:773–775.
22. Benjamin G, Ather A, Bueno MR, Estrela C, Diogenes A. Preserving the neurovascular bundle in targeted endodontic microsurgery: A case series. J Endod 2021;47:509–519.
23. Aktan AM, Yildirim C, Karataşlıoğlu E, Çiftçi ME, Aksoy F. Effects of voxel size and resolution on the accuracy of endodontic length measurement using cone beam computed tomography. Ann Anat 2016;208:96–102.
24. Takei Y, Monzen H, Matsumoto K, Hanaoka K, Tamura M, Nishimura Y. Registration accuracy with the low dose kilovoltage cone-beam CT: A phantom study. BJR Open 2019;1:20190028.
25. Elshenawy H, Aly W, Salah N, Nasry S, Anter E, Ekram K. Influence of small, midi, medium and large fields of view on accuracy of linear measurements in CBCT imaging: Diagnostic accuracy study. Open Access Maced J Med Sci 2019;7:1037–1041.
26. Bornstein MM, Wasmer J, Sendi P, Janner SF, Buser D, von Arx T. Characteristics and dimensions of the Schneiderian membrane and apical bone in maxillary molars referred for apical surgery: A comparative radiographic analysis using limited cone beam computed tomography. J Endod 2012;38:51–57.
27. Velvart P, Hecker H, Tillinger G. Detection of the apical lesion and the mandibular canal in conventional radiography and computed tomography. Oral Surg Oral Med Oral Pathol Oral Radiol Endod 2001;92:682–688.
28. Jonasson P, Kvisr T. Case selection and treatment planning. In: Tsesis I (ed). Complications in Endodontic Surgery: Prevention, Identification and Management. Berlin: Springer, 2014:19–38.
29. Torabinejad M, Sabeti M, Glickman G. Surgical endodontics. In: Rotstein I, Ingle JI (eds). Ingle's Endodontics, ed 7. Raleigh, NC: PMPH USA, 2019:797–834.
30. Kim S, Kratchman S. Modern endodontic surgery concepts and practice: A review. J Endod 2006;32:601–623.
31. Naguib M, Magboul MM, Samarkandi AH, Attia M. Adverse effects and drug interactions associated with local and regional anesthesia. Drug Saf 1998;18:221–250.
32. Daublander M, Muller R, Lipp MD. The incidence of complications associated with local anesthesia in dentistry. Anesth Prog 1997;44:132–141.
33. Matsumura K, Miura K, Takata Y, et al. Changes in blood pressure and heart rate variability during dental surgery. Am J Hypertens 1998;11:1376–1380.
34. Zarei M, Ghoddusi J, Sharifi E, Forghani M, Afkhami F, Marouzi P. Comparison of the anaesthetic efficacy of and heart rate changes after periodontal ligament or intraosseous X-Tip injection in mandibular molars: A randomized controlled clinical trial. Int Endod J 2012;45:921–926.
35. Knoll-Kohler E, Frie A, Becker J, Ohlendorf D. Changes in plasma epinephrine concentration after dental infiltration anesthesia with different doses of epinephrine. J Dent Res 1989;68:1098–1101.
36. Ketabi M, Shamami MS, Alaie M, Shamami MS. Influence of local anesthetics with or without epinephrine 1/80000 on blood pressure and heart rate: A randomized double-blind experimental clinical trial. Dent Res J (Isfahan) 2012;9:437–440.
37. Silvestre FJ, Verdú MJ, Sanchís JM, Grau D, Peñarrocha M. Effects of vasoconstrictors in dentistry upon systolic and diastolic arterial pressure. Med Oral 2001;6:57–63.
38. Cox B, Durieux ME, Marcus MA. Toxicity of local anesthetics. Best Pract Res Clin Anesthesia 2003;17:111–136.
39. Speca SJ, Boynes SG, Cuddy MA. Allergic reactions to local anesthetic formulations. Dent Clin North Am 2010;54:655–664.
40. Batinac T, Sotosek Tokmadzic V, Peharda V, Brajac I. Adverse reactions and alleged allergy to local anesthetics: Analysis of 331 patients. J Dermatol 2013;40:522–527.
41. Torabinejad M, Rubinstein R (eds). The Art and Science of Contemporary Surgical Endodontics. Chicago: Quintessence, 2017.
42. von Arx T, Salvi GE, Janner S, Jensen SS. Scarring of gingiva and alveolar mucosa following apical surgery: Visual assessment after one year. Oral Surg 2008;1:178–189.

43. De Rouck T, Eghbali R, Collys K, De Bruyn H, Cosyn J. The gingival biotype revisited: Transparency of the periodontal probe through the gingival margin as a method to discriminate thin from thick gingiva. J Clin Periodontol 2009;36:428–433.
44. Trombelli L, Roberto F. Flap designs for periodontal healing. Endod Topics 2012;25:4–15.
45. von Arx T, Salvi GE, Janner S, Jensen SS. Gingival recession following apical surgery in the esthetic zone: A clinical study with 70 cases. Eur J Esthet Dent 2009;4:28–45.
46. Velvert P, Peters O. Soft tissue management. In: Torabinejad M, Rubinstein R (eds). The Art and Science of Contemporary Surgical Endodontics. Chicago: Quintessence, 2017:141–153.
47. Velvart P, Ebner-Zimmermann U, Ebner JP. Comparison of papilla healing following sulcular full-thickness flap and papilla base flap in endodontic surgery. Int Endod J 2003;36:653–659.
48. Tsesis I, Rosen E, Tamse A, Taschieri S, Del Fabbro M. Effect of guided tissue regeneration on the outcome of surgical endodontic treatment: A systematic review and meta-analysis. J Endod 2011;37:1039–1045.
49. Grzesik WJ, Narayanan AS. Cementum and periodontal wound healing and regeneration. Crit Rev Oral Biol Med 2002;13:474–484.
50. Metzger MC, Bormann KH, Schoen R, Gellrich NC, Schmelzeisen R. Inferior alveolar nerve transposition—An in vitro comparison between Piezosurgery and conventional bur use. J Oral Implantol 2006;32:19–25.
51. Hitchcock R, Ellis E 3rd, Cox CF. Intentional vital root transection: A 52-week histopathologic study in Macaca mulatta. Oral Surg Oral Med Oral Pathol 1985;60:2–14.
52. Augustin G, Zigman T, Davila S, et al. Cortical bone drilling and thermal osteonecrosis. Clin Biomech (Bristol, Avon) 2012;27:313–325.
53. Tsesis I, Rosen E. Periapical osteotomy and curettage. In: Tsesis I (ed). Complications in Endodontic Surgery: Prevention, Identification and Management. Berlin: Springer, 2014:81–88.
54. Nesari R, Kratchman S, Saad M, Kohli MR. Selective curettage: A conservative microsurgical approach to treating large and complicated lesions. J Endod 2020;46:1782–1790.
55. Love RM, Firth N. Histopathological profile of surgically removed persistent periapical radiolucent lesions of endodontic origin. Int Endod J 2009;42:198–202.
56. Lalonde ER, Luebke RG. The frequency and distribution of periapical cysts and granulomas: An evaluation of 800 specimens. Oral Surg Oral Med Oral Pathol 1968;25:861–868.
57. Block RM, Bushell A, Rodrigues H, Langeland K. A histopathologic, histobacteriologic, and radiographic study of periapical endodontic surgical specimens. Oral Surg Oral Med Oral Pathol 1976;42:656–678.
58. Kuc I, Peters E, Pan J. Comparison of clinical and histologic diagnoses in periapical lesions. Oral Surg Oral Med Oral Pathol Oral Radiol Endod 2000;89:333–337.
59. Karamifar K, Tondari A, Saghiri MA. Endodontic periapical lesion: An overview on the etiology, diagnosis and current treatment modalities. Eur Endod J 2020;14:54–67.
60. Carrillo C, Penarrocha M, Ortega B, Martí E, Bagán JV, Vera F. Correlation of radiographic size and the presence of radiopaque lamina with histological findings in 70 periapical lesions. J Oral Maxillofac Surg 2008;66:1600–1605.
61. Alotaibi O, Alswayyed S, Alshagroud R, Alsheddi M. Evaluation of concordance between clinical and histopathological diagnoses in periapical lesions of endodontic origin. J Dent Sci 2020;15:132–135.
62. Gutmann JL. Parameters of achieving quality anesthesia and hemostasis in surgical endodontics. Anesth Pain Control Dent 1993;2:223–226.
63. al Shalabi RM, Omer OE, Glennon J, Jennings M, Claffey NM. Root canal anatomy of maxillary first and second permanent molars. Int Endod J 2000;33:405–414.
64. Gu L, Wei X, Ling J, Huang X. A microcomputed tomographic study of canal isthmuses in the mesial root of mandibular first molars in a Chinese population. J Endod 2009;35:353–356.
65. de Pablo OV, Estevez R, Péix Sánchez M, Heilborn C, Cohenca N. Root anatomy and canal configuration of the permanent mandibular first molar: A systematic review. J Endod. 2010;36:1919–1931.
66. Khalighinejad N, Aminoshariae A, Kulild JC, Williams KA, Wang J, Mickel A. The effect of the dental operating microscope on the outcome of nonsurgical root canal treatment: A retrospective case-control study. J Endod 2017;43:728–732
67. Wuchenich G, Meadows D, Torabinejad M. A comparison between two root end preparation techniques in human cadavers. J Endod 1994;20:279–282.
68. Peters CI, Peters OA, Barbakow F. An in vitro study comparing root-end cavities prepared by diamond-coated and stainless steel ultrasonic retrotips. Int Endod J 2001;34:142–148.
69. Slaton CC, Loushine RJ, Weller RN, Parker MH, Kimbrough WF, Pashley DH. Identification of resected root-end dentinal cracks: A comparative study of visual magnification. J Endod 2003;29:519–522.
70. Torabinejad M, Hong C U, McDonald F, Pitt Ford TR. Physical and chemical properties of a new root-end filling material. J Endod 1995;21:349–353.
71. Torabinejad M, Chivian N. Clinical applications of mineral trioxide aggregate. J Endod 1999;25:197–205.

72. Hosoya N, Takigawa T, Horie T, et al. A review of the literature on the efficacy of mineral trioxide aggregate in conservative dentistry. Dent Mater J 2019;38:693–700.
73. Parirokh M, Torabinejad M. Mineral trioxide aggregate: A comprehensive literature review—Part I: Chemical, physical, and antibacterial properties. J Endod 2010;36:16–27.
74. Torabinejad M, Parirokh M. Mineral trioxide aggregate: A comprehensive literature review—Part II: Leakage and biocompatibility investigations. J Endod 2010;36:190–202.
75. Parirokh M, Torabinejad M. Mineral trioxide aggregate: A comprehensive literature review—Part III: Clinical applications, drawbacks, and mechanism of action. J Endod 2010;36:400–413.
76. Torabinejad M, Parirokh M, Dummer PMH. Mineral trioxide aggregate and other bioactive endodontic cements: An updated overview—Part II: Other clinical applications and complications. Int Endod J 2018;51:284–317.
77. Nekoofar MH, Aseeley Z, Dummer P. The effect of various mixing techniques on the surface microhardness of mineral trioxide aggregate. Int Endod J 2010;43:312–320.
78. Nekoofar MH, Adusei G, Sheykhrezae MS, Hayes SJ, Bryant ST, Dummer PM. The effect of condensation pressure on selected physical properties of mineral trioxide aggregate. Int Endod J 2007; 40:453–461.
79. Camilleri J. Hydration mechanisms of mineral trioxide aggregate. Int Endod J 2007;40:462–470.
80. Fridland M, Rosado R. Mineral trioxide aggregate (MTA) solubility and porosity with different water-to-powder ratios. J Endod 2003;29:814–817.
81. Fridland M, Rosado R. MTA solubility: A long term study. J Endod 2005;31:376–379.
82. Paños-Crespo A, Sánchez-Torres A, Gay-Escoda C. Retrograde filling material in periapical surgery: A systematic review. Med Oral Patol Oral Cir Bucal 2021;26:e422–e429.
83. Parirokh M, Torabinejad M, Dummer PMH. Mineral trioxide aggregate and other bioactive endodontic cements: An updated overview—Part I: Vital pulp therapy. Int Endod J 2018;51:177–205.
84. Janis JE, Harrison B. Wound healing. Part I. Basic science. Plast Reconstr Surg 2014;133:e199–e207.
85. Parirokh M, Asgary S, Eghbal MJ, Stowe S, Kakoei S. A scanning electron microscope study of plaque accumulation on silk and PVDF suture materials in oral mucosa. Int Endod J 2004;37:776–781.
86. Parirokh M, Asgary S, Eghbal MJ. The effect of different suture removal time intervals on surgical wound healing. Iran Endod J 2006;1:81–86.
87. Kakoei S, Baghaei F, Dabiri S, Parirokh M, Kakooei S. A comparative in vivo study of tissue reactions to four suturing materials. Iran Endod J 2010;5:69–73.
88. Selvig KA, Torabinejad M. Wound healing after mucoperiosteal surgery in the cat. J Endod 1996;22: 507–515.
89. Kim S. Endodontic microsurgery. In: Cohen S, Burns RC (eds). Pathways of the Pulp, ed 8. St Louis: Mosby, 2002.
90. Kim E, Song JS, Jung IY, et al. Prospective clinical study evaluating endodontic microsurgery outcomes for cases with lesions of endodontic origin compared with cases with lesions of combined periodontal-endodontic origin. J Endod 2008;34:546–551.
91. Kim S. Principles of endodontic microsurgery. Dent Clin North Am 1997;41:481–497.
92. Haas DA. Localized complications from local anesthesia. J Calif Dent Assoc 1998;26:677–682.
93. Stone J, Kaban LB. Trismus after injection of local anesthetic. Oral Surg Oral Med Oral Pathol 1979;48:29–32.
94. Lam NP, Donoff RB, Kaban LB, Dodson TB. Patient satisfaction after trigeminal nerve repair. Oral Surg Oral Med Oral Pathol Oral Radiol Endod 2003;95:538–543.
95. Byun SH, Kim SS, Chung HJ, et al. Surgical management of damaged inferior alveolar nerve caused by endodontic overfilling of calcium hydroxide paste. Int Endod J 2016;49:1020–1029.
96. Mohammadi Z. Endodontics-related paresthesia of the mental and inferior alveolar nerves: An updated review. J Can Dent Assoc 2010;76:a117.
97. Pogrel MA, Thamby S. Permanent nerve involvement resulting from inferior alveolar nerve blocks. J Am Dent Assoc 2000;131:901–907.
98. Ericson S, Finne K, Persson G. Results of apicoectomy of maxillary canines, premolars and molars with special reference to oroantral communication as a prognostic factor. Int J Oral Surg 1974;3:386–393.
99. Bhandari PS. Management of peripheral nerve injury. J Clin Orthop Trauma 2019;10:862–866.
100. Leung YY, Fung PP, Cheung LK. Treatment modalities of neurosensory deficit after lower third molar surgery: A systematic review. J Oral Maxillofac Surg 2012;70:768–778.
101. Traeger KA. Hematoma following inferior alveolar injection: A possible cause for anesthesia failure. Anesth Prog 1979;26:122–123.
102. AAE Position Statement: AAE Guidance on the Use of Systemic Antibiotics in Endodontics. J Endod 2017;43:1409–1413.

103. Segura-Egea JJ, Gould K, Şen BH, et al. European Society of Endodontology position statement: The use of antibiotics in endodontics. Int Endod J 2018;51:20–25.
104. Miller PD Jr. A classification of marginal tissue recession. Int J Periodontics Restorative Dent 1985;5:8–13.
105. Kumar A, Masamatti SS. A new classification system for gingival and palatal recession. J Indian Soc Periodontol 2013;17:175–181.
106. Fischer KR, Grill E, Jockel-Schneider Y, Bechtold M, Schlagenhauf U, Fickl S. On the relationship between gingival biotypes and supra-crestal gingival height, crown form and papilla height. Clin Oral Implants Res 2013;25:894–898.

10

Errors During Patient Recall and Outcomes Assessment

MAHMOUD TORABINEJAD
SHANE N. WHITE

Objectives

After reading this chapter, the reader should be able to:

1. Discuss errors related to the definition of success and failure.
2. Understand the meanings of healed, non-healed, healing, and functional.
3. Understand the key contexts of patient history, clinical examinations, and tests.
4. Avoid errors related to radiographic examination and interpretation.
5. Discuss errors related to the timelines of endodontic healing.
6. Discuss errors related to the use of outcome measures and rates.
7. Enumerate alternative treatment options following unsuccessful root canal treatment.
8. Avoid errors in recall and outcomes assessment.

For patients who have been afflicted by pulpal and periapical diseases caused by decay or trauma, the main objectives of root canal treatment are long-term comfort, function, and esthetics. These objectives are achieved by removal of bacteria and their by-products through complete cleaning and shaping, obturation, and restoration to prevent recontamination.[1-3]

As for other phases of root canal treatment, errors can occur during recall and outcomes assessment. Errors during outcome assessment of initial root canal treatment can result in lack of necessary treatment, or inappropriate and unnecessary treatment, along with increased treatment time and cost, patient dissatisfaction, and medicolegal jeopardy.

The purpose of this chapter is to review the errors that may occur during evaluation of the outcomes of initial root canal treatment and discuss their implications. These mishaps can be related to the following: *(1)* defining success and failure; *(2)* the performance and interpretation of clinical examinations and tests; *(3)* the interpretation of radiographic examinations; *(4)* misunderstanding the healing timeline; *(5)* knowledge of outcome rates; and *(6)* knowledge of treatment options for non-healed root-canal-treated teeth. However, the most common error is failure to actively recall treated patients.

Errors Related to Defining the Patient Outcome

Currently, a wide variety of criteria are used for measuring success and failure of endodontic treatment. Some widely used instruments were developed for measuring prognostic indicators for populations,[4,5] but they may not be appropriate for measuring an individual patient's treatment outcomes.

However, concepts from these instruments can be used to categorize success and failure. Success is achieved when an endodontically treated tooth that was previously vital and without a periapical lesion remains asymptomatic and does not develop a periapical lesion after treatment. Using the same concept, development of new symptoms and/or the appearance of a periapical lesion is considered a failure. For a tooth with pulpal necrosis, with or without a preexisting periapical lesion, treatment is considered successful if the tooth remains asymptomatic and its apical lesion heals, as measured in follow-up examinations (see Fig 1-6). The presence of symptoms and/or an enlarging periapical lesion in an endodontically treated tooth is considered a failure.

In order to create a common language and practical understanding among patients, dentists, and other stakeholders, the American Association of Endodontists (AAE) has proposed the following practical and patient-centered criteria for evaluation of the outcomes of endodontically treated teeth:[6]

- **Healed**: Functional, asymptomatic tooth with no or minimal radiographic periradicular lesion.
- **Non-healed**: Nonfunctional, symptomatic tooth with or without radiographic evidence of a periradicular lesion.
- **Healing**: A tooth with periradicular pathosis that is asymptomatic and functional, or a tooth, with or without radiographic periradicular pathosis, that is symptomatic, but for which the intended function is not altered.
- **Functional**: A treated tooth that is serving its intended purpose in the dentition.

A lack of common understanding of these categories among patients, dentists, and third-party payers can cause confusion, disappointment, and distrust. The stakeholders in the dental delivery system have different perspectives and expectations regarding the outcomes of root canal treatment.[7] Patients are usually satisfied if affected teeth are comfortable, functional, and esthetically pleasing. Dentists are usually interested in the delivery of optimal care to their patients, relieving pain and discomfort, and eliminating pulpal and periapical diseases clinically and radiographically, while receiving fair compensation. Third-party payers measure success by access to care, quality of care, cost, and the longevity of the treatment provided. Satisfying all these perspectives and expectations without sacrificing the quality of care can be challenging. Therefore, lack of clarity of the expectations of the parties involved can be considered a mishap following completion of root canal treatment.

Errors Related to Clinical Examinations and Tests

Just like the clinical examinations used during the initiation of the treatment, systematic recall examinations must be performed. Clinical evaluation consists of using a number of methods, history, examination using tests, and radiography to determine the presence or absence of pathologic changes. These tests evaluate the supporting structures using percussion, palpation, mobility, and probing and evaluate the pulp using thermal and electrical tests (see chapter 1). The results of these tests should be compared both with those found in the initial treatment and with current control teeth. The pulpal and apical diagnoses made at recall, using the AAE diagnostic criteria, must be compared with those made at the time of treatment.[6] It must not be assumed, for example, that all canals were identified and that no pulp, vital or non-vital, remains.

A common mistake is not performing these tests systematically. Another is to ignore the tests, while relying solely on the radiographic findings. During a careful evaluation, the clinician often finds that a different tooth is responsible for the patient's signs and symptoms than what was initially assumed.

A common mistake during initial evaluation of a root-canal-treated tooth is ignoring or not paying enough attention to each of these steps. A lack of attention to a systematic approach at this stage can not only result in missing valuable diagnostic information, but it may also cause distrust between the patient and the providers. The clinician should be very careful to report objective systematic findings to the patient, rather than making subjective comments about their perception of the quality of prior root canal treatment.

Although a careful comprehensive evaluation and diagnosis and treatment plan may effectively address disease, this may not address the patient's psychosocial needs.[8] Patients' cognitions are shaped by many inputs and experiences, not just from their dentist's explanations.[9] Patient-centered outcomes have been neglected in dentistry and in endodontics in particular. For patients to be able to make the best decisions, dentists need to think about and address factors such as quality of life, satisfaction, anxiety, fear, pain, tooth survival, and economics when they present treatment plans, communicate, and assess individual patients' outcomes.[9–11]

Errors Related to Radiographic Examination and Interpretation

Radiographic examinations are essential for the evaluation of hard tissues. However, their value is often overestimated by clinicians who habitually rely on radiographic findings without paying sufficient attention to the clinical findings and the patient's chief complaint. Such an attitude is mistaken, and likely to lead to misdiagnosis and inappropriate treatment (see chapter 1). Although cross-sectional data indicates that many root-canal-treated teeth have periapical radiolucencies, a radiograph cannot determine whether the tooth is healing or non-healed.[12]

Based on findings from conventional radiography, history, and clinical tests, as well as the time elapsed, the outcome of a root-canal-treated tooth can be classified as healed, non-healed, healing, or functional. In order to accurately compare radiographs taken at different times, they must be taken at the same angulations and with minimal distortion.

An important shortcoming of conventional radiographic evaluation is that the images are only two dimensional and may not reveal the full picture of the condition of involved structures.

The 3D images produced using CBCT have eliminated the main shortcoming of conventional radiography, making CBCT a valuable tool for diagnosis and outcomes assessment of endodontically treated teeth (see chapter 2). 3D images allow evaluation without the superimposition of surrounding anatomical structures. Like other tools, the CBCT findings can be misused and lead to unnecessary or inappropriate treatment if they are not considered in the context of the patient history and systematic testing. Torabinejad et al examined the prevalence and size of periapical lesions using CBCT imaging in teeth without apparent signs of intraoral radiographic lesions.[13] They reported that the majority of roots (53%) had periodontal ligament widths $\leq$ 0.5 mm; 27% had radiolucency widths of 0.5 mm $< \times \leq$ 1.0 mm; 15% had radiolucency widths of 1.0 mm $< \times \leq$ 1.5 mm; 1% had radiolucency widths of 1.5 mm $< \times \leq$ 2.0 mm; 2% had radiolucency widths of 2.0 mm $< \times \leq$ 2.5 mm; and 3% had radiolucency widths $>$ 2.5 mm. Based on these findings, the authors concluded that periapical features found in CBCT examinations may not be true pathologic conditions, and they cautioned clinicians against overtreatment of endodontically treated teeth without conventional radiographic evidence of periapical lesions, signs from test results, and clinical symptoms. Lack of knowledge regarding the limitations of CBCT can lead to misdiagnosis and inappropriate treatment planning for endodontically treated teeth.

Errors Related to the Timelines of Endodontic Healing

The path to healing and regeneration of bone and periradicular tissues may be long and irregular. Signs of initial healing may appear quickly, but full resolution of a periapical lesion may take years. This is why the diagnostic category of *healing* is needed in addition to those of *healed* and *non-healed*.[14] Recommended follow-up periods have ranged from 6 months to 5 years.[15–20] Six to 12 months is a widely accepted interval for an initial recall evaluation for most patients.[21] If at 6 to 12 months a lesion is still present but is smaller in size, it is likely to be in the process of healing, but additional recall is needed until the lesion has resolved. A radiographic lesion that is unchanged or has increased in size after 1 year is unlikely to resolve, and the treatment may be considered unsuccessful. Larger periradicular lesions take longer to heal than smaller lesions. Unfortunately, apparent successes may revert to failure at a later time, often as a result of reinfection through coronal leakage. However, late healing may also occur. Therefore, an endodontic evaluation, including history, clinical examination, and taking radiographs of treated teeth, must be part of routine patient evaluation. Many asymptomatic treated teeth have varying degrees of radiolucency, even though they may provide comfort and function for decades.[22] The dentist must judge whether these teeth are in progress toward healing or toward failure, and then advise and manage appropriately. A common error during outcomes assessment of initial root canal treatment is taking action too quickly and starting undue nonsurgical or surgical retreatment or extraction of root-canal-treated teeth (see Fig 9-1).

Errors in Measuring and Interpreting Outcome Rates

As with other dental and medical procedures, some endodontic treatments are not successful. Historically, the popular belief has been that the success rates for root canal treatment are between 80% and 95%. However, one must consider the criteria authors use to define "success" as well as the follow-up times used. Historically, instruments such as the Strindberg criteria[4]—developed to identify prognostic indicators, not to measure patient health—were often inappropriately used to measure and report patient outcomes. For example, the Strindberg criteria define a discontinuous or poorly defined lamina dura as "failure," yet vital, healthy, asymptomatic teeth often manifest such features.[4] The widely used Periapical Index (PAI) includes radiographic assessment alone, without the context of patient symptoms or test results.[5] It was designed to be used as a tool in epidemiologic studies, for clinical trials, and for retrospective analyses. Such an instrument is extremely useful in making comparisons between treatment groups or evaluating trends over time, but it is not a measure of the health of individual patients. Success rates using such instruments underestimate the proportion of healing and functional teeth.

Torabinejad et al[13] performed a systematic review of the literature pertaining to success and failure of nonsurgical root canal therapy from 1966 to 2006. Meta-analysis of those studies that all used the PAI suggested an overall "success" rate of 84% over a follow-up period of 4 to 6 years, whereas the same systematic review reported an overall *survival* rate of 97%. Others who assessed the 4- to 6-year outcomes of initial endodontic treatment have reported similar overall rates.[23–25] Survival rates likely overestimate the proportion of teeth that would be categorized as healed, healing, or functional, but at least the meaning is clear and clinically relevant.

Doyle et al used a retrospective cohort study to compare 196 nonsurgical root canal treatment (NSRCT) cases to 196 matched single-tooth implant cases, finding that restored endodontically treated teeth and single-tooth implant restorations have similar failure rates, although the implant group showed a longer average and median time to function as well as a higher incidence of postoperative complications requiring subsequent treatment intervention.[26] Subsequently, Vahdati et al compared the outcome NSRCT teeth with single-tooth implant cases within the same 171 patients at similar intraoral locations.[27] The results of this investigation showed both treatments had a 95% long-term survival rate. However, the number of adjunct and additional treatments, number of appointments, elapsed time before the final restoration, number of prescribed medications, and cost of the treatment were significantly higher for single-tooth implants in comparison to nonsurgical endodontic treatment.

Because most of the other prior studies have used different criteria for "success" and "failure," comparison of results is not meaningful. In addition, historic findings do not include the effects of new advances and innovations in the art and science of endodontics.[8,25–28] Moreover, percentages of "success" or survival are meaningless without a defined minimum follow-up period. A common mistake during outcome assessment of root-canal-treated teeth is comparing the outcomes of disparate studies without considering the confounding factors.

Errors Related to Treatment Options for Non-Healed Teeth

For decades, a primary goal of dentistry has been to preserve the natural dentition. Previously, all efforts would have been made to save teeth with poor pulpal health and periodontal diseases or to extract hopeless teeth and replace them with fixed or removable prostheses. The high survival rates of dental implants have created a paradigm shift in treatment planning. Clinicians are regularly confronted with difficult choices after failure of root canal treatment. Treatment options after failure of initial root canal treatment include nonsurgical retreatment, endodontic surgery, tooth replantation, tooth transplantation, extraction and replacement using a single-tooth implant, extraction and replacement using a fixed dental prosthesis, and extraction without replacement.[29] All these treatment options must be considered, and the appropriate diagnostic data must be collected before advice is given to patients and decisions are made.

Nonsurgical retreatment

The principal indication for nonsurgical retreatment is failure to heal after a reasonable period of time has passed, 1 year or thereabouts, without favorable changes to patient symptoms, signs, and radiographic evaluation. Nonsurgical retreatment is the first-line treatment for NSRCT teeth that have not exhibited healing (see chapter 8). Contraindications to nonsurgical retreatment include poor periodontal or restorative prognosis, vertical fractures, and unmotivated patients. Apical surgery should be considered for teeth that are not amenable to nonsurgical approaches.

10

Potential errors during evaluation of teeth that have had initial root canal treatment are to ignore the indications and contraindications for nonsurgical retreatment or to immediately perform surgical endodontics or extraction, with or without replacement (Fig 10-1).

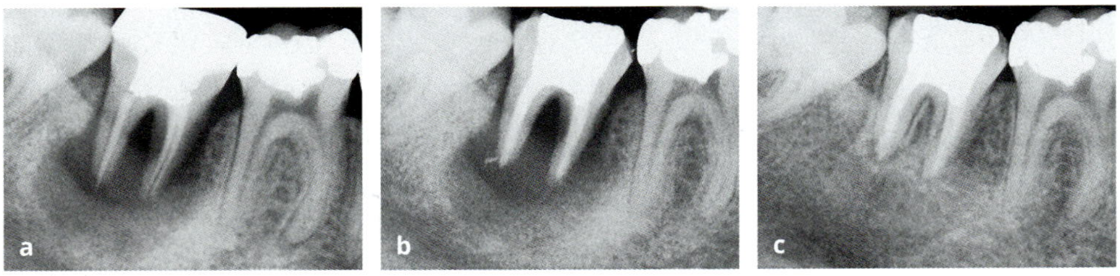

Fig 10-1 *(a)* A mandibular second molar with inadequate root canal treatment, symptomatic apical periodontitis, and a large lesion, scheduled for extraction. *(b)* A postoperative radiograph following nonsurgical retreatment. *(c)* A postoperative radiograph 1 year later, showing complete resolution of the periradicular lesion. (Courtesy of HJS Kang.)

Surgical retreatment

Endodontic surgery has a very high success rate.[30] The main indications for endodontic surgical treatment are teeth that have not exhibited signs of healing after nonsurgical retreatment and follow-up; teeth that are not amenable to a nonsurgical approach due to nonnegotiable calcified canals, irretrievable filling materials, large posts, unusually complex anatomy, etc; and teeth requiring exploratory biopsy. Contraindications for surgical endodontics include teeth with poor periodontal and restorative prognoses, including deep periodontal pocketing, poor crown-to-root ratio, and vertical cracks; health conditions that preclude minor surgery; and jeopardy to adjacent anatomical structures such as the mandibular canal and mental and nasopalatine foramina (see chapter 9).

A potential error during evaluation of teeth that have had initial root canal treatment is to ignore the indications and contraindications for surgical endodontic treatment (Fig 10-2), tooth replantation, or autotransplantation and to perform nonsurgical endodontic treatment or extraction, with or without replacement.

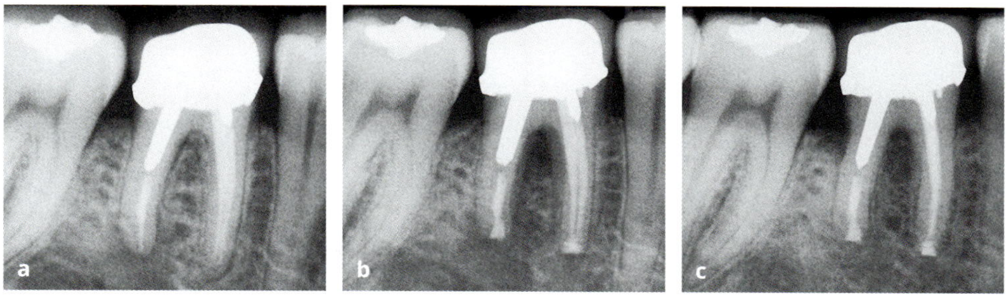

Fig 10-2 *(a)* A mandibular first molar with symptomatic apical periodontitis, a large lesion around the distal root, and a large post in the distal root, scheduled for extraction. *(b)* A postoperative radiograph showing surgical retreatment using mineral trioxide aggregate as a root-end filling material. *(c)* A postoperative radiograph a few months later, showing resolution of periradicular tissues. The tooth was asymptomatic at this time.

Tooth replantation

Tooth replantation is the reinsertion of a tooth into its own alveolus socket after the tooth has been extracted for the purpose of performing root-end surgery in the dentist's hand while out of the socket.[31] Tooth replantation is indicated when there is no other treatment alternative to maintain a strategic tooth where initial NSRCT has not led to healing. Tooth replantation is often successful if careful case selection is performed and the procedure is carried out quickly (Fig 10-3).[32] Ankylosis and resorption are the most common causes of failure for tooth replantation.

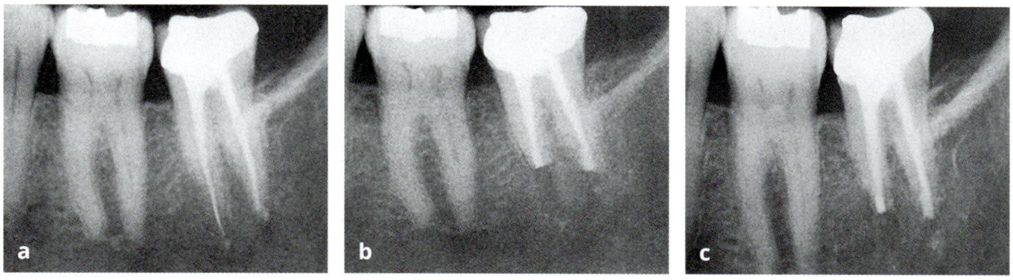

Fig 10-3 *(a)* A mandibular second molar with previously treated root canals and symptomatic apical periodontitis. *(b)* A postoperative radiograph after performing tooth replantation using mineral trioxide aggregate as a root-end filling material. *(c)* A postoperative radiograph 2 years later, showing resolution of the periapical lesion.

Potential planning errors include not considering tooth replantation at all; inadequate evaluation and case selection; inadequate communication with the patient; or immediately performing extraction, with or without tooth replacement. Technical mishaps during tooth replantation include fracture of the tooth during extraction; damaging the periodontium during root-end cavity preparation and root-end filling through mechanical pressure, drying, or the use of non-isotonic irrigation; and keeping the tooth out of the socket for more than a few minutes. To avoid these mishaps, case selection, proper communication with the patient, experience in tooth extraction, and careful organization prior to and during the procedure are all required.

Tooth transplantation

Tooth transplantation, or autotransplantation, is the transfer of a tooth from one alveolar socket to another in the same patient.[33] The clinical procedures involved include socket preparation, extraction, transplantation, and stabilization. Like tooth replantation, tooth transplantation is often successful if careful case selection is performed and the procedure is carried out appropriately and quickly (Fig 10-4).[34,35] Similar to tooth replantation, ankylosis and resorption are the most common causes of failure.

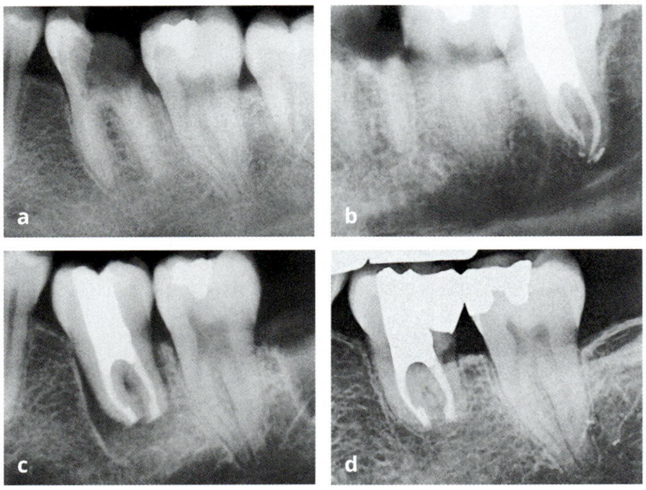

Fig 10-4 *(a)* A nonrestorable mandibular first molar with necrotic pulp and normal periapical tissues. *(b)* Another radiograph showing the presence of a third molar for an autotransplantation. *(c)* A postoperative radiograph after transplantation of the third molar into the socket of the nonrestorable first molar. *(d)* A postoperative radiograph 9 years later, showing excellent results.

Potential planning errors include not considering autotransplantation at all; inadequate evaluation and case selection; failure to ensure that adequate alveolar bone is present; failure to recognize that immature teeth with open apices have the best prognoses; inadequate communication with the patient; or immediately performing extraction, with or without tooth replacement. Technical mishaps during tooth autotransplantation include fracture of the tooth during extraction; damaging the periodontium through mechanical pressure, drying, or the use of non-isotonic irrigation; keeping the tooth out of a socket for more than a few minutes; failure to perform NSRCT in teeth with closed apices ahead of time; and failure to recognize a need for NSRCT after transplantation.

To avoid these mishaps, case selection, proper communication with the patient, experience in tooth extraction, and careful organization prior to and during the procedure are all required.

Tooth extraction and replacement using a single-tooth implant

Only a very small proportion of endodontically treated teeth are extracted. Of these, very few are extracted for endodontic reasons.[14,26,36–38] Common reasons for extraction are caries, periodontal disease, nonrestorability, prosthodontic failure, and root fracture.[22,36–41] Therefore, it is critical that risk factors for all these problems be considered during comprehensive patient assessment and treatment planning.[14,42,43]

Teeth that have a very poor prognosis, for any of the above reasons, should not receive initial NSRCT or second-line endodontic treatment. These teeth should be removed and replaced with an implant (Fig 10-5), or removed and not replaced, as appropriate. The long-term survival rates of single-tooth implants and root-canal-treated teeth are both very high.[8,25]

Potential mishaps related to this treatment are failure to recognize a hopeless periodontal, restorative, or endodontic prognosis; failure to recognize the indications for an implant; and failure to consider grafting procedures and implant placement before tooth extraction.

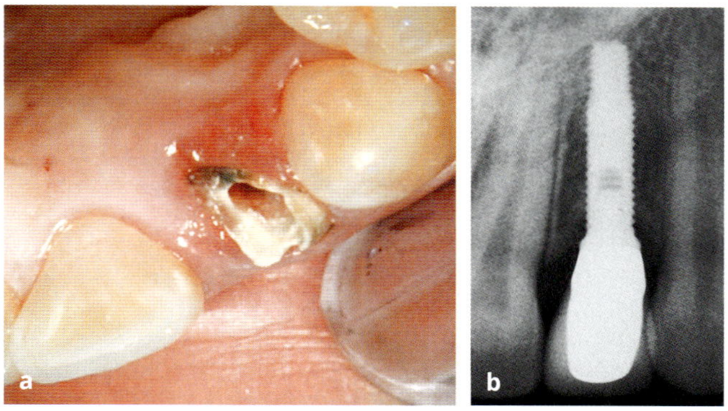

Fig 10-5 *(a)* A maxillary lateral central incisor with inadequate tooth structure to restore. *(b)* After extraction of this tooth, a single implant was placed.

Conclusion

Significant errors can be made in patient recall and outcomes assessment. These errors are primarily of a cognitive nature and can be related to the provider's understanding of outcomes definitions; the endodontic evaluation, with the context of patient symptoms, test results, and radiography; the long healing timeline; the outcome rates over time; and the full consideration of all available options in the event of non-healing. Clear communication with the patient is also vital. Again, the most common error of all is the failure to actively recall treated patients. Errors made in recall and outcomes assessment may often be irreversible, so their avoidance is paramount.

References

1. Sundqvist G. Bacteriological studies of necrotic dental pulps [Odontol Dissertation, No 7]. University of Umeå, Sweden, 1976.
2. Bergenholtz G. Micro-organisms from necrotic pulp of traumatized teeth. Odontol Rev 1974:25:347–358.
3. Kantz WE, Henry CA. Isolation and classification of anaerobic bacteria from intact pulp chambers of non-vital teeth in man. Arch Oral Biol 1974;19:91–96.
4. Strindberg LZ. The dependence of the results of pulp therapy on certain factors. Acta Odontol Scand 1956;14(suppl 21):1–175.
5. Orstavik D, Kerekes K, Eriksen HM. The periapical index: A scoring system for radiographic assessment of apical periodontitis. Endod Dent Traumatol 1986;2:20–34.
6. AAE Consensus Conference Recommended Diagnostic Terminology. J Endod 2009;35:1634.
7. Anderson MH. Use of evidence-based data by insurance companies. J Evid Based Dent Pract 2004; 4:120–124.
8. Torabinejad M, Anderson P, Bader J, et al. The outcomes of endodontic treatment, single implant, fixed partial denture and no tooth replacement: A systematic review. J Prosthet Dent 2007;98:285–311.
9. Hamedy R, Shakiba B, Fayazi S, Pak JG, White SN. Patient-centered endodontic outcomes: A narrative review. Iran Endod J 2013;8:197–204.
10. Pak JG, White SN. Pain prevalence and severity before, during, and after root canal treatment: A systematic review. J Endod 2011;37:429–438.
11. Khan S, Hamedy R, Lei Y, Ogawa RS, White SN. Anxiety related to nonsurgical root canal treatment: A systematic review. J Endod 2016;42:1726–1736.
12. Pak JG, Fayazi S, White SN. Prevalence of periapical radiolucency and root canal treatment: A systematic review of cross-sectional studies. J Endod 2012;38:1170–1176.
13. Torabinejad M, Rice D, Maktabi O, Oyoyo U, Abramovitch K. Incidence and size of periapical radiolucencies using CBCT in teeth without apparent intraoral radiographic lesions: A new periapical index with a clinical recommendation. J Endod 2018;44:389–394
14. White SN, Miklus VG, Potter KS, Cho J, Ngan AY. Endodontics and implants, a catalog of therapeutic contrasts. J Evid Based Dent Pract 2006;6:101–109.
15. Reit C. Decision strategies in endodontics: On the design of a recall program. Endod Dent Traumatol 1987;3:233–239.
16. Ørstavik D. Time-course and risk analyses of the development and healing of chronic apical periodontitis in man. Int Endod J 1996;29:150–155.
17. Adenubi JO, Rule DC. Success rate for root fillings in young patients. Brit Dent J 1976;141:237–241.
18. Byström A, Happonen RP, Sjögren U, Sundqvist G. Healing of periapical lesions of pulpless teeth after endodontic treatment with controlled asepsis. Endod Dent Traumatol 1987;3:58–63.
19. Sjögren U, Hägglund B, Sundqvist G, Wing K. Factors affecting the long-term results of endodontic treatment. J Endod 1990;16:498–504.
20. Molven O, Halse A. Success rates for gutta-percha and Kloroperka N-Ø root fillings made by undergraduate students: Radiographic findings after 10–17 years. Int Endod J 1988;21:243–250.
21. Pirani C, Chersoni S, Montebugnoli L, Prati C. Long-term outcome of non-surgical root canal treatment: A retrospective analysis. Odontology 2015;103:185–193.
22. Lee AH, Cheung GS, Wong MC. Long-term outcome of primary non-surgical root canal treatment. Clin Oral Investig 2012;16:1607–1617.
23. Torabinejad M, Kutsenko D, Machnick TK, et al. Levels of evidence for the outcome of nonsurgical endodontic treatment. J Endod 2005;31:637–646.
24. Friedman S, Abitbol S, Lawrence HP. Treatment outcome in endodontics: The Toronto Study—Phase 1: Initial treatment. J Endod 2003;29:787–793.
25. Iqbal MK, Kim S. For teeth requiring endodontic treatment, what are the differences in treatment outcomes of restored endodontically treated teeth compared to implant-supported restorations? Int J Oral Maxillofac Implants 2007;22(suppl):96–116.
26. Doyle SL, Hodges JS, Pesun IJ, Law AS, Bowles WR. Retrospective cross sectional comparison of initial nonsurgical endodontic treatment and single-tooth implants. J Endod 2006;32:822–827.
27. Vahdati SA, Torabinejad M, Handysides R, Lozada J. A retrospective comparison of outcome in patients who received both nonsurgical root canal treatment and single-tooth implants. J Endod 2019; 45:99–103.
28. Shabahang S. State of the art and science of endodontics. J Am Dent Assoc 2005;136:41–52.
29. Torabinejad M, White SN. Endodontic treatment options following unsuccessful initial root canal treatment: Alternatives to single implants. J Am Dent Assoc 2016;147:214–220.

30. Kohli MR, Berenji H, Setzer FC, Lee SM, Karabucak B. Outcome of endodontic surgery: A meta-analysis of the literature—Part 3: Comparison of endodontic microsurgical techniques with 2 different root-end filling materials. J Endod 2018;44:923–931.
31. American Association of Endodontists. An Annotated Glossary of Terms Used in Endodontics, ed 6. Chicago: American Association of Endodontists, 1998.
32. Torabinejad M, Dinsbach N, Turman M, Handysides R, Bahjri K, White SN. Survival of intentionally replanted teeth and implant-supported single crowns: A systematic review of treatment outcomes. J Endod 2015;41:992–998.
33. Tsukiboshi M. Autogenous tooth transplantation: A reevaluation. Int J Periodontics Restorative Dent 1993;13:120–149.
34. Akiyama Y, Fukuda H, Hashimoto K. A clinical and radiographic study of 25 autotransplanted third molars. J Oral Rehabil 1998;25:640–644.
35. Andreasen JO, Paulsen HU, Yu Z, et al. A long-term study of 370 autotransplanted premolars. Part II. Tooth survival and pulp healing subsequent to transplantation. Eur J Orthod 1990;12:14–24.
36. Wang C, Chueh L, Chen S, Feng Y, Hsiao CK, Chiang C. Impact of diabetes mellitus, hypertension, and coronary artery disease on tooth extraction after nonsurgical endodontic treatment. J Endod 2011;37:1–5.
37. Chen S, Chueh L, Hsiao CK, Tsai M, Ho S, Chiang C. An epidemiologic study of tooth retention after nonsurgical endodontic treatment in a large population in Taiwan. J Endod 2007;33:226–229.
38. Bernstein SD, Horowitz AJ, Man M, et al. Outcomes of endodontic therapy in general practice: A study by the Practitioners Engaged in Applied Research and Learning Network. J Am Dent Assoc 2012;143:478–487.
39. Vire DE. Failure of endodontically treated teeth: Classification and evaluation. J Endod 1991;17:338–342.
40. Fuss Z, Lustig J, Tamse A. Prevalence of vertical root fractures in extracted endodontically treated teeth. Int Endod J 1999;32:283–286.
41. Chen SC, Chueh L, Hsiao CK, et al. First untoward events and reasons for tooth extraction after nonsurgical endodontic treatment in Taiwan. J Endod 2008;34:671–674.
42. Torabinejad M, Goodacre CJ. Endodontic or dental implant therapy: The factors affecting treatment planning. J Am Dent Assoc 2006;137:973–977.
43. Zitzmann NU, Krastl G, Hecker H, Walter C, Waltimo T, Weiger R. Strategic considerations in treatment planning: Deciding when to treat, extract, or replace a questionable tooth. J Prosthet Dent 2010;104:80–91.

Index

Page numbers followed by "t" denote tables; those followed by "f" denote figures

D

E

P